Taking Control Of Your Diabetes

3rd Edition

Steven V. Edelman, MD

Founder and Director of
Taking Control Of Your Diabetes

Professor of Medicine
Division of Endocrinology and Metabolism
University of California, San Diego

Director, Diabetes Care Clinic
Veterans Affairs Medical Center
San Diego, California

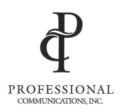

PROFESSIONAL
COMMUNICATIONS, INC.

Published by
Professional Communications, Inc.

Marketing Office:
400 Center Bay Drive
West Islip, NY 11795
(t) 631-661-2852
(f) 631-661-2167

Editorial Office:
PO Box 10
Caddo, OK 74729-0010
(t) 580-367-9838
(f) 580-367-9989

For orders, please call
1-800-337-9838
Or visit our website at
www.pcibooks.com

ISBN: 978-1-932610-29-1

Printed in the United States of America

DISCLAIMER: THE OPINIONS EXPRESSED IN THIS PUBLICATION REFLECT THOSE OF THE AUTHOR. HOWEVER, THE AUTHOR MAKES NO WARRANTY REGARDING THE CONTENTS OF THE PUBLICATION. THE PROTOCOLS DESCRIBED HEREIN ARE GENERAL AND MAY NOT APPLY TO A SPECIFIC PATIENT. ANY PRODUCT MENTIONED IN THIS PUBLICATION SHOULD BE TAKEN IN ACCORDANCE WITH THE PRESCRIBING INFORMATION PROVIDED BY THE MANUFACTURER.

This text is printed on recycled paper.

To my wife, Ingrid, and my two daughters, Talia and Carina, for their never-ending support of my work and living with my diabetes. They are the most important part of my life.

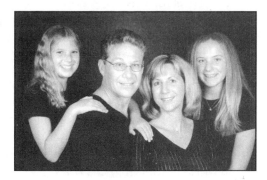

And to my lifelong friend, Ken Facter, MD, MBA, JD, who made a career of fighting for patient's rights in the arena of managed care. For his inspiration and guidance in starting our nonprofit organization *Taking Control Of Your Diabetes* and for being a great friend. May he rest in peace.

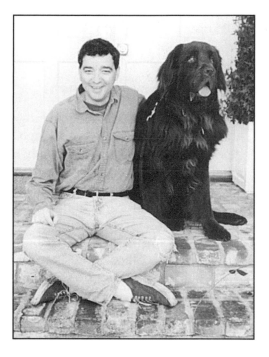

Acknowledgments

The basis for this book embodies the philosophy of the large patient-oriented conferences and health fairs that all of us at Taking Control Of Your Diabetes have been presenting across America for the past 12 years.

I would like to express my appreciation to Sandy Bourdette, Jill Yapo, Michelle Day, Antonio Huerta, and Michele Huie for their hard work and dedicated service to Taking Control Of Your Diabetes. My thanks also go to Malcolm Beasley and Phyllis Jones Freeny of Professional Communications, Inc. for their friendly and expert advice and help in putting together this book and to Nikki D. Merrill for the design concepts and typography. I would like to thank my wife, Ingrid, Sandy Bourdette, Michele and Rob Huie, and Candis Morello for reviewing the third edition of this book. I also wish to acknowledge my sister, Susan, who writes for the *New York Post*, for reviewing parts of my work, and my mother, Joyce, and brother, Barry, whom I love very much.

Special Acknowledgement

A very special acknowledgement goes to Sandy Bourdette for her never-ending devotion to Taking Control Of Your Diabetes and the people we serve. I came to Sandy in 1995 and asked her to help me make my vision of holding a patient-oriented educational conference a reality. That first conference is what ultimately led to TCOYD becoming the organization it is today. Not only did Sandy give up her successful meeting planning business to work solely for a grass-roots, not-for-profit organization, she also sacrificed her home, which served as our office in the early years of the organization's history. Since those early days over 12 years ago, Sandy has maintained the infrastructure of TCOYD, serving as executive director, and has consistently produced the unprecedented high quality programs that have truly made TCOYD the premier, nationwide, patient-education organization.

Contents

Contents

Contributors

Timothy S. Bailey, MD, FACP, FACE, CPI
San Diego, California
Assistant Clinical Professor of Medicine
University of California, San Diego
Dr. Bailey is a practicing clinical endocrinologist in San Diego.

Patrick J. Boyle, MD
Albuquerque, New Mexico
Professor of Medicine, University of New Mexico Health Sciences Division of General Internal Medicine

Sheri R. Colberg, PhD, FACSM
Norfolk, Virginia
Professor of Exercise,
Old Dominion University
Dr. Colberg is an exercise physiologist with a doctorate from UC Berkeley.

Lorena Drago, MS, RD, CDN, CDE
Forest Hills, NY
Lorena Drago is a registered dietitian, a certified diabetes educator, and author of the bilingual book Beyond Rice and Beans: The Caribbean Latino Guide to Eating Healthy With Diabetes.

Cyndee R. Fena, RDH, MT
Carlsbad, California
Cyndee Fena was a certified dental hygienist who had type 1 diabetes. She was also a professional belly dancer and was featured on the cover of Diabetes Forecast *magazine. Sadly, Cyndee passed away before the publication of this 3rd edition.*

Kriss S. Halpern, JD
Santa Monica, California
Kriss Halpern is a trial attorney in Santa Monica, California, specializing in the rights of consumers. He has type 1 diabetes, often contributes to Diabetes Interview *on legal issues, received the Charles H. Best award from the American Diabetes Association as a volunteer with the Diabetes Control and Complications Trial, and is a member of the Diabetes Coalition of California.*

Francine R. Kaufman, MD
Los Angeles, California
Professor of Pediatrics,
Keck School of Medicine, USC;
Head of the Center for Diabetes,
Endocrinology and Metabolism,
Childrens Hospital, Los Angeles

Mayssoun S. Khoury, DDS
Newport Beach, California
Dr. Khoury is a dentist, educator, lecturer, and author.

Rachel Peterson Kim, MD
San Diego, California
Dr. Kim is a rheumatologist and Medical Director of Medikinetics.

Ingrid Kruse, DPM
San Diego, California
Dr. Kruse is an expert in diabetic foot care. She received her training at the prestigious Joslin Clinic in Boston and has set up the high-risk diabetes foot clinic at the Veteran's Hospital, San Diego.

Contributors

Urban Miyares
San Diego, California
President, Disabled Businesspersons
Association
Urban Miyares is a nationally recognized disabled Vietnam veteran, entrepreneur, lecturer, writer, inventor and patent holder, television personality, and world-class athlete. He was diagnosed with diabetes during the Vietnam War.

Aaron B. Morse, MD, FCCP
Santa Cruz, California
Diplomate of the American Board of Sleep Medicine and Medical Director of the Central Coast Sleep Disorders Center

William H. Polonsky, PhD, CDE
San Diego, California
Assistant Clinical Professor in Psychiatry, University of California, San Diego; Founder, Behavioral Diabetes Institute; and author of *Diabetes Burnout: What to Do When You Can't Take It Anymore*

Ruth Roberts, MA
San Diego, California
Director of Diabetes Services, Inc
Ruth Roberts is a medical writer, sales development and training director at financial institutions, and a university and community college writing teacher.

Julia Sarmiento
Santa Cruz, California
Technical Director of the Central Coast
Sleep Disorders Center
Julia Sarmiento is a registered polysomnographic technologist.

Paul E. Tornambe, MD
San Diego, California
Dr. Tornambe is in active practice, limited to medical and surgical diseases of the retina and vitreous.

Janet M. Trowbridge, MD, PhD
Edmonds, Washington
Staff Physician, Northwest Dermatology and Skin Cancer Clinic

John Walsh, PA, CDE
San Diego, California
Clinical Diabetes Specialist, North County Endocrine, Escondida, California
John Walsh has been a pump wearer since 1983 when he began developing protocols to make pumping easier and more effective for his patients.

James D. Wolosin, MD
San Diego, California
Dr. Wolosin is a gastroenterologist and a Staff Physician for Sharp Rees Stealy Health Care System.

Taking Control Of Your Diabetes, or TCOYD, our nonprofit organization, has been in existence now for over 12 years. Through our nationwide series of educational and motivational conferences, we have directly touched the lives of well over 100,000 people with diabetes and their loved ones. I have always known that when it comes to effective self-management of diabetes, there is nothing better than personal interactions with diabetes experts in order to become educated and motivated to do well with diabetes. With over 85 conferences completed to date, more and more people with diabetes continue to attend our programs and tell us what a difference TCOYD is making in their lives and in their ability to take control of their diabetes. With the education and support provided by TCOYD, people with diabetes learn to look at life differently and to appreciate what people who don't have diabetes tend to take for granted. "I can live a normal life and do anything I want to do without letting diabetes get in my way," is the mindset that is encouraged through every TCOYD conference.

This book is written with the same spirit and delivers the same messages as our live events. I was inspired to write this 3rd

Team TCOYD

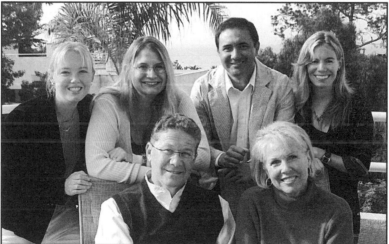

Standing in the back row from left to right are Michele Huie, Jill Yapo, Antonio Huerta, and Michelle Day. Seated in the front are Steve Edelman and Sandy Bourdette.

edition of the TCOYD book because of the many new advances that have become available since the 2nd edition was published and also because of the many joyful and moving experiences I've had during the past several years directing TCOYD. It is my privilege to work side-by-side with so many diabetes professionals who volunteer their time and expertise in order to help TCOYD achieve and maintain our status as the premier patient education organization worldwide. Our super dedicated, talented, and hard-working TCOYD team supports me by continuously transforming the mission and vision of TCOYD into reality. And, of course, without the loving support of my wonderful family, none of this would be possible.

This 3rd edition consists of new and updated chapters written by professionals, many of whom have diabetes and are dedicated to helping people with diabetes live healthier, happier, and more productive lives. I am confident that the material in this book will help you become more educated and motivated to be the most active member of your own health care team.

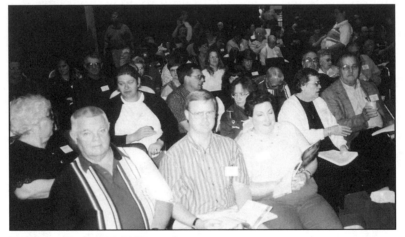

The crowd at a TCOYD conference.

1

Taking Control of Your Diabetes

We Are on the Offensive!

Diabetes: on the Offensive

It dawned on me recently while thinking about my favorite pro football team, the San Diego Chargers, that with all the new advances in diabetes screening, diagnosis, and treatment strategies, those of us living with diabetes can now be on the offensive in terms of our health care. This is quite a different situation than just defending against what seems to be the inevitable dreaded complications of the disease. We can now aggressively tackle diabetes in a more proactive, effective, and safer manner than we have ever been able to do before. However, the big problem, as I see it, is that there is a lack of education, of both the caregivers in this country and the people living with diabetes, about these new advances. The future of diabetes care is here and now, and it is up to you to go after it.

My Personal Story of Living With Diabetes for 37 Years

Everyone wants to know what Dr. Edelman's A1C is because I am supposed to be "the expert." Please do not think that I am the perfect person living with diabetes just because I am a diabetes doctor. I have experienced and continue to deal with the same physical and emotional challenges that many of you experience living with diabetes 24/7. I know it is not an easy task to take control of your diabetes and to stay in control.

I developed diabetes when I was 15 years old. I had the classic symptoms of weight loss, excessive thirst, tiredness, and poor wound healing. I clearly remember at that time I had a scab on my knee that just would not heal. As a teenager, I was disappointed because I was waiting for that big, round piece of "beef jerky" to get hard so I could pick it off (although it never did). In between my classes at Patrick Henry Junior High in Los Angeles, I would run to the restroom to urinate and relieve my distended bladder and then slurp up as much water as possible at the drinking fountain. I could not quench my thirst and I remember all of the kids in line behind me yelling at me because I took so long. Then, halfway through my next class, I would have to urinate again and almost desperately seek out the nearest drinking fountain. My teachers were annoyed with me because I was the only kid to ask for the bathroom pass every single day. I was also reprimanded several times for falling asleep in class. I just could not keep my eyes open and I had hardly any energy at all. By the time that class was over, my bladder was bursting again and I would be dying of thirst. I would come home from school and go to bed at 3 o'clock in the afternoon and sleep until the next morning. I lost 20 pounds in a few weeks, which I loved because I was always a little chunky. My nickname at school was "the stump." I also remember a family vacation in Mexico when I drank nothing but bottle after bottle of soft drinks, which are packed with sugar and, of course, made matters worse. Even if diet drinks had been available, I would not have ordered one because I did not know I was developing diabetes.

Finally, I realized something was wrong and I asked my mother to take me to the doctor. We went to the urgent-care unit of my health maintenance organization (HMO) and had my blood and urine collected for tests. The doctor spent a few minutes with me asking medical questions. After looking at the results of my tests, he called in an army of nurses who urgently wheel-chaired me off to the intensive care unit (ICU) to give me intravenous (IV) fluids and insulin. I was in the hospital for 1 week, and during my stay all kinds of people came to my bedside to tell me about diabetes. Several nurses kept telling me, "You can live a normal life"; I had no clue what they were talking about. When you are first diagnosed and in emotional shock, retaining information is pretty difficult. I do remember attending a diabetes class that first week while in the hospital. There I was, a newly diagnosed, young, naive teenage boy with type 1 diabetes sitting in a room with 25 very obese, older people, all with type 2 diabetes (adult onset). The single fact I remember from that class in 1970 was that ketchup has a lot of sugar in it. I kept thinking, "What am I going to dip my French fries in now?" I had lots of fun practicing how to give insulin injections into an orange, but the fun ended when it got to be my leg.

The other big fiasco that I remember at that time was the first injection I received from a new nurse after I was moved to a regular hospital room from the ICU. She came in with what looked like a horse syringe. It was huge and reminded me of a large pump squirter that I used for water fights with the kids on my block. The nurse proceeded to inject me with this large syringe, which really hurt because of the large volume of insulin that was forced into my thigh. A short time later, the doctor who was assigned to take care of me, who was not a diabetes specialist, came in to see me. I asked him why the shot was so large and he was also puzzled. To make a long story short, the nurse had misread the doctor's order. Instead of giving me 15 units of insulin (handwritten very sloppily as 15U), she gave me

150 units of insulin. Then all hell broke loose. They put me back in the ICU, stuck some more IV lines in me, made me drink very sweet fluids, and tested my blood glucose every 5 or 10 minutes for several hours. All hospitals now have a rule that the word *Units* must be written out completely and not indicated by just a capital U.

Eventually I was discharged to go home on only one shot a day in the morning, and given a strict diet using the old exchange system, by which I would weigh all of my portions of protein, carbohydrate, and fat on a little scale. What a pain! I was also supposed to test my urine for glucose four times a day and keep records of everything. At first, with the help of my mother, I did everything by the book, but eventually I lost interest. I did not realize why it was so important and I certainly was not informed or motivated to take control of my diabetes.

I would see my doctor every 3 months, have my blood and urine collected in the morning, and then wait the usual 2 to 3 hours for the results to come back from the lab. My doctor would come into the room, look at the results, and say the same thing every time, "Steve, you are doing fine. I will see you next time." In addition, I never went to a camp for diabetic kids or spent any time in support groups or classes for young people with diabetes. I was never educated about how to take an active role in my own diabetes care, and as a result, my control started to slip.

I worked at a boys' camp in Los Angeles every summer and almost every weekend during the rest of the school year as a camp aid, cook, and counselor. Every week we had a contest called, for lack of a better term, "The Pissing Contest." The contest was to see who could urinate for the longest period of

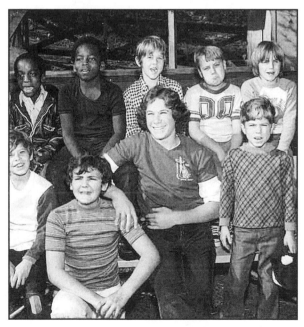

Picture of me at the Griffin Park Boys Camp. No, I am not Spanky in the back row with the double zero on his t-shirt!

time. We took this event seriously. We used a stopwatch that measured to 1/100th of a second. During competition, you had to have one continuous stream and you had to keep your hands behind your back so you could not do any type of weird manipulation to artificially increase your time. Well, I remember winning week after week after week, and I still hold the camp record to this day. Just try urinating continuously for 1 minute and 15 seconds straight, without stopping! Time yourself the next time you go. The not-so-funny thing about this story is that my diabetes was horribly out of control, resulting in excessive thirst and urination. I am sure I also stretched my bladder terribly back then, and I am paying for it now. Home glucose monitors and the hemoglobin A1C test had not been invented at that time.

It took me several years before I realized that I should do something about the fact that I was probably not doing well, despite the repeated comments at every visit from my doctor that I was "doing fine." I truly did not know that I was doing harm to my body. I was not a rebellious teenager who purposely went out of control to gain attention. I simply was never told what my goals of control should be and why it was so important in a way that I understood.

On one occasion, I decided to test my doctor because what he was saying to me at every visit did not make sense. On the morning of my next appointment, I went to Winchell's Donut Shop and ate five donuts including two glazed, two chocolate cake, and one maple bar (my favorite)! I then proceeded to give my urine and blood samples at the office as usual. I remember using my own urine test strips in the hospital bathroom to test the sample I turned in for analysis. The strip turned black in about 3 seconds, indicating that my urine was packed with sugar. I waited the usual 2 or 3 hours, and finally my doctor walked into the examination room holding his clipboard and studying the results of the blood and urine tests. He looked me straight in the eye and said, "Steve, you are doing fine. I will see you next time." From that point onward, I knew I could not trust him to take care of me, and I made a decision never to see that doctor again.

The bad news is that those early years of poor control contributed greatly to my development of several diabetic complications. I have proliferative diabetic retinopathy, an advanced form of diabetic eye disease, and I have received extensive laser surgery to both eyes in order to stabilize the problem. I have diabetic kidney disease, causing protein to spill into my urine and give me high blood pressure, for which I take three different medications to control the situation. I also have some manifestations of diabetic neuropathy (slight numbness in my feet) and problems with my stomach (gastroparesis). The good news is that I sought out good diabetes specialists, such as Doctors

Mayer Davidson and Richard Berkson, and started to receive the appropriate treatment to minimize and slow down the progression of these complications. I feel fortunate that I was able to improve my control at a time when my complications were not extremely advanced.

I was always interested in science and decided to go to medical school. At the University of California at Los Angeles (UCLA), where I did my undergraduate premedical studies, I became more interested in medicine and specifically diabetes. I worked in a diabetes research laboratory with Dr. Mayer Davidson and observed Dr. Richard Berkson treat his patients in his diabetes clinic. During that time, I also realized that one shot a day was totally inadequate, and I improved my regimen to allow for better control. Later, during my last year in medical school, I went on an insulin pump and became "fuel injected." Over the past several years, I have experimented with the new rapid-acting and long-acting designer insulin analogues (Symlin [pramlintide]) and continuous glucose monitoring in trying to find a regimen that fits my lifestyle the best.

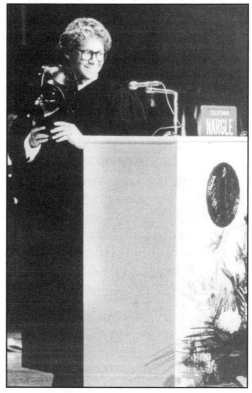

Me at my graduation from UC Davis Medical School as I gave the Valedictorian address.

I remember quite vividly when I studied physiology during my first year of medical school in 1978 at the University of California, Davis campus. The professor was citing statistics from old textbooks about the high death rate in people with diabetes. He stated that 50% of people with diabetes die from diabetic kidney disease within 20 years after the initial diagnosis. During the lecture, my classmates were trying to avoid eye contact with me or attempted to give me some type of visual sympathy from across the lecture hall (both situations made me feel uncomfortable). That afternoon we had a physiology laboratory and had to dissect the cadaver of a 25-year-old male who had died of diabetic kidney disease.

15

At the time, I was 23 years old with 8 years of diabetes behind me. My best friend, Ken Facter, always tried to comfort me by saying that at least I knew what I was going to die of! These early experiences motivated me to take better care of myself and to devote my career to helping people with diabetes.

After my medical residency at UCLA, I did the first part of my diabetes specialty training (fellowship) at the famous Joslin Diabetes Clinic in Boston. It was there that two great things happened to me:

The first was that I met my wife, Ingrid, as she was training to be a podiatrist, specializing in the care of feet for people with diabetes. The second is that I learned a great deal about all aspects of diabetes care as I worked and gained experience in the various departments that dealt with pregnancy, the kidneys, the eyes, young children with diabetes, the feet, the heart, and general care. I also gave lectures to the patients admitted to the Joslin Clinic and spent a lot of time answering questions about diabetes. I was always impressed by how thirsty the patients were for information about their condition.

Ingrid and I eventually ended up in San Diego, where I am a professor at the University of California San Diego School of Medicine, a staff member of the Veterans Affairs Medical Center, and Founder and Director of Taking Control Of Your Diabetes (TCOYD). Ingrid works in a high-risk diabetic foot clinic at the Veterans Affairs Medical Center. Ingrid and I are both involved in many diabetes organizations, and we attend and lecture at conferences across the United States and internationally. Although our two daughters, Talia and Carina, tested negative for diabetes when they were young, I still consider our clan as one big happy diabetes family. If you think about it, they have lived their entire lives in an environment surrounded by diabetes-related products, information,

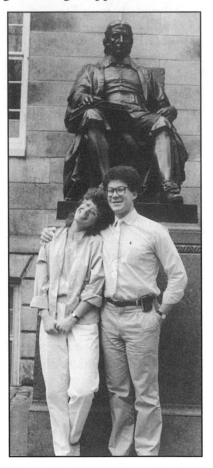

Me and Ingrid in Boston where we met at the Joslin Clinic.

and social events. I can't tell you how many times I have dragged them to a diabetes function that my wife and I were attending or to a TCOYD conference.

The main message I want to convey to you is that you can take control of your diabetes, even if you already have complications. It is never too late to get in control, both mentally and physically. The whole concept of TCOYD embodies the philosophy of self-help and self-advocacy. You cannot help others you love until you have taken care of yourself. It is not a selfish attitude; it is a smart and effective way to live a happier, healthier, and more productive life. You owe it to yourself and your loved ones.

Taking Control of Your Diabetes

Taking control of your diabetes is not easy, physically or mentally. For many people living with this condition, diabetes causes profound suffering and severe hardship. Living with a loved one who has diabetes can be just as difficult. You can take control of your diabetes by becoming educated, motivated, and a self-advocate for your medical care. By educating people with diabetes on the prevention, early detection, and aggressive management of diabetes and its complications, TCOYD strives to reduce the human suffering caused by this condition. This is what TCOYD is all about.

I initially spent a lot of time and energy trying to educate primary-care physicians on how to take care of their patients with diabetes. I organized conferences, gave lectures, and published articles for general practitioners so that they could be knowledgeable about all of the recent advances in diabetes and be able to provide the highest standards of care to the people who had diabetes in their practice. The problem was that it took many years for the information to be translated into clinical practice, and some caregivers were so stuck in their ways they were unable to change their practice habits for the better.

After many years of hard work trying to spread the important messages about diabetes care to other professionals, I realized that diabetes care was not improving fast enough at the community level. I witnessed many situations in which terrible complications due to diabetes could have been avoided by simple tests performed at the right time along with correct therapy. For these reasons, I started to change my focus from educating the medical professionals to translating the important messages directly to the people living with diabetes. Now, as I write this updated edition, I have come full circle. TCOYD also involves my spending time and resources to educate caregivers as well as patients in our new Making the Connection program. It cannot be one or the other, patients or professionals. It must be a dual-pronged approach and TCOYD is now working to close the gap between the patient and the physician in terms of education and communication.

Taking Control Of Your Diabetes, which I founded in September 1995, is a not-for-profit organization that promotes education, motivation, and self-advocacy by presenting large patient-oriented conferences and health fairs across the United States. TCOYD also has an active website, newsletter, and television show.

Mission Statement: To educate and motivate people with diabetes and their loved ones to take a more active role in their condition in order to live healthier, happier, and more productive lives.
Vision Statement: for all people with diabetes and their loved ones to have full access to proper education and therapy to aid in the prevention, early detection, and aggressive management of diabetes and its complications.

I truly believe that the most efficient and effective way to improve diabetes care in this country and around the world is to educate and motivate the people living with diabetes to take a more active role in their health care.

Historically, it takes 10 to 15 years for a pharmaceutical company to develop a new medication and get it officially approved by the Food and Drug Administration (FDA). Once a drug is approved, it normally takes medical institutions and teaching hospitals many more years to educate and change the practice habits of the vast number of caregivers who are taking care of people with diabetes. Once the new information is disseminated, the doctor must then absorb it and begin to implement changes in the way he or she cares for people with diabetes. Changing habits, whether we are talking about caregivers or about you and me, is a difficult thing to do. Furthermore, these primary caregivers in turn have little time to pass on this new information to their patients when they come in for their yearly, biyearly, or quarterly visit. As a result, many patients do not receive optimal care because they rely solely on their caregiver to tell them what is up and coming in the world of diabetes. This approach does not always work, and the losers are the people with diabetes.

People with diabetes must work with their caregivers and not merely trust and wait for the proper care to be delivered. Many physicians are not accustomed to their patients taking an active role in their own condition. If your caregiver seems uncomfortable when you ask a question or suggest a test or therapy that you learned may be of benefit to you, perhaps you should find another physician. I repeatedly tell physicians and medical administrators that the educated patient is the best patient because they help you do your job and, in the long run, save you time and money.

Since the beginning of TCOYD in 1995, we have been pushing these three important themes of Taking Control Of Your Diabetes. They have never lost their importance or magnitude:

1. *You have the main responsibility for taking control of your diabetes.* This is your life and no one should be more interested in getting the most proper health care than you. The responsibility does not lie with your wife, husband, mother, father, sister, brother, or doctor. Your doctor does not bear the main responsibility for your health; that is your responsibility. It is you who will personally suffer if you develop blindness or kidney failure, not your physician.

2. *You are your own best advocate.* In these days of managed care and the shrinking health care dollar, it is becoming more and more difficult to obtain the proper care you deserve and need to stay healthy. You must become knowledgeable about and get involved with the administrative aspects of your health care system so that you have timely access to the proper tests, most effective medications, and latest medical devices. This can be a frustrating and time-consuming process that can wear you down, but in the end, you will win if you are persistent (see Chapter 23).

3. *Be smart and be persistent.* Educate yourself about preventive measures to avoid eye, kidney, nerve, and heart disease. Be knowledgeable about the screening tests used to diagnose diabetes-related problems early so that you can obtain proper treatment in time. Be up-to-date on all of the various treatment options available to aggressively treat any complication that you have so that its progression will be slowed or halted.

The Different Types of Diabetes

I always like to clarify up front what the different types of diabetes are. Many folks become confused about what type of diabetes they have. Knowing and understanding what type of diabetes you have really sets the foundation of what you need to know throughout the rest of the book, because there are important differences in screening, prevention strategies and treatment regimens for type 1 and type 2 diabetes. The classification of the different types of diabetes has changed many times in the past several years, leading to lots of confusion. There are many different types of diabetes, but the most common are type 1 diabetes, type 2 diabetes, and gestational diabetes (**Table 1-1**).

Type 1 Diabetes

Type 1 diabetes was formerly called insulin-dependent diabetes mellitus (IDDM), juvenile-onset diabetes, brittle diabetes, or unstable diabetes. While type 1 diabetes usually develops before the age of 20, one can develop type 1 diabetes at any age, hence the term juvenile-onset is misleading. I do not like the words "brittle" and "unstable." These terms refer to the fluctuation in blood glucose values throughout the day that are commonly experienced by people with type 1 diabetes. At the time of diagnosis, people with type 1 diabetes are usually thin or of normal weight and there are usually no other associated conditions, such as high blood pressure or abnormal cholesterol levels, that are commonly seen in type 2 diabetes (**Table 1-2**). Only about 10% of all diabetics in the United States have the type 1 variety. Type 1 diabetes does run in families, although not nearly as strongly as is observed with type 2 diabetes. There have been case reports of several children in the same elementary school class coming down with type 1 diabetes within a short period of time. One of my female patients has type 1 diabetes and all three of her children developed type 1 diabetes before the age of 7. These later scenarios are less common than the sporadic cases. I am the only person in my family who developed type 1 diabetes, which is the more typical situation. People with type 1 diabetes have "first-degree" relatives (parents, siblings, or children) with type 1 diabetes approximately 4% to 8% of the time.

The cause of type 1 diabetes is not entirely known, but it is believed that for some reason (genetic, viral, or environmental), antibodies are produced that specifically destroy the pancreas. Any condition in which antibodies are produced that attack the body is called an autoimmune condition. Antibodies are the cells in the body that normally attack and destroy anything foreign, and the pancreas is the organ that produces and secretes insulin. Insulin is needed to help the glucose molecules that appear in the blood after eating get into the cells of the body to be used and stored for energy. If there is not

---

Table 1-1

The Different Types of Diabetes*

Type 1 Diabetes
Previously called insulin-dependent diabetes mellitus (IDDM), juvenile-onset diabetes, brittle diabetes, unstable diabetes, and ketosis-prone diabetes

Type 2 Diabetes
Previously called non–insulin-dependent diabetes mellitus (NIDDM), adult-onset diabetes, old-age diabetes, stable diabetes, and non–ketosis-prone diabetes

Gestational Diabetes
Also called diabetes of pregnancy

---

* Although there are many other types of diabetes, they are not as common.

Table 1-2

Main Differences Between Type 1 and Type 2 Diabetes

Characteristics	Type 1 Diabetes	Type 2 Diabetes
Age at onset	Usually less than 20 years	Usually over 35 years
Body habitus	Typically thin or not obese	Typically obese
Other family members also with diabetes	Approximately 4% to 8%	Approximately 70% to 90%
Ethnic groups	Typically white	African American, Asian American, Hispanic, Pacific Islander, Native American
Cause of diabetes	The insulin-producing cells of the pancreas are destroyed by antibodies	The body is resistant to the glucose-lowering effect of insulin—insulin resistance
Type of therapy required	Insulin	Diet alone and/or pills and/or insulin
Associated conditions at the time of diagnosis	Usually none	High blood pressure, high cholesterol levels, heart disease
Total diabetes in the United States	Approximately 10%	Approximately 90%

enough insulin, the glucose stays at high levels in the bloodstream and circulates to all of the organs of the body, including the eyes, kidneys, heart, blood vessels, and nerves. It is the chronic elevation of blood glucose levels over many years that leads to damage of these organs and the classic complications of diabetes.

The main problem in type 1 diabetes is a lack of insulin, not insulin resistance, which is the main cause of type 2 diabetes. This is why people with type 1 diabetes always need insulin and the diabetic pills do not work for them. Insulin must be injected because if it is swallowed, the enzymes in the stomach will digest and inactivate it before the insulin enters the bloodstream. We now have inhaled insulin that will give us old-timer insulin users and people newly needing insulin an option other than injections.

An important subcategory of type 1 diabetes is called LADA (Latent Autoimmune Diabetes in Adults). This is basically when someone is diagnosed with type 1 or autoimmune diabetes later in life as an adult. Barbara is one of my good friends and a patient diagnosed with type 1 diabetes at the age of 64. The destruction of the insulin-producing cells of the pancreas (beta cells) is slower in LADA patients so the symptoms are not as severe as they would be in a newly diagnosed teenager with extreme thirst, urination, and weight loss.

This type of presentation of elevated blood glucose levels in an adult with not-so-severe symptoms can fool the caregiver into thinking the patient has type 2 diabetes. The person may be prescribed oral medication commonly used for type 2 diabetes, which does not work well. Eventually the need to start insulin will arise. I tell practitioners at the medical education lectures that I give around the country to look out for LADA patients and to order a test called the GAD antibodies test. GAD stands for glutamic acid decarboxylase (see why I use GAD instead) and can be easily measured by most laboratories. If positive, the patient most likely has type 1 diabetes. Knowing what type of diabetes you have is important because it has important genetic and treatment implications.

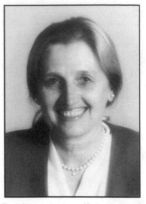

Barbara was diagnosed with type 1 diabetes at age 64.

The ultimate cure for type 1 diabetes will most likely come from stem cell research. Developing a vaccine that allows for immune protection against the autoantibodies that attack the pancreas is another approach being studied. At the time of this edition, there have been no major advances in preventing type 1 diabetes that will affect a large number of people. In the mean time, it is important to stay as healthy as possible so that when a cure comes along, you will be a good candidate.

Type 2 Diabetes

Type 2 diabetes was formerly called non–insulin-dependent diabetes mellitus (NIDDM), adult-onset diabetes, and stable diabetes. This terminology of "non–insulin-dependent" led to confusion because many people with type 2 diabetes are treated with insulin, usually after the oral diabetic mediations have lost their effectiveness. In addition, blood glucose levels of people with type 2 diabetes can be just as unstable or brittle as those of type 1 diabetics. People who develop type 2 diabetes are usually over the age of 35, but one can develop type 2 diabetes at any age, as is the case with type 1 diabetes. People with type 2 diabetes are usually overweight and commonly have high blood pressure and abnormal cholesterol levels at the time of diagnosis. Type 2 diabetes is also commonly found in certain ethnic groups such as African Americans, Native Americans, Asian Americans, Pacific Islanders, and in people of Hispanic descent. In contrast, type 1 diabetes is predominantly a white man's disease. Approximately 90% of all all people with diabetes are of the type 2 variety. In addition, type 2 diabetes runs strongly from generation to generation. Approximately 70% to 90% of people with type 2 diabetes have a family history of diabetes, whereas only about 4% to 8% of type 1 diabetics have someone else in their family with the same type of diabetes (**Table 1-2**).

The cause of type 2 diabetes could not be more different than that of type 1 diabetes. However, many of the complications are similar because both types of diabetes lead to high blood glucose levels. At the time of diagnosis in people with type 2 diabetes, there is usually an excess amount of insulin, which is in striking contrast to what is observed in type 1 diabetics. The problem is that the tissues of body are resistant to the normal glucose-lowering effects of insulin; thus the medical phrase "insulin resistance."

In the early prediagnosis stage, insulin resistance can be found in high-risk individuals who will eventually develop type 2 diabetes. When insulin resistance is present, the blood glucose values start to climb because the insulin is not totally effective at getting the glucose molecules into the cells of the body for energy. As a compensatory mechanism, the pancreas secretes more and more insulin in an effort to overcome this insulin resistance. For many years, this physiologic adaptation works well and the individual's glucose values are near normal. This is why it commonly takes many years to diagnose type 2 diabetes. It is often said that of the estimated 23 million people with diabetes in this country, only two thirds of them know they have the condition. It is important to note that in the early stages of type 2 diabetes there are no symptoms, such as excessive thirst and urination, and this is why screening is so important.

As time goes on, the pancreas gets tired of overproducing excess amounts of insulin to overcome the insulin resistance and eventually burns out or becomes exhausted. When this occurs, the blood glucose levels really go through the roof, and this is normally when the oral medications start to lose their effectiveness and the patient needs insulin and/or Byetta (exenatide) to control the glucose levels (discussed in Chapters 9 and 10). How long does it take for the pancreas to become exhausted? It is different for everybody, but it is usually 5 to 10 years from the time of diagnosis. This scenario of events that occurs in type 2 diabetes is commonly referred to as "the natural history of type 2 diabetes" (**Figure 1-1**). It is my belief that the earlier the diagnosis is made and the better the glucose control from the time of diagnosis, the longer someone with type 2 diabetes can control their diabetes with an exercise program and realistic meal plan with or without medication(s). The various types of therapy available for type 2 diabetes may also influence this "natural history" and will be discussed later in the book. An important point is that

Figure 1-1
The Natural History of Type 2 Diabetes

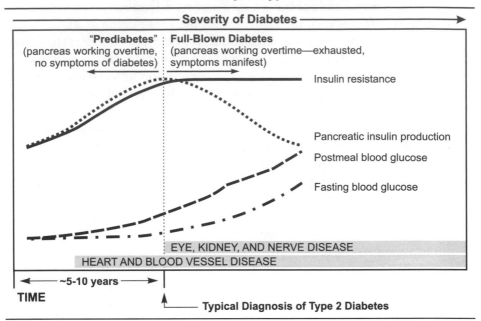

Insulin resistance can be present for many years before the diagnosis of diabetes. Blood glucose levels are not markedly elevated in the early stages of diabetes. Once the pancreas becomes exhausted, the blood glucose values go through the roof. As the pancreas becomes exhausted, the chance of achieving good glucose control with diet and exercise alone or with one oral agent goes down. The need for insulin therapy normally goes up over time as well.

glucose control is the most important issue, even if you need "tons" of medication to achieve your goals. You will be much better off and have less complications than someone who brags that they take no medications and has horrible glucose control.

Gestational Diabetes

Gestational diabetes is another common type of diabetes. It usually occurs in women... (get it?). It refers to the development of diabetes while a woman is pregnant. The cause of gestational diabetes is more closely related to type 2 diabetes in that insulin resistance is present with the added influence of female hormones that fluctuate during pregnancy. Most women revert to normal glucose levels after delivery. However, women with a history of gestational diabetes also have a higher chance of developing type 2 diabetes with subsequent pregnancies and later in life. It is also extremely important to keep blood glucose levels under control during pregnancy to prevent fetal abnormalities and problems with the delivery. One of the problems at delivery is that the baby is too large physically but internally underdeveloped so the rate of C-sections goes up and the length of time that the baby needs to stay in the hospital is longer. If you have type 1 diabetes and you become pregnant, in reality you do not have classic gestational diabetes. You are simply diabetic and pregnant. Treatment for gestational diabetes is somewhat different than it is for type 2 diabetes. In general, insulin is used most of the time; however, use of oral medications such as the sulfonylureas and metformin are being used more and more as their safety in offspring is being monitored closely. As in all types of diabetes, diet and exercise regimens are extremely important. Dr. Lois Jovanivic is an international expert on gestational diabetes. Lois runs the Samsun Research and Treatment Center in Santa Barbara, California, and has been a speaker for TCOYD. (Please see *Diabetes & Pregnancy: What to Expect* and *Gestational Diabetes: What to Expect* by the American Diabetes Association.)

Diagnosis of Diabetes

If you are reading this book, you probably already have diabetes, but I think it is important to discuss how diabetes is officially diagnosed. This may be important for your friends or family members who are at risk for developing diabetes. The criteria for diagnosis were recently changed by the American Diabetes Association and are shown in **Table 1 3**. It is important to note that these criteria are only for the diagnosis of diabetes in people who previously did not know they were diabetic and are not the treatment goals for people already living with diabetes.

The most common and easiest way to make the diagnosis is by measuring the fasting blood glucose (FBG),

Table 1-3

Official Criteria for Diagnosing Diabetes*

- Any individual with the symptoms of high blood glucose (hyperglycemia) and a blood glucose value at any time of the day over 200 mg/dL

OR

- A fasting blood glucose (FBG) test, which is done in the morning before anything to eat or drink other than water, that is 126 mg/dL or higher

OR

- An abnormal oral glucose tolerance test (OGTT), defined as a 2-hour glucose value that is 200 mg/dL or higher (discussed in the text)

---

* These official criteria are from the American Diabetes Association. Available at: *www.diabetes.org*.

which refers to the glucose value in the morning after an overnight fast and before breakfast. If the blood glucose value is 126 mg/dL or higher, the diagnosis of diabetes can be made. FBG levels less than 100 mg/dL are considered normal. It is important to point out that any FBG over 100 mg/dL but less than 126 mg/dL is abnormal and should warrant close follow-up. The official phrase for FBG in this gray zone is "impaired fasting glucose" or "prediabetes" (**Figure 1-2**). Furthermore, the sugar level 1 to 2 hours after eating may be an even better screening test than the FBG for the diagnosis of type 2 diabetes. The reason for this is that the postmeal or postprandial glucose value usually becomes abnormal before the FBG level in the natural history of type 2 diabetes discussed earlier (**Figure 1-1**).

The postmeal or postprandial glucose value is normal below 140 mg/dL in individuals without diabetes. If the postmeal glucose value is consistently above 200 mg/dL, diabetes can be diagnosed. In addition, if one has symptoms of elevated blood glucose values, such as excessive thirst and urination, lethargy, poor wound healing, blurry vision, frequent urinary tract infections, and random glucose values over 200 mg/dL at any time of the day, diabetes is present and no further tests are needed for a diagnosis. If the postmeal glucose value is above 140 but less than 200 mg/dL, we classify these folks as having impaired glucose tolerance or once again prediabetes (**Figure 1-2**). Chapter 25 is devoted to the prevention of diabetes in people who have prediabetes.

The oral glucose tolerance test (OGTT) is an official diabetes diagnostic test, although not commonly needed. After an overnight fast, one swallows 75 grams of glucose (a large glass of very sweet syrup) in the morning and the blood glucose levels are followed over the next 2 hours. The OGTT is mainly used for clinical research purposes. There is a modified OGTT that is now used for screening women who are at risk for developing gestational diabetes; it is performed at 26 weeks into the pregnancy. An individual is defined as being at risk for diabetes if she has had a prior episode of gestational diabetes, has given birth to an infant weighing over 9 pounds, has a family history of diabetes, is overweight, has high blood pressure or cholesterol levels, or is of an ethnic group with a high incidence of diabetes (**Table 1-4**).

Why Is Glucose Control Important?

Why is everyone stressing that your glucose values should be as close to normal as possible? It is simply because high glucose values over an extended period of time can cause damage to the organs of the body. Certain organs seem to be more susceptible to elevated blood glucose

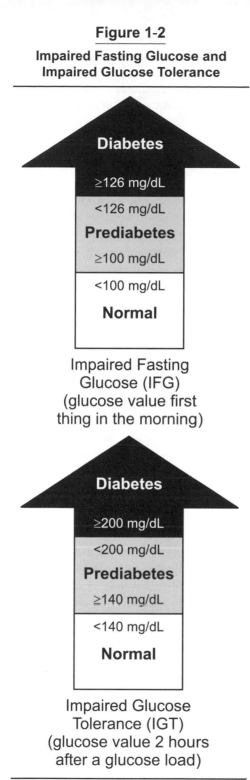

Figure 1-2

**Impaired Fasting Glucose and
Impaired Glucose Tolerance**

Diabetes

≥126 mg/dL

<126 mg/dL

Prediabetes

≥100 mg/dL

<100 mg/dL

Normal

Impaired Fasting
Glucose (IFG)
(glucose value first
thing in the morning)

Diabetes

≥200 mg/dL

<200 mg/dL

Prediabetes

≥140 mg/dL

<140 mg/dL

Normal

Impaired Glucose
Tolerance (IGT)
(glucose value 2 hours
after a glucose load)

levels or hyperglycemia than others, with the eyes, kidneys, nerves, and blood vessels being the most seriously affected. Remember that the blood bathes every organ in our bodies at all times, and anything that is toxic in the bloodstream will have a major impact on the health of our organs. It is also important not to panic if your blood glucose level gets too high occasionally, even if it is high for a few weeks or months. It is the chronic elevation over years and years that causes the real damage, leading to blindness, kidney failure, amputation, heart disease, and stroke. I feel that every diabetic needs to work out an individual treatment plan to get their blood glucose level as close to normal as possible. It is also important that in the quest for normal or near normal glucose levels, the treatment plan should not be so rigid that there are major disruptions of one's lifestyle, including frequent episodes of hypoglycemia (blood glucose levels that are too low). Treatment plans need to be individualized based on your age, risk of hypoglycemia, normal daily eating and sleeping habits, other medical problems, etc. One size does not fit all!

For many years, most physicians did not stress good or "tight" glucose control in their diabetic patients because definitive, long-term clinical studies demonstrating the benefits of tight glucose control had not been undertaken and there was concern that all of the trouble and expense of controlling their patients' glucose values were not warranted until the benefits were proven. I was among a minority of physicians in this country at that time who believed that tight glucose control not only made one feel better on a day-to-day basis, avoiding short-term or acute complications, but that it also reduced the long-term complications. Long-term microvascular complications refer to the eye (retinopathy), kidney (nephropathy), and nerve (neuropathy) diseases commonly seen in people with diabetes.

My beliefs were based on my own experience as a patient and physician and on a fairly large body of medical literature already published supporting the notion that glucose control matters. The government initiated a long-term clinical trial to address this important issue. This study is called the Diabetes Control and Complications Trial (DCCT)

Table 1-4

Risk Factors for Developing Type 2 Diabetes

- Having someone in your family with diabetes, especially a first-degree relative
- Being overweight, especially with central obesity, commonly referred to as a "beer belly"
- Having some or all of the other associated conditions commonly seen in type 2 diabetes, such as high blood pressure or high cholesterol levels (these conditions may appear before the diagnosis of diabetes)
- Being a member of an ethnic group that has a high incidence of diabetes, such as African American, Hispanic, Native American, Asian American, and Pacific Islander
- Developing diabetes during pregnancy (gestational diabetes)
- Giving birth to an infant weighing over 9 pounds. (If a woman has high blood glucose during pregnancy, the infant may be large physically although it is usually developmentally abnormal internally.)
- Being told by a caregiver that you have "a touch of diabetes" or "borderline diabetes." (There is no such thing.)

and was completed in 1993. The DCCT was one of the longest, most extensive and expensive studies in the history of medicine. The DCCT was not the first study to show the importance of glycemic control in preventing and delaying the progression of microvascular complications of diabetes. The DCCT was, however, the most powerful and well-done study and has set the standard of care for the United States and the world. The DCCT, sponsored by the National Institutes of Health, was a 9-year, $160 million, multimember trial that studied over 1400 patients with type 1 diabetes.

The DCCT was designed to answer two main questions:

1. Whether intensive glycemic control could prevent the classic long-term microvascular complications of diabetes
2. Whether intensive glycemic control could delay the progression of microvascular complications already present in people with diabetes. The DCCT also looked at the incidence of hypoglycemia (low blood glucose) and weight gain.

In the DCCT, patients were put into either an intensive treatment group or a conventional treatment group. The people randomized to the intensive treatment group were put on multiple insulin injections or insulin pumps and were required to perform frequent home glucose monitoring. The goal was to lower the glucose values to normal or near-normal levels. The treatment goal for the people in the conventional treatment group (who were put on 1 or 2 injections per day) was to avoid symptoms of extreme low and high blood glucose levels. Home monitoring with glucose meters was not encouraged.

The patients were further subdivided into a primary prevention group (those who had no evidence of microvascular complications when the study began) and a secondary intervention group (those who already had some evidence of eye, kidney, or nerve disease at the beginning of the study).

Figure 1-3 shows the glycosylated hemoglobin (or A1C; a long-term glucose control factor that will be discussed later) and daily average blood glucose values during the 9-year study in the intensively and conventionally treated groups. It is important to note that despite an enormous amount of attention and effort given by the DCCT study personnel and the use of multiple injection regimens, insulin pumps, and home glucose monitoring devices, the patients randomized to the intensive treatment group did not achieve completely normal glucose values or a normal A1C value (a blood test that determined the extent of blood glucose control over the preceding 3 months). The important message here is that it is very difficult to achieve completely normal glucose values in the majority of people with diabetes compared with those who do not have diabetes. We now have designer insulin analogues and continuous glucose monitors, which were not available at the time of the DCCT, that can help people achieve even tighter control.

The average daily glucose value (before and after meals) for the intensively treated group was about 155 mg/dL. The average daily blood glucose value for the conventionally treated group was about 230 mg/dL. These are valuable numbers to keep in mind, especially if

Figure 1-3

Glycosylated Hemoglobin (A1C) and Daily Average Blood Glucose Values During the 9-Year Diabetes Control and Complications Trial

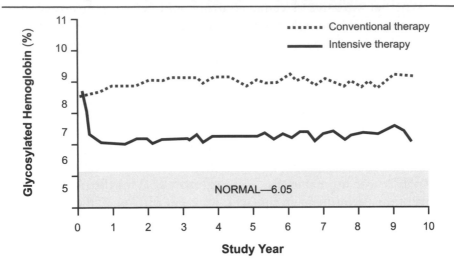

Diabetes Control and Complications Trial Research Group. *N Engl J Med*. 1993;329:977-986.

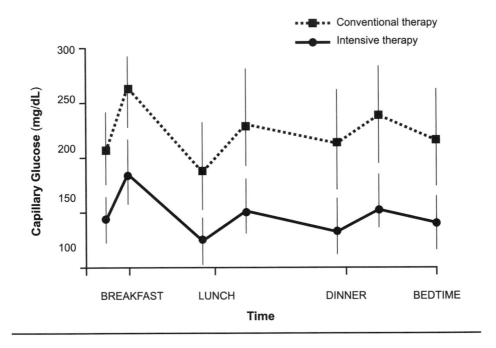

you have a glucose meter that keeps an average of your values. You can always compare your averages with the patients in the DCCT. Despite having poor glucose values in the conventionally treated group, on the average they still had better control than most diabetics in this country at that time. This, in my opinion, represented the sad state of diabetes care in the United States. Unfortunately, diabetes care did not change much during the ensuing years, which is one of the reasons I founded TCOYD. Finally, I feel that diabetes care is slowly improving in this country.

Intensive glycemic control reduced the risk of developing new retinopathy by an impressive 76% and delayed significant progression by 54% in people who already had eye disease. The benefits of intensive glucose control became apparent when the groups were compared after only 3 years of therapy. The reductions in kidney and nerve disease with intensive glucose control were also impressive, showing the same trends as seen with retinopathy.

It is clear that intensive glycemic control can prevent the onset and delay the progression of microvascular complications in type 1 diabetes. Further analysis also revealed that the risk for developing complications increased dramatically when the A1C was greater than two percentage points above the upper limit of normal (greater than 8% in the DCCT). It has been estimated that for every 1% rise in A1C above 8%, there is a 40% to 50% increase in the risk of developing retinopathy or eye disease.

The quality of life of the patients who achieved good glucose control was excellent, although as a group they experienced a small weight gain and a higher incidence of hypoglycemia (low blood sugar) compared with the patients with poor glycemic control. The patients who were intensively treated experienced a threefold incidence of severe hypoglycemic reactions requiring assistance from others, or they experienced unconsciousness. In addition, there were no differences between the two groups with respect to major accidents or deaths.

The gain in body weight (about 5 to 10 pounds) that occurred in patients in the intensive therapy group is commonly observed when people with diabetes markedly improve their blood glucose control. Part of the reason for the weight gain in the well-controlled group is that less glucose was spilling over into the urine and more was available for energy. Both hypoglycemia and weight gain can be minimized by diet control and exercise.

Both groups scored equally on the quality-of-life questionnaire despite the daily study demands imposed on the intensive treatment group. In other words, the group that achieved excellent control did not feel that their lifestyle was adversely affected. I believe that the patients who were performing home glucose testing and going through the rigors of an intensive diabetes regimen felt great and in control, both mentally and physically. A similar study was completed in the United Kingdom that demonstrated the same benefits in people with type 2 diabetes (the United Kingdom Prospective Diabetes Study, or UKPDS). The debate over the importance of good glucose control is over and current studies are aimed at evaluating the various methods used to achieve glycemic goals in type 1 and type 2 diabetes.

In addition to the long-term microvascular complications of diabetes (eye, kidney, and nerve disease) that are minimized by improved glucose control, the acute short-term complications are also lessened. Acute complications, such as excessive thirst and urination, daytime tiredness, poor wound healing, blurry vision, urinary tract infections, and tooth and gum disease, affect how one feels on a day-to-day basis (**Table 1-5**). These acute complications of poorly controlled diabetes reduce the quality of life and adversely affect work performance in adults and school performance in children and young adults. The acute effects of hyperglycemia may manifest as frequent falls and mental impairment in the elderly. Many of the acute complications develop gradually, and it is only when good glucose control is achieved that one realizes how much worse they felt when in poor control of their diabetes. If hyperglycemia were painful, a lot more people with diabetes would be under better control and experience far fewer complications.

Table 1-5

Acute Complications of Poorly Controlled Blood Glucose Levels

- Excessive thirst, especially for cold drinks
- Frequent urination, including during the night
- Daytime tiredness and lack of energy
- Cuts, scrapes, and scratches take a long time to heal
- Frequent urinary tract and vaginal infections
- Tooth and gum disease
- Frequent falling and mental impairment may be seen in the elderly

Achievable Goals of Glucose Control That Protect Us From the Complications of Diabetes

The goals of glucose control for people with diabetes are quite different from the diagnostic criteria or the normal ranges that are seen in nondiabetic people. Glucose control goals, which have changed dramatically over the past few years, are shown in **Table 1-6**. The goals for glycemic control for people with diabetes keep getting lower

Table 1-6

Goals of Glucose Control for People With Diabetes

Test	Typical Glucose Range (mg/dL)	
	Normal (no diabetes)	**People With Diabetes**
Before-meal glucose level (preprandial)	<115	<120
After-meal glucose level (postprandial)	<140	<180
Bedtime glucose value	<120	100-140
A1C*	4% to 6%	<7%

* The normal range for glycosylated hemoglobin (A1C) is not standardized and may vary from lab to lab.

From the American Diabetes Association. Available at: *www.diabetes.org*.

and lower as the clinical researchers find out that we really should be shooting for totally normal blood glucose levels all of the time to avoid 100% of the complications. This is a tough goal to achieve but with all the new advances in diabetes care, a lot more people with diabetes are achieving better A1C values than ever before. Different organizations have different recommendations, but the bottom line is that we should all try to get our numbers as low as possible while avoiding frequent and severe hypoglycemia. An A1C of less than 7% is an excellent start.

Glycosylated Hemoglobin or A1C: The Long-Term Control Factor

The A1C is an important laboratory parameter that gives doctors and patients an idea of what the glucose control has been over the past 2 to 3 months. Remember that there are 1440 minutes in a day and a single glucose test only represents one moment in time and does not reflect the overall glucose control on the average for an extended period of time. I call the glycosylated hemoglobin (also known as A1C or HgbA1c) the "long-term glucose control factor." When the glucose level in one's blood is high for an extended period of time, the excessive glucose molecules stick or bind to many structures in the body, including the red blood cells, which contain an oxygen-carrying substance called hemoglobin and other proteins (**Figure 1-4**). The average life span of red blood cells, which are being produced and cleared from the body continuously, is about 2 to 3 months. When we measure the amount of glucose on the hemoglobin of the red blood cells, for example, it is called the glycosylated hemoglobin, and is indicative of the amount of glucose in the circulation over the past 2

Figure 1-4

A1C Measures Glucose Levels Over a 2- to 3-Month Period

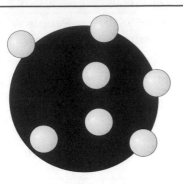

Normal Blood Glucose

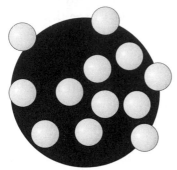

High Blood Glucose

● Red blood cell
○ Glucose

Abbreviation: A1C, glycosylated hemoglobin (a test that measures how much glucose has been sticking to the red blood cells in the last 2 to 3 months).

Glucose irreversibly attaches to red blood cells in proportion to the average glucose concentration in the blood.

to 3 months. We then compare this number with that of nondiabetic individuals. You can look at a chart to determine what your blood glucose average has been over a 2- to 3-month period by knowing your A1C values (**Figure 1-5**).

The Bayer Diagnostic Division has developed a home kit so you can measure your A1C with a drop of blood in the privacy of your own home. The test kit will give you an accurate value in 8 minutes. You do not have to wait a few days for the results, and best of all, you do not have to fight the usual medical office bureaucracy to get your own result. There is another long-term glucose control factor called fructosamine, which gives you an idea of the average blood glucose value of the past 2 to 3 weeks. It is normally used in women with diabetes

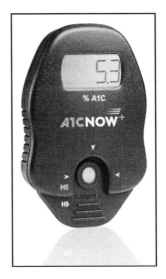

The A1CNow home glucose monitoring (HGM) device.

Figure 1-5

A1C and HGM Results

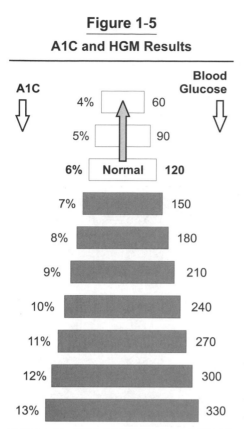

Abbreviations: A1C, glycosylated hemoglobin; HGM, home glucose monitoring.

This chart shows the relationship between A1C levels and average blood glucose readings; A1C measurement is presented as a percentage of glycosylation. A 6% A1C corresponds with a 120 mg/dL blood glucose level on average over the past 2 to 3 months.

during pregnancy because of the need to keep tight control during this important time period. Home glucose monitoring is probably the most important test to do when you are pregnant and have diabetes. GlycoMark (*www.glycomark.com*) is another very short-term glycemic control marker that gives you an idea of what your average blood glucose has been over the past several days and in addition correlates well with your postprandial glucose values.

It is extremely important to realize that unlike the glucose value, the A1C value is not measured the same way everywhere in the United States. This is why there are different normal ranges depending on the laboratory technique used. Always compare your A1C value with the nondiabetic ranges. The normal ranges that are usually preprinted next to your value represent the ranges that nondiabetic people have. In general, your value should be less than 1 percentage point above the upper limit of normal. For example, if the normal range is 4% to 6%, your first goal would be to get below 7%.

Don't you love it when the front office clerk says, "You cannot have your results"? You can sign a release-of-information form that should allow them to release your lab results to you. Make sure you ask the office staff about this requirement at your next appointment. Do not trust others to interpret your laboratory values. You need to know your numbers and know what the numbers mean. Ask questions and do your own investigation and research. Remember that you are your own best advocate. Be smart and be persistent!

Home Glucose Monitoring: A Personal Laboratory in the Palm of Your Hand

Home glucose monitoring (HGM) has been one of the more important advances in the field of diabetes since the discovery of insulin in the 1920s. People with diabetes have been able to test their own blood sugar levels with these hand-held devices for almost the past 30 years. Before the availability of HGM devices, people with diabetes tested their urine for glucose, which is terribly inaccurate. When the glucose in the blood is too high, the kidneys try to filter it out in the urine, which can be measured either by test strips or chemistry pills that you put in a test tube with water. The results of these archaic urine tests do not give you an actual number but rather a very rough guide depending on the color change of the urine strip or test tube concoction. The problem is that when you measure glucose in your urine, it actually is a reflection of what your blood glucose was several hours prior to the test and does not reflect what is happening at the time of

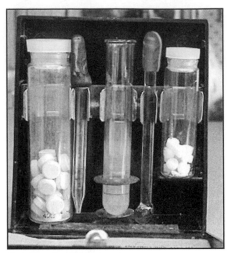

A urine test kit.

the test. Urine testing cannot be used effectively to make day-to-day decisions on insulin dosage and other self-management techniques. In addition, as one grows older, the ability of the kidneys to filter out the glucose in the blood declines so that the urine test may look good when the blood has excessive amounts of glucose.

In the old days before home glucose monitoring and the availability of the A1C test, patients would go to the doctor's office early in the morning, have their blood drawn and urine collected, and then wait… wait… and wait some more. It took a long time to get the results back from the laboratory. To make matters worse and delay things further, the office staff would schedule everyone at 8 o'clock in the morning in order to get everyone's specimens collected early. Eventually, the doctor would see you and make decisions on your treatment plan based on one blood glucose level at one point in time.

Many people with diabetes, including me, would do everything possible to make sure that all blood glucose values were good ones on the morning of our appointments. I would eat a well-balanced dinner low in carbohydrates with absolutely no "cheating" the night before my appointment. I remember seeing my nondiabetic sister, Susan, indulge in chips, ice cream, and cookies while we watched TV… and it almost killed me. I would then get up really early the next morning and exercise, skip breakfast, and take extra insulin before my appointment. If I experienced a low blood glucose reaction before my blood was drawn, I would take just enough sugar or orange juice to reduce my symptoms of sweating, shaking, and heart pounding, and not the usual entire package of Oreo cookies! The real problem was that my blood glucose was too high most of the time. I only did this sort of thing for a short time when I was young because I quickly realized that I

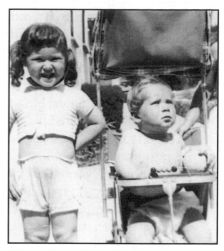

Me and my sister, Susan.

was only fooling myself. Believe it or not, I have adult patients who are intelligent professional people who do this type of thing all the time! It is basically a reflection of the emotional issues that accompany a chronic illness such as diabetes. I have devoted a separate chapter to these emotional barriers, written by my good friend Bill Polonsky, because the majority of people with diabetes can relate to these problems.

Should all people with diabetes test their own blood levels at home? In my opinion, the answer is a strong, loud, and resounding YES! Some individuals who are elderly with consistent daily schedules and whose diabetes is quite stable on oral medications may only need to test once or twice a week at the most. On the other hand, others may be on a multiple injection insulin regimen or an insulin pump, running around like a wild man or woman, working long hours, and exercising and eating at different times. These active people with diabetes, trying to lead normal lives, may need to test as often as 8 to 12 times a day in order to stay in good control. Continuous glucose monitoring (CGM) now is available and can be a tremendous asset to folks on insulin. I have devoted an entire chapter to this topic.

It is not enough to merely test your blood glucose at home or during daily activities. It is of utmost importance that you know what to do with the numbers and then act on those numbers. Don't test and just write the number down in your logbook for your caregiver to review. You should be thinking about what that number means, why you are at that glucose level, and what you should do to correct the number, if needed. You should also be thinking about how to avoid problems again in the future. If you are on insulin, you can always give yourself extra insulin (only if you have been educated to do so) to bring down a high blood glucose level. In addition, there is a whole list of nonpharmacologic maneuvers that do not involve pills or insulin adjustments that can help bring the glucose level into a more normal range. Techniques used to adjust for high premeal blood glucose levels are listed in **Table** 1-7. These techniques are important to minimize extreme hyperglycemia after eating and give you the power to act on the results of HGM, even if you are taking pills alone and not on insulin.

Even with HGM and the knowledge and ability to act on the results, it is difficult to mimic the metabolism of a nondiabetic individual. A normally functioning pancreas is a sophisticated organ with complicated and precise physiologic mechanisms to keep the blood glucose level in a tight range 24 hours a day, no matter what type of food is ingested. In a normal individual, the cells of the pancreas (beta cells) not only can detect changes in glucose on a second-to-second basis, but they can also identify and react to the rate of change of glucose during meals (how fast the blood glucose is rising or falling). There are other important glucose regulatory hormones such as amylin, glucagon, GLP-1, etc, that also play an important role and will be discussed in detail later in the book. This is one reason nondiabetic people can eat

Table 1-7

Techniques Used to Adjust for High Premeal Glucose Levels

- Increase the time interval between consumption of the meal and the insulin shot (if you are on insulin)
- Eat less than your usual amount of food
- Eliminate or replace foods containing simple or refined sugars, such as fruits
- Delay your meal if possible
- Exchange the milk, or any beverage with calories in it, for a noncaloric drink
- Do not eat all of your meal at once if possible. Spread the calories over an extended period of time. For example, save the fruit or bread for later
- Do mild exercise, such as walking, after eating
- If you recognize a consistent trend of high glucose values at a particular time of day, you should notify your caregiver to make the appropriate change in your oral medication or insulin. You can also make the appropriate changes yourself if you have been properly educated to do so

a hot fudge sundae and their blood glucose will never go above 140 mg/dL… those S.O.B.s!

If your physician does not offer you an HGM device, you need to be your own advocate and ask for one or get one on your own. Many patients do not like to prick their finger and test on a daily basis. I have heard many caregivers say, "I can't get my patients to test." I know why this is so; the patients may not have been given the knowledge to analyze and act on each individual number at the time of the test. I would give up testing myself if I could never do anything with the number. Many patients become frustrated when their blood glucose level are always high and they are not given any instructions about how to bring them down. "So why test? It is always high!" is a common complaint. Throughout the rest of the book, and especially in the chapters on therapy, I will be explaining how I manage my diabetes and the diabetes of my patients using HGM and CGM results. In addition, there are definitely proper techniques to make the fingerstick less painful.

In people with diabetes, emotional issues also play a big role in not utilizing this valuable tool of HGM to control their diabetes. We all want to "do good" for our doctors and are ashamed that we did not test often enough or that our glucose values were too high. I have collected some of my favorite and most common excuses that my patients have used when they "forgot" to bring their HGM logbook to clinic… once again!

- "My meter was stolen." (The Rolex watch was next to the meter but the thief just took the meter… give me a break.)
- "Oh, gosh, I forgot it again!"
- "My dog ate it."
- "Darn… I left it in the car." At this point, I usually tell my patient to go out to the parking lot to get it. Then there is the usual reply, "I took the bus today."
- "Oh, I didn't think you wanted to see it!" This one really bugs me. My usual reply is, "I am the diabetes doctor, this is a diabetes clinic, I am the one who asked you to test your blood glucose at home, and I would really be interested in seeing the results. Now why wouldn't you think I wanted to see it?"
- "My wife was supposed to bring it." This excuse gets back to one of my three main themes of this book: You have the main responsibility of taking control of your diabetes.
- "I went on vacation and did not take my meter." She also left her diabetes at home too? I would think that one of the more important times to test is while on vacation when you are not eating, exercising, and sleeping as you normally do.

To make life easier and more comfortable, many companies have developed meters that require a very small amount of blood. This means that the traditional and sometimes painful "fingerstick" can now be done on the forearm or thigh, which turns out to be a gentler, more preferred area from which to obtain blood. There are many glucose meters and you can find one that best fits your needs. There are very simple ones with large easy-to-read screens. There are meters with lots of bells and whistles that help you analyze and track your numbers at different times of the day. There are meters that do not require coding with each package of strips that you use and meters that communicate with other devices like insulin pumps. Please see the reference guide on the various meters in the Appendix.

I have observed many children and adults "dry lab it." "Dry labbing" is when a person fills up his or her logbook with falsely normal or near-normal glucose values (smart patients will put an occasional high level in to throw off the caregiver). The numbers are written with the same colored pen, there is no food or blood on the sheets, and there is not much variation in the numbers, which is unusual in real life. In addition, certain numbers repeat themselves too often, which is statistically highly unlikely. Now that long-term glucose control factors such as the A1C are widely available to caregivers, it is difficult to avoid getting caught faking your results (darn it!). **Figure 1-6** is the logbook of someone who has been dry labbing it. The funny

Figure 1-6

Glucose Logbook Example of Dry Labbing by an Adult Patient With Type 2 Diabetes

DATE	INSULIN			BREAKFAST		LUNCH		DINNER		BED TIME	OVER NIGHT	COMMENTS
	TYPE	AM	PM	BEFORE	AFTER	BEFORE	AFTER	BEFORE	AFTER			
3				160		135		121				
4				157		144		135				
5				149		—		130				
6				162		150		147				
7				155		144		150				
8				144		160		133				
9				162								

Usual Target Before Meals: 70-130 — BLOOD GLUCOSE — Usual Target 1-2 Hours After Meals: 70-180 thing about this guy is that the clinic date was in the afternoon on the 8th and when he was making up the numbers he went past the 8th and when he realized it, he simply crossed off the number on the 9th and did not think I would notice it. Look how many times he logged a value of 144 or numbers ending in zero or 5.

Whenever I mention this problem of dry labbing at one of our patient-oriented educational conferences, a large majority of the 1000-plus participants start to laugh. My next comment is, "Those of you who laughed have done this before!" It is important to emphasize that people who falsify their results or who seem to consistently forget their logbooks are not bad people. It simply means that there are emotional barriers that have not yet been broken down. It is an important challenge to me as a diabetologist and to other caregivers to be able to develop a good enough doctor-patient relationship so that the patient feels comfortable or is not afraid or ashamed to tell the truth (either did not test at all or changed the numbers). Part of the solution to this problem definitely lies with the attitude of the physician, certified diabetes educator (CDE), primary care physician, or any professional working with that person.

Home glucose monitoring and the knowledge to act on the results are the keys to freedom for people with diabetes. It allows you to have a more flexible lifestyle, while achieving tight glucose control at the same time. HGM and CGM makes you feel in control of your condition both physically and mentally. They allow you to take control of your diabetes. (See Chapters 9 and 10 for more details.)

Continuous Glucose Monitoring Is Here: Technology That Will Dramatically Change the Lives of People With Diabetes

"Continuous glucose-sensing devices will revolutionize the treatment of diabetes. It will also be a blessing for the unfortunate people with diabetes who have hypoglycemic unawareness and are in constant fear of passing out due to low blood sugar levels." This excerpt is from the last edition of the TCOYD book published in 2001. It is now a reality!

People living with diabetes have many day-to-day struggles, and this is especially true with type 1 and insulin-requiring type 2 diabetes. There are so many factors that go into insulin-dose decisions several times each day, 7 days a week, 12 months a year, year after year. Some of these factors include type and amount of food to be ingested, prior type and intensity of exercise, anticipated type and intensity of exercise, other illnesses and stresses, the blood glucose level at the time, *and* the trend of blood glucose levels preceding the current test (important information that too few people currently have). In addition, the way we are given insulin is not physiologic; subcutaneous insulin delivery can be inconsistent and lead to unpredictable blood glucose results.

Home glucose monitoring has been one of the more important advances in diabetes care, but it does have limitations. Even when people are testing frequently, they see only a partial snapshot of what is happening. We do not lack knowledge about how to treat the disease, but rather, we lack constant information about what our blood glucose levels are doing in order to effectively respond. CGM can now fill those wide and potentially dangerous gaps.

Like millions of Americans living with diabetes, for the past 36 years, I have struggled to control my blood glucose level as best I could while avoiding the lows. I personally have avoided unconsciousness from hypoglycemia but at a price. I have diabetic retinopathy, kidney dysfunction, and neuropathy. The best way to describe how I felt when I used CGM technology for the first time was like finally being able to see clearly after 36 years of partial blindness.

The challenge now is to get this technology into the hands of the people who could benefit the most. This will take a concerted effort to educate the people living with diabetes, the professional community, and the insurers. At the current time, several companies are working on CGM devices as discussed in detail in Chapter 9.

Summary

Who should take care of the people with diabetes in this country? I say anyone who is interested, and the most interested person should be you! Taking control of your diabetes is simply being an informed health care consumer. The first step is to become motivated to take care of yourself so that you can live a happier, healthier, and more productive life. You have a responsibility to yourself and to your loved ones to take the best possible care of yourself. The second step is to become informed about what you need to do to get in control of your diabetes and stay there. Education is the key to survival both mentally and physically, and you must not rely on anyone else to do this for you. If the proper therapy is not instituted in a timely manner, the person who will suffer is you. The third step is to be a self-advocate. In the current times of managed care and the shrinking health care dollar, you may need to fight for what you need and deserve.

Taking control of your diabetes requires a healthy mind-set that you can live a normal life and do anything that you want to do without letting diabetes get in your way. You must take the attitude that by having diabetes, you will look at life differently and appreciate the things that others take for granted. Don't be afraid to learn as much as you can about diabetes, and please do not hesitate to be aggressive in order to obtain the medications, tests, devices, and examinations that you will need to stay healthy. Teach others, spread the word about diabetes, and motivate your friends and family members who have any chronic condition to take an active role in their health care. Please see Chapter 26 to learn about all the new programs that TCOYD is doing to help you take control of your diabetes. Remember that you have the main responsibility for taking control of your diabetes. You are your best self-advocate, so be smart and be persistent. Take control of your diabetes—you owe it to yourself and to your loved ones.

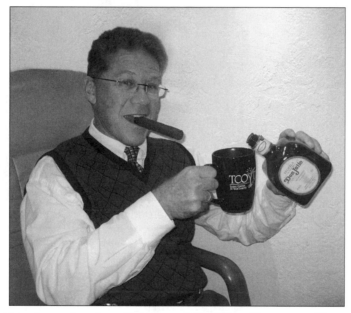

Here I am showing off the new TCOYD coffee mug with fake tequila and a sugar free, chocolate cigar (yeah, right!).

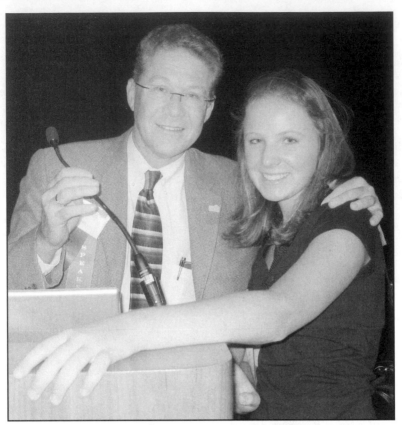

My oldest daughter, Talia, joining me on the podium at a TCOYD conference.

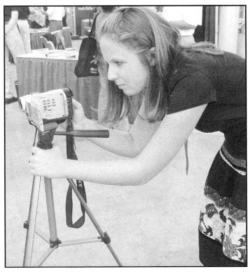

Talia filming a TCOYD conference.

2

The Emotional Side of Diabetes

by William H. Polonsky, PhD, CDE

Diabetes is easy. When you first developed diabetes, perhaps some of your friends, your family members, or even your health care providers told you that. After all, you just need to make some small changes in your everyday behavior. For example:
- Exercise regularly
- Check your blood glucose frequently
- Take your new medications and don't ever forget them
- See your health care provider regularly
- Make sure your blood glucose never gets too high or too low
- Lose some weight (but not too much)
- Don't forget to check your feet regularly
- Pay attention to your blood pressure and cholesterol
- Pay attention to your portion sizes when you eat
- Make sure you are consuming the correct amount and type of carbohydrates (there are good carbohydrates and bad carbohydrates)
- Eat more fruits and vegetables
- Try to eat less of the bad fats (but remember to eat enough of the good fats)
- And on and on and on…

Don't worry if you start to feel confused, because you have a 10-minute appointment with your doctor sometime next month. Certainly you will get all of your concerns and questions addressed then. See, just like you were told, diabetes is easy!

Of course, you know that's not the way it really is. Diabetes can be tough, even though friends, family, and even some health care providers may not realize this. Not surprisingly, many people with diabetes are struggling. Take Ralph, for example. He is a middle-aged man who has been living with type 2 diabetes for more than a decade. While he has always taken his diabetes medications regularly, he stopped checking his blood glucose several years ago. When asked why, Ralph explained, "Trust me, whenever I check, it is always too high. So what's the point?" He started walking regularly after he was first diagnosed, but life has gotten busier and busier and walking began to seem increasingly boring, so now Ralph hardly gets any exercise. He had made some healthy changes in how he eats, but he is only able to maintain those healthy habits until dinnertime. After dinner, Ralph starts to snack, and he keeps snacking until bedtime. This is not an uncommon problem; we call it the "werewolf syndrome." Diabetes werewolves are seemingly normal people who are able to follow a fairly diabetes-friendly way of eating but only while the sun is up. When the moon rises in the sky, they are transformed. It is almost as if hair begins to sprout on their face, their eyes grow large, and beware to any food that can't jump out of their path. Sound familiar?

Ralph was labeled by his physician as "in denial," but that was an inaccurate and unhelpful diagnosis. Ralph certainly knew he had diabetes, and he had lots of thoughts and feelings about it. While he wanted to manage his diabetes effectively, he felt overwhelmed and defeated. Nothing seemed to work. He was angry and frustrated with himself, and he felt alone with his diabetes. He knew his wife and his kids cared about him, but they didn't understand diabetes and why he had become so discouraged. Feeling defeated, Ralph decided to try and stop thinking about his diabetes. He was avoiding seeing his doctor (since she would be certain to remind him about his diabetes), was no longer checking his blood glucose (since that would make him think about diabetes), and was not talking about it with his family and friends (so they would not bring up the subject). What a mess!

There are many people like Ralph. In a survey of more than 600 people with diabetes around the United States, my colleagues and I found the majority had tough feelings about diabetes (**Table 2-1**). For example, more than two thirds reported feeling at least somewhat hopeless about serious long-term complications, believing that there was nothing they could do to avoid them. More than half reported being somewhat angry, scared, or depressed about diabetes.

Studies have also shown that many people are not taking perfect care of their diabetes—not even close. It is likely that the majority of patients are struggling with following a diabetes-friendly meal plan, are not getting enough physical activity, and are not checking blood

Table 2-1

Diabetes Is *Not* Easy!

Emotional reactions to having diabetes can include:

- Worrying about complications (82% of patients)
- Feeling hopeless about complications (69% of patients)
- Feeling that diabetes takes too much energy (66% of patients)
- Feeling angry, scared, or depressed (58% of patients)

glucose frequently enough. Many are not taking their medications as prescribed. The result? Too many people never achieve the metabolic goals needed to stay healthy and avoid complications. Therefore, if you have ever felt down, discouraged, or aggravated about diabetes, know that these are very common feelings. If you are concerned that you're not giving your diabetes the attention it needs, welcome to the club. You are not alone.

Why is managing diabetes so tough? In a large survey conducted by Dr. Edelman and me, we found that health care providers commonly think the reason is that their patients don't have enough willpower or aren't scared enough about complications (**Table 2**-2). The evidence, however, doesn't support these beliefs. In fact, almost no one is unmotivated to live a long, healthy life. But diabetes care, day in and day out, is difficult. It can be a lot of work. It is tough to change one's habits. High blood glucose and high blood pressure don't really hurt, and they may not even be noticeable. Plus there are common, often unconscious obstacles that can dampen your enthusiasm to manage diabetes. Following are the top six.

Table 2-2

Physician's Beliefs About Poor Treatment Adherence

Percentage of physicians that strongly endorse the following reasons for their patients' poor adherence to diabetes treatment plans:

- Poor self-discipline (53.2%)
- Poor will-power (50.0%)
- Not scared enough (36.9%)
- Not informed enough (16.3%)

Polonsky WR, Boswell SL, Edelman SV. *J Diabetes.* 1996;45(suppl 2):14A. Abstract.

Obstacles That Can Dampen Your Enthusiasm to Manage Diabetes

Depression

People with diabetes are almost twice as likely to develop a serious problem with depression as people who don't have diabetes. And no one is quite sure why. One recent scientific review suggested that 20% or more of people with diabetes may be suffering from a clinically significant depressive disorder right now. Of course, everyone feels down or blue from time to time, but a clinically significant problem—such as the diagnosis of major depressive disorder—means that depression is actively interfering with your ability to function effectively in your life. In addition to a chronically depressed mood, other worrisome signs of a possible depressive disorder are:

• Lasting fatigue (your "get up and go" has got up and went)

- Diminished ability to experience pleasurable events (things that used to bring joy—such as friends, food, favorite activities, and sex—no longer do)
- Chronic sleeping problems
- Difficulty with concentration
- Significant changes in appetite.

Depression is especially worrisome in diabetes because it can interfere with your ability and your interest in following diabetes self-care recommendations. Exercise, for example, can seem a lot more difficult, or even impossible, when depression looms. Not surprisingly, depression is associated with poorer blood glucose control, more frequent hospitalizations, and higher rates of long-term complications and mortality.

Harmful Beliefs

How you think about diabetes has a big influence on how you feel and what you do—there are two common beliefs that can be problematic. They are problematic because they are just plain wrong. The first is "diabetes is no big deal." Perhaps your health care provider told you this. Perhaps you have type 2 diabetes and all you know is that at least you don't have the bad kind (type 1). Perhaps you think that since you aren't taking any medication, or not too many different medications, or not using insulin, your diabetes doesn't really need to be of great concern. Since long-term complications typically come on slowly over the course of years, it is seductive to think that you can start worrying about them sometime later. It is, therefore, easy to conclude that diabetes isn't that important… at least not right now. As one of my patients said, "Look, I promise you that I'll be ready to get serious about this disease, just as soon as something falls off."

The second belief is that diabetes is a death sentence. You have probably heard about the many long-term complications associated with diabetes. Perhaps you have known people who have been hit hard by the disease—losing their eyesight, ending up on dialysis, undergoing amputations, and more. Scary stuff. If you hear enough stories like these, it is easy to begin thinking that this will be your fate as well. Once you become convinced that complications are inevitable and that there is nothing you can do to stop them from occurring, who wouldn't get discouraged about their own diabetes care?

Vague or Unreasonable Ideas About What to Do

Even people who have been through comprehensive diabetes education programs may not be entirely clear about what they need to do to manage their diabetes. There is a lot to learn and a lot to do, and it can be confusing. Some people have overly demanding ideas about what needs to be done. Said one of my patients, "I know I am supposed to give up all of my favorite foods, eat perfectly, and never cheat." She believed that she needed to be perfect with her diabetes care, but since this was impossible to achieve, she ended up feeling like a failure every day. Other people have notions about what to do that are too vague or incomplete. Consider the following quotes from patients, "I was told I have to start eating healthy" and "I've gotta lose 10 pounds before my next doctor visit, which is tomorrow!" It is difficult to be successful when you don't have a clear, concrete, achievable plan.

Why do so many people end up being confused? This is embarrassing to admit, but often it is our fault—health care providers just like me. We get so enthusiastic about wanting to be helpful that sometimes we try to tell you everything all at once. Without meaning to do so, we may overwhelm you with facts, stories, and things to do. It can be hard to know where to start when your head is full of a zillion healthy changes you should make in your diet, new rules about foot care, physical activity, blood glucose monitoring, and the like.

Poor Social Support

If you are alone with diabetes, it is tougher to deal with the disease. When you have people in your life who are rooting for you, making and maintaining some of the tough changes that diabetes demands may become more doable. For example, trying to make diabetes-friendly changes in how you eat is easier when your family decides to join you in that endeavor. Making the time for regular exercise might be less difficult if your spouse volunteers to go with you.

But sometimes friends or family members provide you with too much support, taking on the role of the "diabetes police." Sound familiar? The diabetes police are loved ones who have decided that they have been deputized to help you manage your diabetes, whether you like it or not. They frequently say things like "Should you be eating that?" "You seem upset, maybe you should check your blood glucose." "Ya' know, you really should get some willpower." "Gee, your numbers are high again. What did you do wrong this time?" When friends and family act this way, they are usually coming from a place of love. They mean well and they are trying to help—even though they are driving you crazy. The more they try and offer help in this manner, the more you may bristle. In fact, since most people don't like being nagged, there is a tendency to act out, to do the opposite of what has been suggested.

Life Gets in the Way

Most of us live in a challenging environment for managing diabetes. If you have a lot of stress in your life, your diabetes care can suffer. If you are terribly busy, it can be difficult to find the time to exercise or even to check your blood glucose. Most of us lead very busy lives, with many competing demands on our time. Money is another big issue. Many people can't afford their medications, and many don't have the money for health insurance. Perhaps the biggest culprit is the culture in which we live. In the United States, life is sedentary and food is served and sold in very large portions, both in restaurants and at home. And, as you know, these are not necessarily the healthiest foods in the world. You may not notice it, but portion sizes can influence you, even if you don't like the foods you are eating. The bigger the portion on your plate, the more likely you are to eat. Americans grow heavier and heavier as the years go by. However, this doesn't mean you are helpless. As discussed later, you can fight back.

Discouraging Results

Here are some representative comments from my patients: "I did everything I was supposed to and my blood glucose is still all over the place!" "I tried that new medication and I don't feel any better." "I've been walking regularly for 2 months now, but I haven't lost an ounce of weight!" When you feel like you've made your best efforts and you still don't see the results you expect, it can be hard to stay enthusiastic about controlling your diabetes. Coping with errant blood glucose results is probably the most aggravating aspect of this problem. Many people, in fact, can start to develop an unusual relationship with their blood glucose meters. Once they start thinking of their numbers as good or bad, their meter can start to influence how they feel. Blood glucose running too high or too low in the morning? Then you are a bad person, a failure. When you start letting your meter determine your self-worth as a human being, you may eventually start to hate your meter. And who wants to check their blood glucose then?

So diabetes is tough because there are a lot of obstacles that make it tough. But that doesn't mean there isn't something you can do about this! Following are five solutions to consider.

Fight Back Against Depression

If any of the symptoms of depression described previously sound familiar, don't waste a moment. You can feel good again. There are a number of effective strategies for overcoming depression, so talk to your physician and find out what you can do. There is no need to blame yourself for your feelings (as if you aren't depressed enough). Depression is not the result of a weak mind. In fact, your doctor can help you discover whether there might be a physical cause to your depression (certain medications may contribute to depression, for example).

There is solid scientific evidence that brief forms of counseling (especially one form in particular, known as cognitive-behavioral therapy)

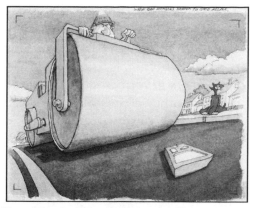

Your blood glucose meter readings yo-yo up and down... discouraged, your meter becomes your enemy!

can help many people with diabetes to recover from depression. It is also well established that commonly prescribed antidepressant medications can reverse depression in diabetes. In addition, remember that regular physical activity (like daily walking) is an antidepressant! All by itself, exercise will not be enough to cure a problem like major depression, but as one part of a comprehensive treatment plan, it can work wonders. Don't let depression get you down or keep you down. Take the first step today.

Challenge Your Own Discouraging Beliefs About Diabetes With Facts

The most important step you can take is to become educated about diabetes. And since you are reading this book, you have already started! If you are feeling frightened and hopeless about diabetes, please remember this one fact: While poorly controlled diabetes is the leading cause of many serious problems (like blindness, nontraumatic amputations, kidney damage, and more), well-controlled diabetes is the leading cause of... nothing! With good care, odds are good that you can live a long, healthy life with diabetes. Of course, no guarantees are possible, but the scientific evidence is overwhelming.

Your risk of running into long-term complications of diabetes can be dramatically lowered when you are working closely with your doctor to keep your blood glucose, blood pressure, and cholesterol levels within safe ranges. In fact, you may find that following a diabetes-friendly lifestyle that includes regular activity and a healthy way of eating can even extend your life. Yes, diabetes is a serious disease, but you are not doomed.

Frustrated that you haven't seen positive results from your self-management efforts? Maybe it is time to reconsider how you measure success. For example, many people judge how well or how poorly they are doing with diabetes by how much medication they are taking. The more pills they are taking, the sicker they must be. And if insulin is needed, that must mean their diabetes is now very serious. When people think this way, discouragement is almost inevitable. Said one of my patients, for example, "This just isn't fair; I've been doing everything I was supposed to do, and now I have to start insulin! Why have I even bothered trying?" But let's consider this carefully: The individual who is on no medication and has an A1C of 9% is at a much higher risk of developing complications than the person who is on multiple shots of insulin and has an A1C of 7%. In other words, it is the blood glucose levels that determines your risk, not the number or kind of medications being taken. And remember that no matter what you do, diabetes changes over the years and can get harder to handle, requiring more and different medications. This is not your fault, and it doesn't mean that your diabetes is now worse.

Other common ways that people measure their diabetes success is by how well how they are eating, or how they are feeling, or whether or not they ever see a blood glucose level higher than, say, 200 mg/dL. But none of these are appropriate ways to judge how well or how poorly you are doing. In fact, you can drive yourself crazy this way!

So what to do? Find out about the major medical tests that can help you to really determine your diabetes health. The most important ones are those that measure your A1C (a blood test typically done at your doctor's office that measures your average blood glucose level over the past 10 to 12 weeks—also referred to as glycosylated hemoglobin), blood pressure, and cholesterol. When the results of these tests are in a safe range, you can be assured that you are doing well and your risk of complications is pretty darned low.

You, not your doctor, need to make sure these tests are done regularly (blood pressure and cholesterol at least once yearly, A1C every 3 to 6 months). And you need to know the actual numerical results of these tests and what they mean. If your doctor tells you that you are fine, that is not sufficient. As my friend and colleague, Dr. Richard Jackson says, "Imagine going up to a bank teller and asking how much money you have in your account. The teller looks up your records and tells you, 'Not to worry, you are fine.'" Would you be satisfied with this response? Of course not. You need to know your numbers.

Develop a Sensible, Personalized, Action-Oriented Plan for Self-Management

To manage your diabetes more effectively tomorrow, what exactly should you do? If you were going to make one positive change in your diabetes management over the next week, what would it be—and why? And what is stopping you from taking this step? These are not easy questions to answer, but they are critical. To succeed with diabetes, you need a plan... steps for taking action.

First of all, as you think about what first steps you might take, make sure that they are specific and are truly actions to start. Many people make the mistake of focusing on vague and unachievable actions, such as "I'm definitely going to get myself some will power." Others commit the error of focusing on actions they want to stop, like "Starting tonight, I'm going to quit eating ice cream." But few people are successful in the long term when their chief goal is to deprive themselves. Instead, if the goal is to give up ice cream, then consider what action you could take that will help you achieve that end. It doesn't have to be an enormous step, but it should be a first step, and it should be very specific. For example, "When I get home tonight, I am going to throw out all the ice cream in my freezer."

Plans are best when they are personally meaningful (you must have a good reason for wanting to take control of your diabetes, not just because your doctor thinks it is a good idea), when the action steps you have chosen are very specific, and when the steps chosen are achievable and reasonable (given the other stresses and priorities in your life). Don't try to change everything at once; the best approach is one small healthy step at a time. So talk with your doctor about developing a plan for immediate action. For more helpful examples and specific strategies, see my book *Diabetes Burnout: What to Do When You Can't Take It Anymore* (American Diabetes Association, 1999).

Seek Out Rewarding Relationships

If you only have time to make one change, this is it! If at all possible, don't do diabetes alone. Reach out to the people in your life for the love and support you need. At a practical level, invite one or more of your loved ones to join you in making a healthy change. For example, you will be more successful at diabetes-friendly dietary changes if you can convince your family and/or friends to take those same healthy steps along with you.

Regular physical activity is much easier when you have an exercise partner. Don't know anyone who might join you in, say, taking a walk around the park each morning? Then perhaps it is time to knock on a neighbor's door. Make a new friend and help someone else to make a healthy change in their life as well.

When you are looking for loving support, remember that the key is to be as specific as possible. Don't just ask your spouse to be more supportive; instead, explain that you would like him or her to, for instance, sit with you at the kitchen table every morning when you check your blood glucose.

Consider attending a diabetes support group. It is always nice to meet other people who are going through some of the same or similar experiences. Your doctor or local hospital may be able to help you find one that is right for you.

If your loved ones are acting like diabetes police, select a quiet, dispassionate moment to discuss this matter with them (or perhaps consider writing them a letter). Let them know that you understand they mean well, but they must realize that their nagging is not helpful. Remember, since they love you, odds are good that they will never stop trying to be helpful. Therefore, you must give them something to do. You might explain, for example, that always asking you "Should you be eating that?" is not useful, but if they could please remember to keep the refrigerator stocked with diet soda, that would be terrific.

Summary

Remember that diabetes is *not* so easy. Diabetes care is a job, and it is not a job you volunteered for! There are many reasons why managing diabetes can be tough, but there are many solutions as well. So don't give up. With effort and support, you can live well with diabetes. And for more information about the emotional side of diabetes, please come visit us on the Internet at the Behavioral Diabetes Institute, *www.behavioraldiabetes.org*.

3

The Diabetes Warranty Program and Sick-Day Rules

Developing a Diabetes Warranty Program

One of the more powerful and simple tools that you can use to take control of your diabetes is to follow a diabetes warranty program. The concept is simple and is similar to the warranty program that accompanies a new automobile. If you follow the regularly scheduled maintenance program that is recommended by an automobile manufacturer, your new car will run better and last longer. I designed the diabetes warranty program in order to prevent the onset and delay the progression of the complications of diabetes. If you follow the regularly scheduled maintenance program that is recommended by leaders in the field of diabetes, you will feel better and last longer!

All people with diabetes need a maintenance record book that lists the recommended tests with dates and results (**Figure 3-1**). This information is vital, primarily to those of us with diabetes, and secondarily to our caregivers, in order to diagnose and track the common problems that occur with diabetes. In many cases, your record will be more orderly and complete than the one in your medical chart. It is also not uncommon to change physicians, so your record keeping takes on an even greater importance. The individual items in **Figure 3-1** will be discussed in the appropriate chapters throughout the book. Remember to keep updated and organized records. If you can, it would be very helpful to make a file on your computer so that you can easily update it and print it out for your health care visits. As a physician who cares for people with diabetes, I love it when my patients keep good records of their medical problems, list of medications, tests, etc. It helps me take better care of them.

How Often Should You Be Seen by Your Caregiver?

The official recommendations state that if you are currently on insulin, your physician should see you approximately every 3 to 4 months. If you are not on insulin, you should been seen approximately every 3 to 6 months. The frequency of visits obviously depends on how well or how poorly you are doing and on whether you have taken control of your diabetes. For example, if your home glucose monitoring (HGM) values

Figure 3-1

Diabetes Warranty Program

What Should Be Done at *Every Visit*

	Date	Result	Normal Range or Goal
Weight			
Blood pressure			
Glycosylated hemoglobin* (know the normal range)			
Foot examination†			

What Tests/Examinations Should Be Done at Least *Every Year*

	Date	Result (recommendations)	Normal Range
Cholesterol levels (fasting):			
▪ Total cholesterol			
▪ Triglycerides			
▪ HDL			
▪ LDL			
Urine protein (microalbumin)			
Serum creatinine			
Thyroid function test (TSH)			
Eye examination (dilated)			
Dental examination			
Other tests/examinations (depending on individual needs):			
▪ Cardiologist (for heart disease)			
▪ Podiatrist (for foot problems)			
▪ Gastroenterologist (for stomach problems)			

* Glycosylated hemoglobin (A1C) is a long-term diabetes control factor (see Chapter 1).
† This may not be necessary, since you should examine your own feet as discussed in Chapter 13.

are consistently in the desirable ranges and your diabetes regimen is stable, you do not need to see your caregiver as often as someone who never tests blood glucose levels at home and has no clue how he or she is doing. If you are really on top of your diabetes and know that you are doing well via HGM and/or continuous glucose monitoring (CGM) data, then in reality you only need to be seen once a year to renew your

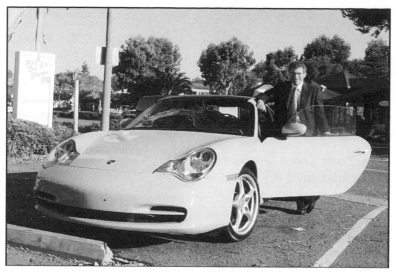

A Diabetes Warranty Program is like the warranty program that accompanies a new car. Famous diabetes specialist, Irl Hirsch, who is a Professor of Medicine at the University of Washington in Seattle, has been living well with diabetes for a long time.

prescriptions and to make sure all of the appropriate tests and exams are done according to your diabetes warranty program.

When you visit your physician, be prepared to discuss any issues that you have questions about. **Table 3-1** lists some of the areas that you may want to discuss with your caregiver. There is obviously not enough time at any one visit to discuss all of these issues; however, you should decide which ones are the most important to you at the time of your visit. Please do not come in with a list so long that it freaks out your caregiver even before starting your visit. Also, mention to your doctor that you have a list of questions when he or she first walks in the room so that the limited time of your visit can be used to get to the issues most important to you. If you need new prescriptions, try to coordinate them so they can all be done at once with a 1-year supply of refills. I have to say that filling out prescriptions is one of the biggest pains in the medical

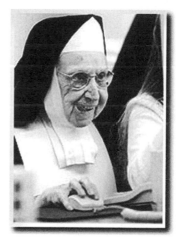

If an 80-year-old nun can be online, why can't prescription refill requests be made easier?

profession. The system is archaic and should be totally revamped. Even if they make refill requests available via email, that would be a huge improvement in efficiency and convenience for the doctor and the patient!

Write Up Your Own Diabetes History Sheet and Keep It Updated

It is also helpful to have a basic information sheet about your medical history (**Figure 3-2**). Write up your own diabetes history sheet. Much of your medical history does not change and is easy to update periodically. You can then bring a copy of your medical history, along with your diabetes warranty program sheet, to any health care professional, such as your dentist, physician, nurse, or pharmacist. It will also allow time for other important issues during your appointment. I have listed my medical information in **Figure 3-2** as an example. As you can see, I spilled my guts by telling my medical problems to the world!

Table 3-1

Potential Topics to Discuss With Your Caregiver

- Home glucose monitoring (HCG) results
- Continuous glucose monitoring (CGM) results
- Problems with hypoglycemia
- Medication questions
- Test or examination results and when necessary, options for therapy
- Pregnancy issues
- Exercise routine
- Meal planning
- Sexual dysfunction issues
- Immunization requirements (ie, yearly flu shot)
- Sick-day rules
- Any tests or examinations not completed that are recommended by your diabetes warranty program

If you discover that a test or examination has not been done that is needed in order to comply with your diabetes warranty program, you should discuss this with your caregiver and request the test or examination. Phrase your comments and questions constructively and not too aggressively (for example, "Is it possible to please check my cholesterol levels next visit? My last values were done over a year ago and I am concerned about them.") You must work with your caregiver in order to maintain your health and quality of life. Staying healthy is much easier when preventive measures are taken early, especially with diabetes. Most caregivers will be glad to help with your requests if they are correct and reasonable.

What Should Be Done at Your Office Visits?

The standards of care call for certain things to be done at your office visits, including measurement of your weight (I know this may be

Figure 3-2

Sample Diabetes Medical History

Last updated	June 2007
Name	Steven V. Edelman
Date of birth	September 6, 1955
Date of diabetes diagnosis	1970 (15 years old)

Type of diabetes therapy	1971-1976: One injection per day (NPH/Regular)
	1976-1982: Two or three injections per day
	1982 to 2000: Insulin pump (basal rate 0.7 units/hour),
	  carbohydrate-to-insulin ratio (15:1), correction factor
	  1 unit rapid-acting will lower my blood glucose ~50 mg/dL
	2000-present: The untethered regimen (75% of my basal
	  requirements from Lantus and 25% via the insulin pump)

Incidence of hypoglycemia	Once or twice a week, not at any consistent time, with symptoms of light-headedness and dizziness; I no longer experience palpitations or getting sweaty
Other medical problems	1. 1979: Retinopathy diagnosed (received laser treatment of both eyes; Dr. Paul Tornambe is my ophthalmologist) 2. ~1985: Kidney disease diagnosed (see diabetes warranty sheet for most recent kidney tests; Dr. David Ward is my kidney doctor) 3. ~1985: High blood pressure diagnosed, take three different medications (see list below) 4. ~1989: High cholesterol levels diagnosed (see below for list of medications I take) 5. Gastroparesis, heartburn, and constipation 6. The syndrome of limited joint mobility/trigger fingers
Recent hospitalizations	None
Surgery or operations	1. 1997: Right middle trigger-finger repair 2. 1999: Left middle trigger-finger repair 3. 2000: Left knee surgery (ACL repair) 4. 2002: Left ring finger trigger-finger repair 5. 2003: Frozen shoulder treated with physical therapy
Medications	1. Rapid-acting insulin analogue (Apidra, Humalog, or Novolog) in my pump or pen (~45 units/day) 2. Lantus (glargine) 15 units subcutaneously each night 3. Symlin (pramlintide) 10 units before each meal 4. Lozol (indapamide) 2.5 mg twice a day 5. Monopril (fosinopril) 20 mg twice a day 6. Cardizem CD (diltiazem HCl) 180 mg twice a day 7. Lipitor (atorvastatin) 20 mg once a day at bedtime 8. Aspirin 81 mg once a day (enteric coated) 9. Vitamin C 1000 mg twice a day (2 total)
Allergies	None

Continued

Important family history (heart disease, cancer, diabetes)	1. Great uncle (mother's side) and grandmother (father's side) had type 2 diabetes 2. Grandfather (mother's side) died of a heart attack at the age of 65 years 3. Several relatives on my father's side of the family died of stomach cancer 4. Uncle (mother's side) with Alzheimer's disease at the age of 67 years

painful and embarrassing for some of you) and blood pressure (BP), a discussion of your HGM results, your CGM results (if appropriate), and laboratory values, blood for which should have been drawn a few days before your appointment. A foot exam is also in order, especially if you are experiencing a problem or have loss of sensation (neuropathy).

As is true with all official recommendations, certain items may not be as pertinent in your case. For example, if you examine your own feet and have no current problems, this part of your office visit is not necessary and not a good use of the limited time you may have with your caregiver. In addition, if you have a home BP device and take your own reading at home in your natural environment, keep a log of your BP measurements. It may make the reading performed in the caregiver's office not as valuable, especially if you have the "white coat" phenomenon—your blood pressure goes up when you get it measured at the doctor's office.

How to Make Your Doctor's Appointment a Success

Recommendations from Dr. Ian Blumer—diabetes specialist and advocate from Ontario, Canada

Have you ever left a doctor's appointment feeling that the visit was not a resounding success? Maybe you felt that you spent too much time in the waiting (and waiting… and waiting…) room? Or maybe you had a question that never got answered? Or you felt rushed? Or you did not get part of you checked that should have been? If this rings a bell, then you have come to the right place, because here (with apologies to David Letterman) I present my Top Ten ways to make your next family doctor or diabetes specialist appointment a success.

Number 10: Think of your doctor as being your guidance counselor, not your school principal. Your doctor gives advice; that is all. You can choose to accept this advice or you can choose to reject this advice. Thank goodness we live in a society where the decision is yours! (But, of course, if you are rejecting your doctor's advice because you do not trust it, you will have to ask yourself whether it is time to change doctors.)

Number 9: Imagine, if you will, that you have your entire life's savings invested in the stock market. Every hard-earned dollar. Now imagine you call your broker and ask how your investments are doing. What would you think if your broker said to you, "They're fine!" and then hung up? Does "fine" mean you are making lots of money? Or does "fine" mean you are having an average rate of return? Or does it mean you have lost some money, but from your broker's perspective it could have been worse? Who knows? I sure wouldn't. So when your doctor checks your BP or your kidney urine test or your A1C, do not accept being told the result is "fine" or "good" or "okay" or some such thing. Make sure you find out the exact result. Ask if the result is above target. If it is, ask how you can work with your doctor to improve it. Your doctor will not be offended. Quite the opposite. In fact, your doctor will be thrilled to have such a keen partner with which to work toward attaining a common goal—keeping you healthy!

Number 8: If you have had a lab test and you do not subsequently receive a call from your doctor's office, do not for one moment conclude that "no news is good news." Maybe no news means that the result got lost in the mail, got accidentally thrown out, or went to the wrong doctor. (Just ask my wife who shares the same name as three other doctors in Toronto and regularly has their patients' results mistakenly sent to her!). I would suggest that when you see your doctor, you ask how you will find out your results. Can you call the office to get them? Should you book a follow-up appointment to review them? Can you have the lab or the office send you a copy of the results? (Heck, it's your body fluid after all).

Number 7: If you are being prescribed a drug, be sure to ask your doctor some crucial things about the medicine. For example, why is it being prescribed, how will it help you, what possible side effects can be expected, and what should be done if side effects occur? For a helpful way to record this key information, feel free to download a "Cheat Sheet" from my web page (go to *www.ruleyourdiabetes.com* and click on the link that says "Rx drug essentials").

Number 6: Tired of waiting (and waiting… and waiting… and waiting…) in the "waiting room?" Try booking your appointment for the first slot of the day or the first slot in the afternoon. Dollars to donuts, your wait will be a lot less.

Number 5: Need more time with your doctor than you are getting? Feeling constantly rushed during appointments? Next time, when you book your appointment, ask the doctor's secretary to book you in for a longer time slot. If that does not work, ask for the last slot of the day. Most likely if you are the last patient the doctor has to see that day, he or she will not feel as rushed (which means more time for you).

Number 4: Want to get preferred appointment times? Longer appointment times? Want to get squeezed into an already-full schedule? Then remember, the doctor's secretary is a VIP! So be sure to be extra nice. Nice helps. Trust me! Better yet, trust my secretary!

Number 3: Your doctor should be checking your feet regularly, but this important part of one's anatomy often gets overlooked at the time of routine appointments. Not any more! Because now as soon as you go into your doctor's examining room you are going to take off your shoes and socks and present your beautiful (or not so beautiful as the case may be) tootsies to your doc for an examination.

Number 2: Almost everyone with diabetes should be testing their blood glucose readings and keeping a written record of the values in a logbook. Doing this will help keep you on the up and up regarding your status and progress, and will similarly help your doctor help you. So be sure to bring the logbook to each and every appointment with your family doctor and diabetes specialist. And remember: Your logbook is not a report card! It should never be used to judge you and should never be something that is used in a punitive or judgmental way. It is a tool to help you and your doctor monitor and adjust your therapy; nothing more, nothing less. On the subject of writing things down, I would also suggest that you write down any questions you have before you see your doctor and then pull them out of your pocket or purse during your appointment to double check that you have had all your questions addressed. So many people end up remembering a question they had meant to ask only after they have left the office! I would also suggest that you write down your doctor's answers or bring a loved one or trusted friend with you to hear your doctor's replies. (You know what they say about two sets of ears, eh?)

Number 1: Now, as much as I hope that you have found the preceding nine tips helpful, I have saved the absolutely, positively, most important tip for last. Forget about waiting-room lineups, log books, guidance counselors, and secretary VIPs. No, when it comes to the truly essential, number-one tip for making your doctor's appointment a success it is this: Whatever you do, never honk or yell (or worse) at the guy that cut you off in the doctor's parking lot; he could be the guy wearing the rubber gloves that you will be seeing in 5 minutes!

For more information on Ian Blumer, please visit his web site at *www.ianblumer.com.*

What Tests or Exams Should Be Done at Least Annually?

Certain tests and exams must be done every year in order to initiate aggressive therapy when needed to avoid the complications of diabetes (**Figure 3-1**). A yearly cholesterol panel, a test of how your kidneys have been affected by diabetes, and thyroid levels are a few of the important ones and are discussed in subsequent chapters. The yearly dilated eye exam is a must for all people with diabetes and, depending on your list of other medical problems, you may need to see a dentist, cardiologist, podiatrist, stomach specialist, etc on an annual or more frequent basis.

What Should Be Discussed With Your Caregiver?

Please do not go into your doctor's office with a list of questions that is half a mile long! This will put the usually hassled caregiver immediately on edge. Decide what issues listed in **Table 3-1** are the most important to you. Try to do your homework first and look up the topic of the question so that you can get the most out of your office visit. It is like going to an auto mechanic for a particular problem; if you know a little about cars and how they work, you will understand the explanation of what is wrong with your car a lot better. Please, do not wait until the end of your appointment time to mention that you have a list. Mention it early so that there is enough time allotted to discuss each issue during your visit.

Sick-Day Rules

Every person on this planet living with diabetes must know his or her sick-day rules. What exactly do I mean by sick-day rules? It is basically having a game plan on how to manage your diabetes when you are sick. Sick-day rules are especially important for people using insulin to treat their diabetes.

One of the most common situations is when someone gets the flu or a bad cold. The way *not* to handle it is to withhold your diabetes medication because your appetite is down and you are eating a lot less than normal. In times of illness or stress (emotional or physical), your body normally becomes resistant to the glucose-lowering effects of insulin and/or oral medications, thus increasing the medication requirements.

If you are on insulin and you become ill, the key is to do a lot of testing of your blood glucose levels (as often as every 2 or 3 hours) and know what to do with the results. For people taking rapid-acting insulin, such as Humalog (lispro), Novolog (aspart), or Apidra (glulisine), taking small-to-medium amounts of extra insulin throughout the day may be in order to keep the blood glucose level from climbing above 200 mg/dL. The amount of insulin needs to be individualized according to your sensitivity and normal amounts that you take when you are not sick (insulin therapy is discussed in Chapter 7).

If you have type 2 diabetes and are on oral medication only, your sick-day rules will probably not include insulin injections. Drink plenty of noncaloric fluids, test your blood glucose frequently (approximately 3 or 4 times a day), and please do not stop your medications without talking to your caregiver.

In certain circumstances when you have been really sick with vomiting, you may need to test a substance in your body called ketones, which indicates a more severe illness and calls for closer monitoring, aggressive insulin therapy, or a visit to the emergency room. Ketones can be measured by a strip that you dip into a urine sample or by a drop of blood on some home glucose meters using a different type of strip. They can also be measured in most laboratories and are a commonly ordered test in the emergency room.

Treatment of Hypoglycemia

On May 27, 2006, I attended a memorial service for Cyndee Fena. Cyndee was a friend, patient, and TCOYD volunteer. She was found dead in bed from severe hypoglycemia. She lived alone and was discovered by her neighbor. The paramedics documented a blood glucose level of 20 mg/dL for her. Cyndee did have hypoglycemia unawareness and had been found unconscious from hypoglycemia in the past, but I could not convince her to back off on her control because she was determined to not become blind, lose a leg, or go on dialysis… complications she fought so hard to avoid all of her life. Unfortunately, this is not an uncommon scenario. Prevention and proper treatment are especially important for any person with diabetes taking oral medication and insulin. Hypoglycemia unawareness is discussed in more detail in one of the cases in Chapter 11.

Treatment of hypoglycemia is another "taking control" topic that is super important. For people on insulin or taking oral medications that can cause hypoglycemia (discussed in Chapter 11), awareness of low blood glucose is crucial for early treatment and avoidance of passing out. Unfortunately, this happens too frequently while people are at work, caring for young children, or driving an automobile. The results can be disastrous. In addition, the proper treatment of hypoglycemia is important in order to bring your blood glucose back into the normal range swiftly without overshooting to the other extreme of hyperglycemia.

First of all, you must always carry something sweet with you if you are at risk for hypoglycemia. Many drug stores sell special glucose tablets to treat low blood glucose levels. There is also an excellent under-the-tongue gel that rapidly elevates the blood glucose level. You can buy a roll of Lifesavers or some type of hard candy that is mostly sugar with no fat, such as Skittles or Mentos. Candy bars with chocolate and fat, such as Snickers, Milky Way, and 3 Musketeers (my favorite), do not raise your blood glucose as quickly and have a ton of calories compared with 4 to 6 ounces of apple juice or a regular soda, both of which are also good for treating acute low blood glucose reactions. The faster you raise your blood glucose to normal, the faster you will lose that incredible craving to eat and eat and eat.

What *not* to do at night (or any other time for that matter) is what I used to do all the time. I would wake up in a sweat and shaking like a leaf, go downstairs, and eat everything in the fridge... cookies, leftovers, peanut butter and jelly sandwiches, and cold cereal! I would then go back to sleep and wake up a few hours later feeling terrible with a blood glucose level over 400 mg/dL. This is not to mention all of the excess calories you can rack up. Ten ounces of juice is about 150 calories with no fat; a huge handful of Oreo cookies is at least 300 to 400 calories with lots of saturated fat. When your blood glucose is low, your body signals to you to eat as much as possible and, if you do not pick the quick-acting foods, you will overdo it. I now keep small cartons of apple juice or glucose tablets at my bedside so that I do not even have to go near the fridge! It should go without saying that if you are experiencing hypoglycemia on a regular basis, you should really try to figure out what adjustment in your treatment regimen is warranted.

Summary

In addition to following the diabetes warranty program, you must be knowledgeable about the available tests and be aware of the kinds of therapy that are available for any abnormality or problem. Remember, it is not enough to just know your results. Be as prepared as possible for your health care visits so you can get the most out of those precious moments. You must also understand them, and when necessary, seek out the best available therapy. Knowing what to do when you get sick or when you experience hypoglycemia is crucial to avoid serious and unnecessary problems. This is what taking control of your diabetes is all about.

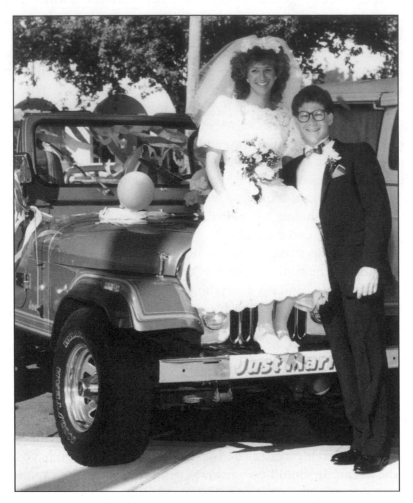

My wife, Ingrid, and I by the get away car at our wedding in San Diego, California, August 16, 1987.

4

If Eating in Moderation Is the Key, I Must Have the Wrong Lock!

by Lorena Drago, MS, RD, CDN, CDE

Introduction

Most people with or without diabetes hope to find low-calorie, delicious foods that have no impact on their blood glucose levels, cholesterol, blood pressure, or any of the other numbers doctors talk about during health care visits. I believe that most people have basic nutrition knowledge and they know that it is better to eat an apple than to eat a slice of apple pie. They also know that a vegetable salad will nutritionally slam-dunk the mayonnaise-lathered potato salad and that steamed is better than fried. Super-sizing, unless you are talking about your bank account, cannot possibly be that good for you. You get the picture.

The most common question my patients ask is "What can I eat now that I have diabetes?" I will say it again. I believe that most people know what foods are better for them, but what they are really asking is how to desire the apple with the same enthusiasm they desire the apple pie. What do they need to do in order to crave the spinach salad the same way their eyes devour the potato salad? People want to know how to eat right, and they also want to know how to have an intense desire to eat right. The challenge is in the action process. How do you do it? I want to share my personal tips and my own struggles with portion control.

Do not bring home what you cannot control. There are certain foods that have magnetic appeal. If you bring them home, you are going to eat more than just one portion. Altoids Sours and Mentos have an overwhelming magnetic effect for me. I seldom buy them. I have fooled myself too many times trying to convince myself that the next time would be different.

Buy the smallest portion available. When I crave ice cream, I buy the smallest size available, which nowadays is not really that small. I have outsmarted the super-sized friendly servers, and ask them to give me a scoop the size of a lemon.

When eating out, wrap before you grab. Your plate is on the table, and it is overflowing with spaghetti, chicken, and a miniscule vegetable. I know that there is way too much spaghetti. With the fork, I separate what looks like about 1 cup and push the rest to the side. All of a sudden

I question whether I truly have the correct portion and I allow my fork to wander to the neatly stacked pile waiting to go home for another meal and slowly pull some of the noodles to my "eat now" pile. I outsmart my wandering fork by asking for a container before I even eat the first bite in order to avoid the temptation. Wrap before you grab.

Nutrition Information Diagnosed With Multiple Personalities

At one time, you heard that butter was bad, so you switched to margarine. Later on, you heard reports that margarine was lethal. You realized after eating too many dry toasts that disregarding the latest nutrition discovery was the smartest solution to multiple-personality nutrition information.

Behind the Scenes

The science of nutrition is an evolving process of discovery. Butter has saturated fat. Excess consumption of saturated fat has been shown to negatively affect cholesterol levels, hence the recommendation to avoid the use of butter. At the time, no emphasis was placed on the effects of trans fats on cholesterol levels. Further studies revealed that trans fats were not heart-friendly either. Margarine was low in saturated fat but contained trans fat. The movement shifted to shun margarines with trans fats.

The media tantalizes health news. It is impossible to package complex information into a 30-second sound bite. The next time you are summoned to stay tuned for killer broccoli, do not rush to quarantine your green fuzzy ally. Talk to a registered dietitian.

How Many Calories Should I Eat?

Patients frequently ask, "What foods can I eat?" I need to know you a little better before I can answer this question. If you asked me what you could wear at a wedding, I could not give you a specific answer before I knew the time of the event, location, and even your favorite colors. Get the picture now? However, most likely you will be able to eat at least 50% of the foods you eat now. They will also ask, "How much can I eat?" Probably not as much as you would like.

"How many calories do you need?" I ask my patients. The majority of women, who have experienced more weight loss diets than options on a company's automated voice phone system, answer 1500 calories and men answer 1800. If you have ever been in a hospital, the 1800-calorie diet reigns supreme. To simplify matters, I use this rule of thumb:

- Adult women:
  - Manage weight: 1200-1500 calories/day
  - Maintain weight: 1500-1800 calories/day
  - Underweight or are very active: 1800-2200 calories/day
- Adult men:
  - Manage weight: 1500-1800 calories/day
  - Maintain weight: 1800-2200 calories/day
  - Underweight or are very active: 2200-2500 calories/day

These are just estimates. Consult with your registered dietitian to obtain your individualized calorie budget.

How Much Should I Weigh?

Health professionals use a trendy term, body mass index (BMI), that measures your weight in proportion to your height. A BMI between 19 and 24 indicates a healthy weight. A BMI under 19 indicates that you are underweight and between 25 and 29 indicates that you are "Ruben-esque" (overweight). The big "O" (obesity) occurs when your BMI is over 30. Blood glucose, blood pressure, and cholesterol are harder to manage as the BMI increases.

What Is My BMI?

Refer to the BMI chart (**Table 4-1**). Find your height in inches and your weight in pounds. Look at the number at the top of the column where these two numbers intersect. That is your BMI.

What You Must Know First: Which Foods Raise Your Blood Glucose (Sugar) Levels the Most

Think of the foods you have for breakfast. Go over them in your head. Write them down. Identify the foods that have carbohydrates, because carbohydrates are converted into blood glucose (sugar). **Table 4-2** lists foods that have carbohydrates. Identify the amount of carbohydrates in the meal. If you eat more carbohydrates than you can process, your blood glucose levels will be higher than desired. If you eat too little, your blood glucose levels may be lower than desired, especially if you take certain medications and/or insulin.

How do I know how much carbohydrate is in the food that I am going to eat? Refer to **Table 4-3** to familiarize yourself with carbohydrate counting. For the Internet savvy, *www.calorieking.com* and *www.nu-tritiondata.com* offer a comprehensive list of foods and corresponding carbohydrate count. For those who prefer the book form, read *The Dia-*

Table 4-1
Body Mass Index Table

Height (inches) / BMI	Normal						Overweight					Obese										Extreme Obesity														
BMI	19	20	21	22	23	24	25	26	27	28	29	30	31	32	33	34	35	36	37	38	39	40	41	42	43	44	45	46	47	48	49	50	51	52	53	54
	Body Weight (pounds)																																			
58	91	96	100	105	110	115	119	124	129	134	138	143	148	153	158	162	167	172	177	181	186	191	196	201	205	210	215	220	224	229	234	239	244	248	253	258
59	94	99	104	109	114	119	124	128	133	138	143	148	153	158	163	168	173	178	183	188	193	198	203	208	212	217	222	227	232	237	242	247	252	257	262	267
60	97	102	107	112	118	123	128	133	138	143	148	153	158	163	168	174	179	184	189	194	199	204	209	215	220	225	230	235	240	245	250	255	261	266	271	276
61	100	106	111	116	122	127	132	137	143	148	153	158	164	169	174	180	185	190	195	201	206	211	217	222	227	232	238	243	248	254	259	264	269	275	280	285
62	104	109	115	120	126	131	136	142	147	153	158	164	169	175	180	186	191	196	202	207	213	218	224	229	235	240	246	251	256	262	267	273	278	284	289	295
63	107	113	118	124	130	135	141	146	152	157	163	169	175	180	186	191	197	203	208	214	220	225	231	237	242	248	254	259	265	270	278	282	287	293	299	304
64	110	116	122	128	134	140	145	151	157	163	169	174	180	186	192	197	204	209	215	221	227	232	238	244	250	256	262	267	273	279	285	291	296	302	308	314
65	114	120	126	132	138	144	150	156	162	168	174	180	186	192	198	204	210	216	222	228	234	240	246	252	258	264	270	276	282	288	294	300	306	312	318	324
66	118	124	130	136	142	148	155	161	167	173	179	186	192	198	204	210	216	223	229	235	241	247	253	260	266	272	278	284	291	297	303	309	315	322	328	334
67	121	127	134	140	146	153	159	166	172	178	185	191	198	204	211	217	223	230	236	242	249	255	261	268	274	280	287	293	299	306	312	319	325	331	338	344
68	125	131	138	144	151	158	164	171	177	184	190	197	203	210	216	223	230	236	243	249	256	262	269	276	282	289	295	302	308	315	322	328	335	341	348	354
69	128	135	142	149	155	162	169	176	182	189	196	203	209	216	223	230	236	243	250	257	263	270	277	284	291	297	304	311	318	324	331	338	345	351	358	365
70	132	139	146	153	160	167	174	181	188	195	202	209	216	222	229	236	243	250	257	264	271	278	285	292	299	306	313	320	327	334	341	348	355	362	369	376
71	136	143	150	157	165	172	179	186	193	200	208	215	222	229	236	243	250	257	265	272	279	286	293	301	308	315	322	329	338	343	351	358	365	372	379	386
72	140	147	154	162	169	177	184	191	199	206	213	221	228	235	242	250	258	265	272	279	287	294	302	309	316	324	331	338	346	353	361	368	375	383	390	397
73	144	151	159	166	174	182	189	197	204	212	219	227	235	242	250	257	265	272	280	288	295	302	310	318	325	333	340	348	355	363	371	378	386	393	401	408
74	148	155	163	171	179	186	194	202	210	218	225	233	241	249	256	264	272	280	287	295	303	311	319	326	334	342	350	358	365	373	381	389	396	404	412	420
75	152	160	168	176	184	192	200	208	216	224	232	240	248	256	264	272	279	287	295	303	311	319	327	335	343	351	359	367	375	383	391	399	407	415	423	431
76	156	164	172	180	189	197	205	213	221	230	238	246	254	263	271	279	287	295	304	312	320	328	336	344	353	361	369	377	385	394	402	410	418	426	435	443

Source: Adapted from Clinical Guidelines on the Identification, Evaluation, and Treatment of Overweight and Obesity in Adults: The Evidence Report. Available at: www.nhlbi.nih.gov/guidelines/obesity/bmi_tbl.pdf.

Table 4-2

Foods With Carbohydrates

- All breads (and I mean *all*—even whole-wheat and 9-grain breads)
- Rolls, crackers, bagels, baguettes, breadsticks
- All cereals (cold and hot cereals, including "healthy" oatmeal)
- All beans (yes, healthy beans such as kidney beans, chick peas, black-eyed peas, etc)
- All starchy vegetables (white and sweet potatoes, green peas, and corn)
- All fruits (even fruits that are not sweet, such as grapefruit; and fruits in every form: juice, canned, frozen, and dried)
- All grains (from the exotic to the traditional: amaranth, barley, buckwheat, corn, emmer, granola, kammut, millet, oats, quinoa, rice, rye, sorghum, spelt, teff, triticale, wheat, wild rice) and foods made with these grains, such as pasta, tortillas, couscous, etc
- Milk and yogurt (whole milk, low-fat milk, and fat-free milk)
- Candy, baked goods, regular sodas, and beverages
- Seasonings and sauces: barbeque sauce, marinades, mayonnaise, ketchup, etc

betes Carbohydrate & Fat Gram Guide, 3rd edition (American Diabetes Association, 2006).

Who eats ⅓ cup of rice? One peanut? One potato chip? Unfathomable. One third cup of cooked rice has 15 grams of carbohydrate; ⅔ cup has 30 grams, and 1 cup has 45 grams. You can eat the quantity that fits your budget. Most "carbohydrate budgets" allow more than 15 grams per meal, so you can probably have a more realistic amount of rice on your plate.

How much carbohydrate can I eat? Are you a male? You can probably eat more. Are you inactive? You probably need to eat less (**Table 4-4**). Identify which foods and behaviors need modification. When it comes to carbohydrates, *profile and discriminate*. Profile dubious-looking carbohydrates and select those with high nutritional value. For example, a glass of soda and a glass of orange juice contain about the same amount of carbohydrate but they are *not* nutritionally equal.

What does it mean to change my behavior? Healthy eating goes beyond selecting the "right" foods and counting carbohydrates. Knowledge does not always precede change in behavior.

Why Is My Head Disconnected From My Stomach? (When You Know What to Do, but the Stomach Does Not Cooperate)

A typical scenario is that you are too busy to prepare breakfast so you eat the wrong choices and end up feeling guilty. Why is this happening? In order to find a solution to this problem, identify the barriers to the right behavior. They could include:

- Waking up late
- Not having anything healthy to take on the run
- Not being hungry early in the morning

Ask yourself what can realistically be changed in order to accomplish the goal of getting a healthier nutritional start to your day. A possible plan of action could include:

- Setting the alarm earlier
- Preparing foods the evening before
- Preparing a breakfast kit and leaving it at work. It can include such things as oatmeal packages, nuts, dried fruits, fresh fruits, low-fat milk, whole-grain cold cereals, boiled eggs, ready-to-eat shakes or bars (ie, Glucerna)
- Eating breakfast on the go in the car: fruit, ready-to-eat shakes or bars (ie, Glucerna), dried fruit/nut combination, whole-grain bread

Table 4-3

What Are Grams of Carbohydrate?

You are eating 15 grams of carbohydrate every time you eat *one* of the following foods:

- 1 slice of bread
- ½ cup cooked cereal
- ¾ cup cold cereal
- ½ cup starchy vegetable (corn, peas)
- ½ plantain – ½ cup cooked taro, cassava, or tannier
- ⅓ cup cooked rice, pasta
- ½ cup beans
- 1 small potato
- 1 small fruit
- 4 oz (½ small glass) juice
- 1 glass milk
- 6 oz plain yogurt

Carbohydrate bargains are ½ cup of cooked vegetable or 1 cup of raw vegetable. These have only 5 grams of carbohydrates!

Examine other troublesome areas that are hindering your progress, such as eating too much at night. Possible solutions might include:

- Do not leave leftovers; freeze food after eating to avoid temptation
- Eat a mint and/or brush your teeth after dinner
- Eat a snack mid afternoon to avoid overeating at dinner
- Wrap food in opaque containers to avoid temptation—out of sight, out of mind!

Table 4-4

How Much Carbohydrate Can I Eat in One Meal?

	Grams of Carbs *(per meal)*	
	Woman	Man
You need to manage your weight...	50	60
You have a healthy weight...	60	75
You are very active...	75	75

How important is it for me to change this situation? On a scale of 1 to 10, any number above 5 indicates that changing the current situation is important to you.

How confident are you that you will be able to change this situation? On that same scale, a number below 5 indicates that you are uncertain that you can accomplish the change. You need more tools to help you move forward. You have a better chance of succeeding when the levels of importance and confidence are high. If you think it is important to make a change but have low confidence to do so, you will feel frustrated. Enlist the help of a certified diabetes educator to provide you with tools to boost your confidence level.

Do not make too many changes at once. Small victories lead to greater accomplishments. Anticipate obstacles to minimize relapses. Even careful planning can result in behavioral relapses. Everyone slides. Resume your program and continue moving forward.

How do I know what is the right amount of carbohydrate for me? Test your blood glucose levels 2 hours after the beginning of your meal for 1 week. If the numbers are consistently high, eat fewer foods with carbohydrates. If the numbers are consistently low, eat a little more. If your blood glucose levels are consistently above or below the recommended range, talk with your doctor or educator for help in achieving levels that remain more constant with your target range.

Can I save some carbohydrates from one meal and add them to another? It is not a great practice to save, let's say, 50 grams from lunch so you can have 100 grams at dinner. Unfortunately, your body is not going to remember your midday sacrifice, and it will have to process a larger amount at dinner.

I thought that vegetables such as spinach and broccoli did not have any carbohydrates? Nonstarchy vegetables have carbohydrates but at a "bargain carb price" compared with rice or pasta. One cup of spinach has 5 grams of carbohydrates. One cup of cooked rice has 45 grams of carbohydrates. Vegetables are a carbohydrate deal!

Breakfast Is on the Table—What Am I Supposed to Eat?

Eggs, bacon, ham, donuts, bagels, toast, oatmeal... What are you eating? Let's go over the following four steps to be used in determining your carbohydrate budget:

1. Identify foods that have carbohydrates (carbohydrates translate into higher blood glucose levels).
2. Estimate the amount of foods with carbohydrates on your plate. Is it 1 cup? 2 cups?
3. Determine how much carbohydrate you can have in one meal. This is your carbohydrate budget.
4. Identify how you will modify this meal. Can you make healthier substitutions? Are you eating certain foods out of habit?

Deal or No Deal?

In all of the meal examples to follow, I have asked my patient detailed questions concerning food items typically eaten and preferred for any given meal. This helps to establish a routine eating pattern. Each patient's carbohydrate budget is based upon the individual's height, weight, blood glucose levels, and medical history.

Meal Deal #1

Joe's Breakfast (carbohydrate budget = 60 grams)

The Interview: What do you typically eat for breakfast?

- Oatmeal (Which one? Old-fashioned rolled oats, instant oats, oats with added fruits? How much do you eat?)
- Milk (Which kind of milk do you use? Whole? Low-fat? How much?)
- Banana (What is the size of the banana? Indicate length using your hands.)
- Coffee with milk (How much milk do you add to your coffee?)
- Noncaloric sweetener (Which one do you use? The pink, blue, or yellow packets?)

The Menu

1½ cups of cooked instant oatmeal made with water

½ cup of 2% milk

1 medium banana

Coffee with 2% milk (mostly dark)

Prefers yellow packets of sweetener, but will have what is available

Carbohydrate Load of the Menu
  Oatmeal = 45 grams
  Milk = 6 grams
  Banana = 30 grams
  Coffee = carb-free
  Total carbs = 81 grams (21 grams over budget)

Meal Modifications

Joe loves oatmeal, so he is not confident that he can cut back on his usual breakfast portion. He is willing to eat half of the banana or skip it altogether. I would supplement Joe's modifications with the following recommendations:

- Use old-fashioned oatmeal or steel cut oats. Minimally processed foods are digested more slowly, resulting in a gradual and steady rise of blood glucose levels
- Switch to 1% or fat-free milk to reduce saturated fat
- Eat a lower-carbohydrate fruit, such as strawberries. Five medium-sized strawberries (2 oz) have about 5 grams of carbohydrates while a medium-sized (7 inches long) banana has 15 grams

Meal Deal #2

Rosa Maria's Lunch (carbohydrate budget = 60 grams)

The Interview: Rosi buys her lunch at the salad bar where she enjoys the potpourri of choices.

The Menu
  4 oz salmon
  ½ cup beans
  2 small flour tortillas
  1 cup mixed green salad with tomatoes, peppers, cucumbers
  (Rosi tells me that she avoids carrots, because they have a lot of sugar.)
  2 to 3 tablespoons fat-free Ranch salad dressing
  1 can diet soda

Carbohydrate Load of the Menu
  Beans = 15 grams
  Tortillas = 30 grams
  Ranch salad dressing = 16 grams
  Total carbs = 61 grams

- Beans have protein and carbohydrates. They are an excellent source of soluble fiber which can help manage cholesterol levels
- Corn tortillas are a better choice than flour tortillas, since corn meal has more fiber and less hydrogenated fat than flour
- Salad greens are "carbohydrate cheap." Dark vegetables are excellent sources of vitamins A and C
- Carrots and beets have a reputation for having "lots of sugar." Although they might have slightly more carbohydrates than a cucumber or a cup of spinach, they are still a carbohydrate bargain. A cup of cooked carrots has about 10 grams of carbohydrate. A cup of cooked rice has 45 grams. See the difference?
- Fat-free salad dressings have added carbohydrates. Two tablespoons of some fat-free Ranch dressings contain as much as 11 grams of carbohydrate. Remember to check the carbohydrate content of fat-free salad dressing on all labeling

Meal Modifications

Rosi almost met her carbohydrate quota! However, she has learned that she can add carrots to her salad without breaking the carb bank, and she will check the labeling for carbohydrate content of all salad dressings and sauces.

Meal Deal #3

Tony's Dinner (carbohydrate budget = 75 grams)

The Interview: Tony loves to cook and enjoys fine wines. He cooks with a lot of garlic and uses olive oil in his recipes. I ask him to tell me what some of his favorite foods are.

The Menu

- 1 bowl (about 1½ cups) homemade minestrone
- ½ plate linguini and broccoli rabe prepared with garlic and olive oil
- Lemon shrimp prepared with olive oil, garlic, and parsley
- Italian bread (about 4 inches long)
- 1 glass (5 oz) Pinot Grigio

Carbohydrate Load of the Menu

Minestrone soup = about 20 grams
Linguini = 45 grams
Italian bread (1½ oz) = 21 grams
Total carbs = 86 grams (11 grams over budget)

Meal Modifications

Tony could reduce the amount of linguini to ²/₃ cup for a savings of 15 grams of carbohydrate, adding more broccoli rabe to compensate for the reduction in pasta. Reducing the amount of bread by half would save another 10 grams.

Food Tip

■ When cutting back food portions, it is wiser to reduce the carbohydrate with the least "nutritional power." For example, minestrone with its beans and vegetables is more nutritious than Italian bread, so it makes more nutritional sense to reduce the bread rather than to reduce the soup (I apologize to all bread aficionados!)

■ Soups vary in their carbohydrate content. To make a low-carbohydrate soup, add more nonstarchy vegetables and less pasta, potatoes, or rice. Measure your foods until you become an expert in "eyeballing" portions. Wine does not count as a carbohydrate choice, and on an empty stomach, it may lower blood glucose levels

---

Protein: Beef, Pork, Poultry, Fish, Cheese, and Eggs—How Much Can I Eat?

I have talked extensively about carbohydrates, because carbohydrates impact blood glucose levels the most. I will now talk about two other important nutrients: Protein and fat.

Protein foods seldom travel solo. They are often accompanied by fat. Beef, pork, goat, chicken, turkey, fish, eggs, and cheese are frequently consumed protein choices. Super-sizing protein and fats leads to added calories, which translates into weight gain and poor diabetes control. Because diabetes increases the risk of heart disease, it is important to manage blood glucose levels in addition to blood pressure and cholesterol levels.

Saturated and hydrogenated fats (trans fats) increase blood cholesterol levels. Most animal protein sources, such as beef, chicken, pork, etc, contain saturated fat. Your best bet is to select leaner cuts most days of the week, reserving high-fat choices for occasional treats (**Figure 4-1**).

Lean Protein Foods

- Remove skin from chicken and turkey
- Trim all visible fats
- Select cheese with less than 2 grams of saturated fat per ounce
- Select lean cuts of meat

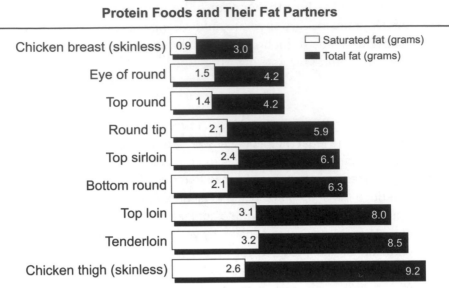

Figure 4-1

Protein Foods and Their Fat Partners

	Saturated fat (grams)	Total fat (grams)
Chicken breast (skinless)	0.9	3.0
Eye of round	1.5	4.2
Top round	1.4	4.2
Round tip	2.1	5.9
Top sirloin	2.4	6.1
Bottom round	2.1	6.3
Top loin	3.1	8.0
Tenderloin	3.2	8.5
Chicken thigh (skinless)	2.6	9.2

All values are based on 3-oz cooked servings of meat cuts.

Adapted from: Michigan Beef Industry Commission. Available at: www.mibeef.org /conleancuts.htm.

How much protein can I eat? You probably have heard that the amount of a protein portion should not be bigger than the palm of your hand or a deck of cards. For most people, this holds true. The daily protein requirement is 6 ounces. Yes, 6 ounces *per day*, not *per meal*.

High-Fat Protein Foods

Medium-fat protein foods contain 7 grams of protein and 5 grams of fat per ounce. Some examples are:
- 1 oz ground beef (most cuts of beef, pork, lamb, or veal)
- 1 oz low-fat cheese
- 1 egg

High-fat protein foods contain 8 grams of fat per ounce. Some examples are:
- 1 oz pork sausage
- 1 oz spare ribs
- 1 oz cheese (American, Swiss, etc)
- 1 oz lunch meat
- 1 oz frankfurter or bratwurst

What do these numbers mean? You can reach your fat quota very quickly if most of your protein foods come from the medium- and high-fat category.

If milk has carbohydrates, why is cheese listed as a protein food? American, Swiss, cheddar and other hard cheeses do not have over 1 gram of carbohydrate per ounce. Cheese is a high-fat protein food. If you have cheese-dependency issues, minimize portions. Select low-fat cheese if you are unable to eat just one half ounce.

Lorena's Cheese Tip

I find Cabot's low-fat cheeses quite palatable. Grated cheese is always a welcome illusion. When I grate 1 ounce of cheese, it appears voluminous compared with a slice. I also mix and match. High-quality grated Romano or Parmesan cheese combined with sliced cheese will make grilled cheese go a long way. I place ½ oz of cheese on a slice of bread, then sprinkle 1 tablespoon of Romano cheese over the top. Another trick is to heat a pan and place about 1 tablespoon of grated Romano or Asiago cheese on it. Let it melt and harden. This cracker-like piece of cheese can be added to salads for extra crunch and lots of taste with less fat. See **Table 4-5** for fat grams in 1 ounce of some common types of cheese.

Fat: How Much Should I Eat Daily?

Limiting saturated fats and hydrogenated fats can lower your risk for cardiovascular complications. When using fats and oils, select monounsaturated fats, such as olive oil and avocado (**Table 4-6**).

Table 4-5

Fat Grams in 1 Ounce of Cheese

	Total Fat (grams)	Saturated Fat (grams)
American	7	4
Cheddar	9	6
Low-fat cheddar	2	1
Mozzarella	6	4
Low-fat mozzarella	4	3
Muenster	8	5
Provolone	8	5
Swiss	8	5
Cottage cheese (½ cup)	5	3

Table 4-6
Daily Fat Budget

Calorie Budget	Total Fat (grams)	Saturated Fat (grams)
1200	40	9
1500	50	12
1800	60	14
2000	67	16
2200	73	22

Show Me the Food! (Do Not Show Me Fat Numbers)

I will use as an example Rebecca's daily budget:
- Calories: 1500
- Total fat: 50 grams
- Saturated fat: 12 grams

Let's take a look at two Meal Deals that are based on a daily fat budget of 1500 calories.

Meal Deal #4
3 oz roasted chicken leg (with skin)
1 medium baked potato
1 tablespoon sour cream
1 dinner roll
2 pats (teaspoons) of butter

1 bowl of green salad
1 tablespoon Ranch salad dressing
Calories = 609
Carbohydrates = 54 grams
Total fat = 31 grams
Saturated fat = 12 grams

Meal Deal #5
3 oz roasted chicken leg (skinless)
1 medium baked potato
1 teaspoon sour cream
1 dinner roll
1 teaspoon rosemary flavored olive oil
1 bowl of green salad
2 teaspoons vinegar with 1 teaspoon olive oil
Calories = 530
Carbohydrates = 54 grams
Total fat = 19 grams
Saturated fat = 5 grams

Meal Deal #4 will provide Rebecca with more than half of her daily fat allowance (31 grams) and all of her daily saturated fat allowance (12 grams), while Meal Deal #5 will provide her with less than half of her daily total fat and saturated fat allowances.

- A teaspoon of olive oil has the same amount of fat (5 grams) as a teaspoon of butter, but olive oil has less saturated fat than butter
- Select clear salad dressings. Creamy salad dressings have twice the fat and saturated fat compared with clear ones
- Omega-3 is a heart-healthy fat. Eat salmon, tuna, sardines, herring, and other fatty fishes a few times per week
- Alternate a high-fat meal with a very low-fat meal to achieve balance
- Select margarines that have less than 2 grams of saturated fat and less than 1 gram of trans fats

Cholesterol: How Many Eggs Can I Have Weekly?

The egg yolk has about 280 mg of dietary cholesterol. The recommendation is not too exceed 300 mg of cholesterol daily. Reducing dietary cholesterol to less than 300 mg per day may result in a 3% to 5% reduction in your LDL (bad cholesterol) levels. If your LDL is high (recommended goal is less than 100), then have no more than 3 egg yolks per week.

Eggs are not the only food with dietary cholesterol. Other foods with cholesterol include:

- Butter: 1 tablespoon = 30 mg
- Peanut butter: 2 tablespoons = 0 grams
- Broiled hamburger patty: 3 oz (75% lean/25% fat) = 76 mg
- Broiled hamburger patty: 3 oz (90% lean/10% fat) = 70 mg
- Broiled hamburger patty: 3 oz (95% lean/5% fat) = 65 mg
- Frankfurter (5 inches long): 1 = 24 grams
- Chocolate ice cream: 1 cup = 44 grams
- Whole milk: 8 oz = 24 grams
- Mozzarella cheese: 1 oz = 22 grams

Five Steps to Lower Your Cholesterol

1. Reduce weight (even a 10-lb loss can help lower your LDL cholesterol 5% to 8%).
2. Stay within your fat and saturated fat budget (see **Table 4-4**).
3. Eat very little trans fats (read the food labels, and select foods with "0" grams).
4. Eat more foods rich in soluble fiber (5 to 10 grams per day can help reduce your LDL cholesterol 3% to 5%):
   - Cooked oats: 1 cup = 4 grams
   - Cooked pearled barley: 1 cup = 6 grams
   - Cooked kidney beans: 1 cup = 6 grams
   - Strawberries: 1 cup (8 berries) = 3 grams

- Cooked okra: 1 cup = 4 grams
- Apple: 1 large = 3 grams.
5. Eat a handful of almonds or walnuts (about 23 pieces); nuts are healthy but "calorie-expensive," so if you add nuts to your diet, cut back on other foods to achieve "calorie balance."

Lowering Your Blood Pressure

Cutting back on salt is just one step up the ladder of blood pressure management. My advice is to continue taking your medications and check those numbers frequently. It is not uncommon to take more than one medication to control your blood pressure. Read more about controlling your blood pressure in Chapter 12.

You can also greatly assist the lowering of too-high blood pressure with the following lifestyle changes:

- Reduce weight until you achieve a level that is realistic for you (see **Table 4-1**)
- Try the DASH diet: A food-combination program that encourages the consumption of fruits, vegetables, and low-fat dairy while cutting back on saturated fat (DASH is an acronym for Dietary Approaches to Stop Hypertension [high blood pressure])
- Increase physical activity: don't squirm—just move, move, move about 30 minutes most days of the week
- Drink alcohol in moderation: That means men should have no more than two drinks and women no more than one drink per day
- Cut back on salt: Look at the sodium content on the food label (a low-sodium food has less than 140 mg of sodium per serving)

Frequently Asked Questions: The Top Ten List

1. *Which fruits have less sugar?* It depends on the serving size. A banana, a pear, a mango all have about 30 grams of carbohydrates; ¼ of a cantaloupe and 1¼ cup of strawberries each has about 15 grams of carbohydrates. *Remember:* All fruits have carbohydrates, which can raise blood glucose levels.
2. *Which foods cut fat?* The only foods that help you lose weight are those that remain uneaten on the plate. Low-calorie options, such as vegetables, allow you to eat more with fewer calories. Whole grains and beans are rich in fiber and increase satiety level. In general, eating less and moving more is the consistent—yet unexciting—message that still holds true to this day.
3. *What are the best cereals?* I will give you some of my favorites, although this is not an all-inclusive list: Nature's Path Optimum

Slim and Flax, General Mill's Fiber One, Kashi Go Lean and Friends, All Bran and Bran Buds, Oats, Uncle Sam, and Glucerna Crunchy Flakes.

4. *Aren't nuts loaded with cholesterol?* Nuts have fats but they have no cholesterol. Only foods that are animal-based have cholesterol. Plant foods may have fat but no cholesterol.

5. *How much sugar can I have?* Let me clarify: There are naturally occurring sugars in foods with carbohydrates. The sugar listed on the food label is the sum of added sugars and naturally occurring sugars. To find out if the food has added sugar, look at the ingredient label. Common names for added sugars are brown sugar, high-fructose corn syrup, corn syrup, and maltose.

6. *Should I use butter or margarine?* Butter is high in saturated fat and low in trans fats. Margarine is lower in saturated fat yet high in trans fats. Look for spray/liquid margarines and avoid stick margarines. If you still prefer to use butter, try whipped butter, and use it sparingly.

7. *Should I take vitamins?* A multivitamin may be beneficial. Do not think, however, that a multivitamin will redeem you from a multitude of food sins!

8. *Is coffee bad?* Some studies have suggested that there is a temporary rise in blood pressure with coffee consumption. If you like it, and it does not make you anxious/nervous or cause you to lose sleep, enjoy it!

9. *Should I eat sugar-free (fill in the blank)?* Sugar-free cookies and cakes contain slightly less carbohydrates than their regular counterparts. The sugar is replaced with sugar alcohols which have minimal impact on blood glucose levels. Nevertheless, they contain other carbohydrate sources, such as flour. Sugar-free is neither calorie-free nor carbohydrate-free. Proceed with caution and still count the carbohydrates.

10. *Can you give me low-carbohydrate options?* If you cringe at the thought of eating 1/3 cup of cooked rice or pasta, try jicama (Mexican potato), winter squashes, rutabaga, parsnips, or turnips.

Summary

1. Eat small portions except for nonstarchy vegetables.
2. Carbohydrates turn into glucose about 15 minutes after eating, and it is the nutrient that affects blood glucose levels the most.
3. Testing your blood glucose level will let you know if the meal plan is working for you.

4. Carbohydrates are found in all fruits, breads, cereals, starchy vegetables, pasta, rice, tortillas, potatoes, corn, crackers, milk, yogurt, and sweets.
5. Nonstarchy vegetables are carbohydrate bargains.
6. Protein and fats do not have much of an impact on blood glucose levels unless you super-size. Trim the fat from your meats and poultry, and select lean cuts. Use olive oil, avocado, and nuts in moderate amounts.
7. Read all food labels, and stay within your calorie, fat, saturated fat, trans fat, and sodium budgets.
8. Select foods high in soluble fiber.
9. Eat vegetables and fruits daily.
10. Get a diabetes coach—a health care professional who can help you put a plan into action that is realistic and makes sense to you!

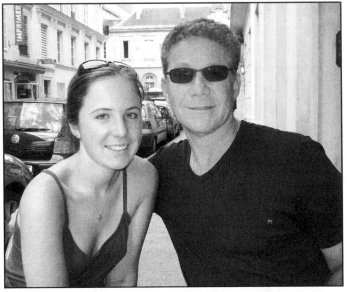

Steve Edelman and his daughter, Talia, in Italy in 2005.

5

Exercising for Life With Diabetes

by Sheri R. Colberg, PhD, FACSM

Introduction

Although exercise has long been one of the three cornerstones of diabetes management—along with diet and medications—it has generally been and continues to be the most overlooked and underutilized of the three. Why? My opinion, as an exercise physiologist and a person living with type 1 diabetes myself, is that people are less likely to exercise regularly because they just don't know enough about how, when, where, and why to fit physical activity into their daily lives. The reality of exercising with diabetes is that regardless of what type you have,

being more active is just one more variable that you have to take into account when you're trying to take control of your blood glucose level. Whether you're just contemplating starting to exercise or you're already a regularly training athlete, by learning more about exercise, you will soon understand why it is so important to living well with diabetes and how to make it work best for you and your unique situation.

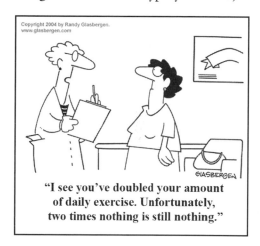

"I see you've doubled your amount of daily exercise. Unfortunately, two times nothing is still nothing."

Why Exercise Is So Important to Your Health

Not only can regular exercise make you fitter, it can also help you lose weight (or at least not gain any more), enhance your mental health, decrease your blood pressure, and lower your risk of heart disease, cancer, other chronic health problems, and your chances of dying from any cause. What is more, people with diabetes experience similar or even greater health benefits from being active than the average nondiabetic person.

We already know for certain that people who exercise regularly really do live longer. A recent study looked at the effect of different levels of physical activity (ie, low, moderate, or high) on the total life expectancy of more than 5200 middle-aged and elderly people, most already older than 50 years. The study concluded that if you get in a vigorous workout almost daily (such as running 30 minutes 5 days a week), you can add nearly 4 years to your life. If you only engage in moderate exercise—the equivalent of walking instead of running for those 30 minutes—then you're likely to live 1.3 to 1.5 years longer for males and females, respectively, likely due to delaying the onset of heart disease, our nation's leading killer and a major cause of death and disability in people with diabetes.

I have to admit that when I first read about this study, I thought, "Doing moderate exercise 5 days a week will allow me to live only a year and a half longer?" To gain this extra time, you would have to walk moderately for at least 2.5 hours a week, 52 weeks a year, for most of your adult life (55 years beyond the age of 21, on average), meaning that you would end up spending over 7000 hours exercising, or about 300 24-hour days, in exchange for only 550 extra days. So, basically, you would have spent over half of your "extended" lifespan exercising the equivalent of 24 hours a day. I guess if you really enjoy exercising, that's not a bad thing (and there are some avid diabetic exercisers out there who wouldn't mind), but if you're like the majority of people, you're probably thinking that for no more than you gain, it's just not worth the extra effort.

Before you stay on that couch and vegetate some more, though, let me try to talk you out of it. What is likely much more important is that exercise can increase your health-related quality of life. Regular physical activity affects not only how long you live but also how long you live a healthy life. Being more active can give you more time in a healthy state, free from a host of chronic illnesses that can make it hard for you to really enjoy living. It can prevent your developing heart disease, regardless of any other risk factors you have… and just by having diabetes, you already have one strike against you. Even if you have not been diagnosed with heart disease, diabetes gives you the equivalent or greater risk of dying from a heart attack as someone without diabetes who has diagnosed heart disease. If exercising moderately can reduce your risk for dying even sooner from a heart attack because of diabetes, then you may have far more to gain from exercising than your nondiabetic friends and relatives.

Diabetes has the potential to rob you, on average, of more than 12 years of your life, not to mention that it can also dramatically reduce your quality of life for more than 20 of those lesser years. A lower quality of life can result from many physical ailments, but in people with poorly controlled diabetes, it often results from a compromised physical capacity, partial limb amputations, lesser mobility, chronic pain, blindness, and kidney dialysis, in addition to heart disease. What's the point of living longer if you aren't living well?

Maybe you've avoided exercising for years, and now you figure it's too late to start. If that's what you think, then you are just plain wrong (or maybe just misinformed)! It's never too soon to start following a healthy lifestyle, and it's never too late to start exercising. Even for people who are already middle-aged, exercising more can add years to their lives. Conversely, remaining sedentary is the most devastating thing you can do to your long-term health, longevity, and hope of avoiding or delaying the onset of chronic diseases and diabetic complications.

How Exercise Helps Improve Blood Glucose Control

Frequent, regular exercise is the key to good blood glucose control if you have any type of diabetes. The glucose-lowering effects of exercise are mainly due to a heightened sensitivity to insulin in exercised muscle, an effect that persists for no more than 1 to 2 days following the activity and that appears to be mostly related to the replenishment of stored carbohydrates (glycogen) in the muscles that you exercised. Thus in order to maximize exercise's positive effects on your blood glucose, you have to exercise regularly and use up as much glycogen as possible.

How does exercise help with blood glucose control? In the short term, any physical activity generally causes your muscle cells to take up more blood glucose, thus resulting in lower glucose during and following the activity. The only exception is really intense exercise (such as sprinting or heavy weight lifting), which can temporarily raise your blood glucose level. Following almost every type of physical activity, though, your muscle cells generally remain more sensitive to any insulin in your body (your own or injected insulin) for a period of time afterward usually for anywhere from 30 minutes to 48 hours. This enhanced insulin action can result in your body requiring less insulin to process the foods that you eat, which in turn improves blood glucose control for most people with type 2 (or gestational) diabetes and oftentimes for type 1s and other insulin users as well. For type 1 exercisers, though, regular exercise will only improve their overall glycemic control if they also make appropriate changes to concurrently balance their insulin doses with their food intake and exercise.

It appears that exercise helps improve your blood glucose levels even if you lose little or no weight. In middle-aged men with prediabetes, an hour and a half of weekly exercise reduced their insulin resistance, whether or not they restricted their calorie intake or lost any weight.

Furthermore, people with diabetes participating in studies conducted by the Pritikin Longevity Centers, who have followed diets that were higher in fiber and complex carbohydrates and very low in refined sugar, cholesterol, fat, and salt, and engaged in 30 minutes or more of daily exercise have also experienced remarkable improvements in their diabetes control in only 3 weeks. For instance, almost 75%

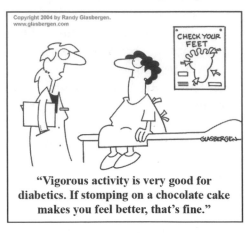

"Vigorous activity is very good for diabetics. If stomping on a chocolate cake makes you feel better, that's fine."

of people taking oral medications to control blood glucose levels were able to discontinue them, and close to 40% on insulin injections were also able to control their blood glucose levels without any extra insulin. Although modest weight loss resulted from their lifestyle changes, their postprogram body fatness was far from ideal after only 3 weeks, and yet their diabetes control vastly improved.

If you have type 2 or gestational diabetes, daily or near daily activities are better for optimizing your blood glucose control and weight maintenance or loss. With type 1 diabetes, regular, predictable exercise makes your blood glucose easier to predict and manage effectively. With any type of diabetes, though, regular blood glucose monitoring will help you control your blood glucose when you participate in an exercise program, but it's easiest when your physical activity is consistent.

How to Be More Active

Luckily, becoming physically active doesn't require a daily trip to the gym or doing physical activities that you detest. It also doesn't mean that you have to be able to complete a marathon or a triathlon, although there are plenty of people with both type 1 and type 2 diabetes who do successfully complete and compete well in such events. It simply means that if nothing else, you will be able to go through your daily life without becoming unduly fatigued, even when doing such physical activities as walking up multiple flights of stairs, caring for your kids or grandkids, working, running errands, volunteering, or doing any other activities without resting. Remarkably, once you become more active, it is likely that you will have more energy throughout the day rather than less.

Getting started is simpler than you think. It's important that you realize that all physical activity you do during the day counts toward your daily total. Until recently, vigorous exercise was believed to be required for optimal health and fitness. While you may stand to gain more health benefits from harder workouts, we now know that almost any activity (including golfing, gardening, mowing the lawn, moderate walking, etc) done for 30 to 45 minutes per day is beneficial to your health. Furthermore, lower-intensity exercises are beneficial even if you do them for only 10 minutes at a time.

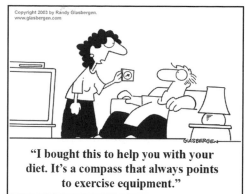

"I bought this to help you with your diet. It's a compass that always points to exercise equipment."

If you haven't been very active lately, you may need to see your doctor before you begin exercising more (**Table 5-1**). Medical clearance prior to easy exercise (like slow walking) is usually not necessary; however, if you plan to do more vigorous exercise, seeing your doctor beforehand is generally a good idea. The more risk factors that you have for heart disease, the greater your chance of having a cardiovascular problem during exercise, and simply knowing what you need to watch out for could be crucial to preventing more serious problems. For instance, if you have any symptoms like shortness of breath when you walk or pain in your lower legs, you may already have cardiovascular issues. It is usually still possible to exercise, but it pays to know what your safe limits are. In fact, regular moderate to vigorous activity can actually reduce your risk of a heart attack.

When it comes to being more active, if you're overweight, you may have special concerns about doing exercise routines. In particular, being overweight may make you acutely aware of your larger body size and self-conscious during certain activities or prevent you from wanting to participate at all. If you fit this profile, it is especially important for you to find activities that are enjoyable for you. For example, swimming or aquatic classes may be a viable alternative. Extra fat stored under your skin acts to insulate and keep you warmer in the pool. Also, the water serves to mostly hide your body, which may decrease any inhibition that you may feel when your figure is more plainly visible during other activities.

Your new goal is simply to be as physically active as possible to maximize your caloric expenditure and blood glucose use, and you don't

Table 5-1

You May Want to See Your Doctor First Before Starting Your Exercise If You...

- Are planning on participating in moderate to strenuous activities, not just mild ones
- Are over 35 years old
- Have been diagnosed with type 1 diabetes for more than 15 years or type 2 for more than 10 years
- Know you have heart disease, a strong family history of heart disease, or high cholesterol or lipid levels
- Have poor circulation in your feet or legs (or lower-leg pain while walking)
- Have diabetic retinopathy (eye disease), nephropathy (kidney disease), or neuropathy (numbness, burning, tingling, or loss of sensation in your feet and/or dizziness when going from sitting to standing)
- Have not consistently been in good control of your blood glucose level

necessarily have to join the nearest gym! Instead, just take the stairs instead of the elevator, park your car at the far end of the lot from where you're headed, walk in place during all the TV commercials, and then take the dog out for a walk! For motivation, you may want to invest in an inexpensive pedometer (step counter) and try to add at least 2000 steps a day (ie, the equivalent of about 1 mile) to your current activity level.

Other Important Physical Activities

Once you can simply start moving more throughout the day, you may feel more able to add in some other forms of more structured exercise while maintaining your new higher level of unstructured physical activity. These more-planned forms of exercise include aerobic, resistance, and flexibility training. While anyone can benefit from these activities, the strength and not just the endurance of your muscles will become more important as you age in maintaining your ability to care for yourself and to balance well enough to stay on your feet.

Structured Aerobic Exercise

The recommendation for everyone choosing to participate in more structured exercise programs is a minimum of 3 to 5 days per week of aerobic exercise (walking, jogging, cycling, swimming, rowing, etc), done for 30 to 60 minutes. When you begin a program of planned exercise, start out slowly, exercising a minimum of 3 days a week for 20 to 30 minutes a day, and gradually work up to 45 to 60 minutes per day and/or 5 days per week. The Surgeon General recommends moderate amounts of daily, aerobic physical activity consisting of 30 minutes of moderate activities (like brisk walking) or shorter sessions of more intense exercise, including jogging or playing basketball for 15 to 20 minutes. Running, tennis, and aerobic dance classes are examples of higher-impact forms of cardiovascular workouts, while lower-impact aerobic exercises include mild walking, swimming, cycling, tai chi, and the like. Moderate walking, though, is much more sustainable over a lifetime than many other activities, making it one of the best "medicines" for both the prevention and treatment of type 2 diabetes and for maintenance of your overall health. You can also make your workouts more taxing simply by adding faster intervals in them occasionally, like temporarily picking up your walking speed between two mailboxes.

Ideally, your chosen activities should be ones that allow you to move your whole body over the greatest distance possible to maximize your energy expenditure, especially if your weight is a continuing issue. However, although both walking and jogging fall into this category of activities, most overweight adults will find jogging and running either too difficult or simply not enjoyable. As an alternative, you can trick yourself into walking more, simply by incorporating it into other activities—such as walking farther than you need to when you go shopping. Walking can be the gateway to more vigorous exercise (not necessarily running, though) and can further increase your overall health benefits. As a bonus, your self-confidence may improve once you start a walking program, which may lead you to start including additional physical activities in your life. You might even want to try out ballroom dancing, cycling, low-impact aerobics classes, or other forms of aerobic exercise.

Resistance Training

Strength or resistance training is imperative to maintain the amount of muscle you currently have, to gain more, and to prevent loss of muscle and strength as you age. Resistance training is just as important as—and possibly even more so than—aerobic exercise for diabetes control as well. Such training can increase your body's insulin sensitivity, along with lowering your risk for thinning bones and loss of muscle mass with aging. The current recommendation is to train 2 to 3 nonconsecutive days per week and include all the major muscle groups of your body. Some examples of strength exercises are biceps curls, triceps curls, overhead press, bench press, leg press, lunges, calf raises, and abdominal crunches.

If you are a novice at resistance work, you can start out with lighter weights, flexible resistance bands, or items that you find around the house (like water bottles or soup cans held in your hands) to complete one to two sets of 12 to 15 repetitions ("reps") on each exercise. When two to three sets of 15 reps are easy for you to do, make your workouts progressive by adding a little weight or resistance to each exercise and drop the number of reps back to 12. If all you can manage to fit into your schedule is one set once a week, don't despair—you'll still experience some strength gains!

When you have completed this elementary stage of your weight program for 6 to 8 weeks, you should be able to handle heavier weights and perform fewer reps per set. It appears far less important, however, to focus on how much weight you lift than to make sure that you are lifting any. By way of example, a study on postmenopausal women showed that both high-load (heavy weights, low reps) and high-repetition (lighter weights, more reps) resistance training were effective in increasing muscular strength and size, indicating that even easy resistance training is beneficial for older women. Likewise, muscular endurance and strength improved similarly in older adults doing only one set of twelve resistance exercises at either 50% of their one-repetition maximum (the maximal amount they could lift one time) for 13 repetitions or 80% for 8 repetitions, which they did three times weekly for 6 months.

You can choose either resistance-training regimen and have similar gains. For variety, you may even decide to have easy days where you do more reps with lighter weights and hard days when you lift heavier weights fewer times, depending on how motivated you feel. The only resistance-training principles you must follow are to work a particular area of your body (ie, upper body) no more frequently than every other day; to equally train muscles with opposite actions on a joint, such as the biceps and triceps muscles of your upper arm or the quadriceps and hamstring muscles of your thigh; and to breathe in and out smoothly while lifting (no breath holding).

Flexibility Training

Working on your flexibility also helps prevent injuries and is doubly important for anyone with diabetes. Everyone is becoming less flexible over time; some loss of flexibility is to be expected. However, poor diabetes control by itself can speed up this loss of flexibility by causing glucose to bind to joint structures (collagen and the like), making them more brittle and less flexible. A loss of flexibility leads to a reduced range of motion for your joints, an increased likelihood of orthopedic injuries and a greater risk of developing some of the joint-related problems often associated with diabetes, such as diabetic "frozen shoulder," tendonitis, trigger finger, carpal tunnel syndrome, and others.

It is recommended that you work on your flexibility a minimum of 2 to 3 days per week, but I recommend stretching before and/or after any exercise session or any other time that your muscles start to tighten up as well. It doesn't appear to matter when you stretch, as long as you do it, but it's usually easier to do once you've warmed up a little. Also include stretching exercises a minimum of 2 days per week to maximize strength gains and minimize the loss of flexibility caused by aging and accelerated by diabetes.

Risks and Precautions Associated With Exercise

Of course, although the benefits are immense, physical activity is not completely risk free. Both diabetes regimens and any potential complications can decrease your ability to exercise safely and optimally. To get the most out of your physical activities, it is important to know the risks and precautions and to take the steps necessary to minimize them.

Hypoglycemia

The greatest risk associated with exercise is the possibility of developing hypoglycemia, usually defined as a blood glucose level less than 65 mg/dL. As you know, insulin causes your muscles and fat cells to take up blood glucose. However, muscle contractions by themselves increase uptake of blood glucose through a separate mechanism without insulin. When you're exercising, your muscles are actually taking up glucose due both to contractions and to insulin circulating in your bloodstream.

Symptoms of hypoglycemia are varied but include shakiness, sudden fatigue, irritability, mental confusion, inability to do simple math, elevated heart rate, sweating, dizziness or light-headedness, poor physical coordination, and visual spots. If you experience hypoglycemia, treat it immediately with small amounts (5 to 10 grams) of readily absorbed carbohydrates, such as glucose tablets, hard candy, regular soft drinks (4 ounces), or sports drinks (8 ounces). Rest 5 to 10 minutes before rechecking your glucose level. Consume the same amount of carbohydrate again only if your symptoms have not begun resolving. Do not overtreat it by eating too much, though, or you'll end up battling a high blood glucose level instead.

Your training state is important in accurately predicting your glycemic response to an activity and lowering your risk of developing hypoglycemia. Becoming more trained increases the proportion of fat your body uses for similar low- or moderate-intensity activity done after training. Using a greater proportion of fat spares both your muscle glycogen and your blood glucose and allows you to more easily control your blood glucose level during physical activities. You will likely find that your blood glucose level drops less when you do the same activities after training for several weeks.

Insulin Use and Hypoglycemia Risk

If you normally take insulin (whether you have type 1 or type 2 diabetes), whatever insulin you have injected through a syringe, infused with an insulin pump, or inhaled, may raise your insulin blood level and elevate your risk of low blood glucose during or following an activity. For most people with type 2 diabetes not using insulin, this risk is minimal. For insulin users, the risk is much higher, and they will have to either eat extra carbohydrates, lower their pre-exercise insulin doses, or both to compensate and prevent lows. Generally, when no more than basal levels of insulin are circulating in your body during exercise, your physiologic response will be more normal, more like that of someone who doesn't have diabetes. If you exercise when your insulin levels are peaking or higher, however, you'll have an increased risk of hypoglycemia.

Oral Diabetic Medications and Hypoglycemia Risk

Use of certain oral diabetic medications may also increase your hypoglycemic risk associated with exercise. Some of the sulfonylureas increase your risk of developing hypoglycemia. For instance, Diabinese (chlorpropamide) and Orinase (tolbutamide) cause insulin release from the pancreas and somewhat decrease insulin resistance, but typically have a longer duration (up to 72 hours) and, therefore, can potentially cause your glucose levels to go too low during and/or following exercise. Amaryl (glimepiride), DiaBeta (glyburide), Micronase (glyburide), and Glucotrol (glipizide) generally don't last as long and carry a smaller risk; of these, DiaBeta and Micronase carry the greatest risk due to their slightly longer duration (24 hours versus only 12 to 16 hours for the others). You will have to frequently monitor your glucose when exercising if you take any of the sulfonylureas that stay in your system longer and, when your exercise becomes regular enough, you may need to check with your doctor about lowering your doses of these medications if you are frequently experiencing hypoglycemia during or following exercise.

Other medications usually have less of an effect on exercise. Insulin sensitizers, such as Avandia (rosiglitazone) and Actos (pioglitazone) mainly affect the action of insulin at rest, so the risk of these medications causing exercise hypoglycemia is almost nonexistent. Similarly, Glucophage (metformin) is unlikely to cause exercise lows. Prandin (repaglinide) or Starlix (nateglinide) only potentially increase your risk of a low blood glucose level if taken immediately before prolonged exercise as they increase insulin levels only temporarily when taken with meals. Finally, medications that slow down the absorption of carbohydrates (Precose [acarbose] and Glyset [miglitol]) would not directly affect your exercise blood glucose, but could slightly delay your treatment of low blood glucose, as could either of the newer injectable medications, Symlin (pramlintide) and Byetta (exenatide). If you plan on exercising, it would behoove you to not take any of these latter medications within 2 hours of when you are going to start being active, just in case you need to treat a low blood glucose.

Hyperglycemia

Technically, any blood glucose level in excess of 125 mg/dL qualifies as hyperglycemia, but your exercise responses will likely be normal up until your glucose level is twice as high or higher, or above 250 mg/dL. Although very uncommon in type 2 diabetes, ketosis (ie, acidosis detected by ketones in the bloodstream and urine) may develop in people with limited or no insulin production. If it does, you should not exercise until you get rid of the ketones, as they indicate that your body is insulin deficient, which will likely cause your blood glucose level to rise even more if you exercise. If you're somewhat hyperglycemic right after eating and you took an insulin injection (maybe just not a high enough dose), though, your blood glucose will likely still decrease during extended exercise because enough insulin will be in your body during the activity.

Dehydration

If you're exercising with any elevation in your blood glucose level, take care to drink enough water as it will be easy for you to become dehydrated. Elevated glucose can increase your water loss through excessive urination, and your risk of losing extra fluids is greater with poorly controlled diabetes. Exercising itself compounds the risk by increasing sweating (thus loss of water), which can rapidly compound a dehydrated state. Since exercising during hot weather can be especially dangerous for older individuals who may not release heat as effectively as younger adults, adequate fluid replacement and frequent rest are needed.

Interestingly, despite the emphasis on proper hydration, it appears that you're more likely to harm yourself with excessive fluid intake than with dehydration during exercise. If you drink too much of anything during exercise, you increase your risk of diluting the sodium content of your blood, potentially causing a medical condition known as water intoxication and putting you at risk for seizures, coma, and even death. While adequate hydration prior to exercise with fluids consumed early (17 ounces of fluid taken 2 hours before exercise) is recommended, in order to avoid overhydrating, it is more prudent to start drinking only when you actually feel thirsty. The only exception is in people with poorly controlled diabetes, since they may have an elevated thirst threshold (meaning that they don't feel thirsty as quickly, even when dehydrated). If that applies to you, start drinking small amounts of water as soon as you start sweating.

Orthopedic Injuries and Arthritis

Simply by having diabetes, you already have a high risk of both joint-related injuries and overuse problems like tendonitis. You may, therefore, find that adopting a more moderate exercise like walking rather than a more vigorous one like running makes more sense, since you'll have less potential for joint trauma with the former type of exercise. The best defense is to prevent all of these injuries with good diabetes control, flexibility exercises that help emphasize and maintain a full range of motion around your joints, and moderate amounts of exercise training.

Arthritis is also more common in people with type 2 diabetes due to the extra body weight most of them are carrying around. Lower extremity joints (the hip, knee, and ankle) are most often affected, and, when present, osteoarthritis can severely limit your ability to exercise. However, exercise is an effective means of managing arthritis, even the more severe rheumatoid type. Get started with some basic range-of-motion exercises to increase your joint mobility, and then move on to specific resistance work. If you have arthritic knees or hips, walking may be uncomfortable or painful. Your best option is to try non–weight-bearing activities, such as walking in a pool (with or without a flotation belt around your waist), aqua aerobics, lap swimming, recumbent stationary cycling, upper-body exercises, seated aerobic workouts, chair dancing, and resistance activities.

Exercising With Diabetic Complications

Finally, there are some exercise risks that may arise if you have certain diabetes-related complications. If you have had diabetes for a number of years, it is likely that you may develop some complications, particularly if your blood glucose control is less than optimal. You can still exercise (and you should!), but you will have to take any health problems into account to exercise as safely and effectively as possible.

Peripheral Neuropathy and Peripheral Arterial Disease

If you have lost some of the feeling in your feet due to nerve damage (neuropathy), consider switching to activities such as swimming or stationary cycling to minimize potential trauma to your feet. On the contrary, if you experience pain in your lower legs when moving around, a symptom of peripheral arterial disease, walking may actually be good for you. A recent study showed that people may actually experience symptom relief and lesser decline in their ability to walk when they participate in walking at least 3 days a week, either in a supervised exercise program or on their own. In either case, to protect your feet, choose athletic shoes with silica gel or air midsoles (the middle section of the shoe that provides the most stability and shock absorption), as well as polyester or cotton-polyester socks to prevent the formation of blisters and to keep your feet dry during physical activities. You or someone else (if you are not able to) should check your feet daily for signs of trauma and treat them aggressively.

Autonomic Neuropathy

If you have damage to your central nervous system known as autonomic neuropathy, this complication may make it harder for you to change your body position without experiencing light-headedness or fainting. You're also more likely to overheat and become dehydrated. If it affects your ability to digest (known as gastroparesis), any carbohydrate you eat may be more slowly absorbed, and hypoglycemia during exercise can become more severe as a result. It may cause an elevated heart rate at rest, but a lower heart rate than normal during exercise. Thus avoid making rapid changes in movement that may result in fainting and spend more time warming up and cooling down. Drink extra fluids, avoid being continuously active for long periods during hotter weather, and eat only smaller meals and snacks before exercise. Last, monitor your exercise by some means other than your heart rate alone.

Diabetic Eye Disease

While exercise itself has not been shown to accelerate proliferative diabetic eye disease (retinopathy), certain precautions may be needed to prevent intraocular hemorrhages or retinal tears. If your eye disease is only mild or moderate with no active bleeds, you should simply avoid activities that dramatically increase the blood pressure inside your eyes, such as heavy weight lifting or activities during which your head is lower than your heart. If your retinopathy is moderate to severe, avoid all jumping, jarring, or breath-holding activities as they increase the pressure inside your eyes and can cause more bleeding and increase your risk of blindness, retinal tears, or retinal detachment. If you have an active retinal hemorrhage or notice sudden, dramatic changes in your sight, stop any activity you are doing immediately and check with your ophthalmologist before resuming your exercise.

Kidney Disease

Intense or prolonged exercise would not usually be recommended for you if you have severe kidney disease, but only because your exercise capacity is likely to be limited. Light to moderate exercise is fine, and even patients requiring dialysis can exercise with no ill effects. If you are undergoing dialysis, exercise would only be advised against if the levels of certain substances in your blood (hematocrit, calcium, or potassium) become unbalanced as a result of the treatments.

Cardiovascular Disease

If you have diagnosed heart disease, you can still participate in most forms of exercise. In fact, resistance training is now recommended for everyone (in addition to aerobic activities), even for people who have had a heart attack or stroke. Be aware that a heart attack can potentially have symptoms other than pain localized in your chest, such as pain that radiates down one arm or shoulder or your neck or that feels like bad heartburn. If you experience any unusual pain or other symptoms during or following exercise, get checked out by your doctor as soon as possible. Diabetes can also potentially cause you to experience silent ischemia, a reduction in blood flow to the heart muscle through the coronary blood vessels that is painless and symptom free. If you ever experience a sudden, unexplained change in your ability to exercise, without any other symptoms, immediately stop exercising and consult your physician as soon as you can to rule out silent ischemia.

When in doubt, follow the exercise guidelines published by the American Diabetes Association with regard to exercising with diabetic complications (**Table 5-2**). Always include proper warm-up and cool-down periods (3 to 5 minutes of a lesser-intensity activity before and after your planned exercise session) to ease the cardiovascular transition and minimize your risks.

Special Exercise Concerns for Insulin Users

Once you learn how your body responds to different types of exercise and what type of regimen changes you need (particularly if you take insulin), you can effectively control your blood glucose. Many insulin users (with both type 1 and type 2 diabetes) employ a combination of short- and long-acting insulins (varying by time to peak action and total

Table 5-2

Precautions for Exercising With Diabetes and/or Its Complications

- Have a blood glucose meter accessible to check your glucose level before, possibly during, and/or after exercise, or if you have any symptoms of low blood glucose

- Immediately treat any hypoglycemia during or following exercise with quickly absorbed carbohydrates like glucose tablets or regular soft drinks

- Inform your exercise partners about your diabetes, and show them how to give you glucose or another carbohydrate should you need assistance

- Stay properly hydrated with frequent intake of small amounts of cool water

- Consult with your physician prior to exercising with any of the following conditions:
  - Proliferative retinopathy or current retinal hemorrhage (diabetic eye diseases)
  - Neuropathy (nerve damage), either peripheral or autonomic
  - Foot injuries (including ulcers)
  - High blood pressure
  - Serious illness or infection

- Seek immediate medical attention for chest pain or any pain that radiates down your arm, jaw, or neck and for serious indigestion, any of which may indicate a lack of blood to your heart and a possible heart attack

- If you have high blood pressure, avoid activities that cause it to go up dramatically, such as heavy weight training, head-down exercises, and anything requiring breathholding

- Wear proper footwear, and check your feet daily for signs of trauma, such as blisters, redness, or other irritation

- Immediately stop exercising if you experience bleeding into your eyes caused by active proliferative retinopathy

- Wear a diabetes Medic Alert bracelet or necklace with your physician's name and contact information on it

duration) given 1 to 4 (or more) times daily. Others receive a continuous infusion of insulin through an insulin pump, which delivers self-programmed basal amounts of insulin and boluses for food via a subcutaneous catheter. The insulin regimen that you use, along with the type, duration, intensity, and timing of exercise, will determine what changes you will need to maintain control over your blood glucose.

When only minimal levels of insulin are circulating during exercise, your body's metabolic responses will be closer to normal. If you choose to exercise during peak times of injected insulin, however, you will experience an increased risk for hypoglycemia unless you cut back your insulin doses or eat extra carbohydrates. For example, if you normally use NPH (isophane), an intermediate-acting insulin, at breakfast, it will peak around noon to cover your lunch and into the afternoon. In contrast, Lantus (glargine) and Levemir (detemir) are designed to last 12 to 24 hours and provide only basal insulin coverage, making a separate dose of shorter-acting insulin (such as Humalog [lispro], Novolog [aspart], or Apidra [glulisine]) needed to provide enough insulin for lunch. If you use NPH, you are much more likely to experience low blood glucose during when exercising in the late morning (if you don't adjust for it) compared with a Lantus or Levemir user with no insulin peaks and whose breakfast rapid-acting insulin has peaked and waned in 2 or so hours, well before pre-lunch exercise. Alternately, if you use an insulin pump, you can lower your risk of lows by either disconnecting your pump or reducing your programmed basal rates before, during, and/or after physical activity.

A multitude of other variables affecting insulin action can confound your glycemic response to exercise as well. For instance, prebreakfast exercise is less likely to make your blood glucose level drop than the same activity done later in the day (even just after breakfast) because in the morning before you eat, your body has higher levels of hormones that make you more insulin resistant. Thus early-morning exercise usually requires less changes in your diabetic regimen. Exercising in the late evening can cause you to develop hypoglycemia during your sleep, but it still can be done safely if you take the proper precautions (eg, eating a bedtime snack and/or lowering bedtime insulin dose).

Moreover, your glucose response can be altered by the type, intensity, and duration of the activity; your starting blood glucose level, when you last ate or took any insulin (and how much), whether the activity is a new or unusual one, if you exercised recently, and many more factors that experience and trial and error can help you figure out. Keep in mind that during higher-intensity, prolonged activities such as moderate-paced running (or faster), carbohydrate is almost exclusively your muscles' fuel of choice, and depletion of both muscle glycogen and blood glucose is inevitable if you exercise at that level for long. For shorter-duration and more-intense activities, carbohydrate supplementation alone can work effectively for glycemic control, but for more prolonged exercise sessions, you will likely need to reduce your insulin doses as well.

If you consume some carbohydrate within 30 minutes after exhaustive exercise, your muscles will restore their muscle glycogen more rapidly, and you will be less likely to experience late-onset hypoglycemia that can occur up to 24 hours after exercise. Your insulin sensitivity is generally heightened immediately after a workout, and during that time, you don't need much insulin to take up glucose into your muscles for glycogen replacement. Good blood glucose control during this period is essential, though, for optimal glycogen replacement.

To learn your body's unique response to different exercise situations, you will need to go through some trial and error to find the best way to handle your diabetes for each one, and you will need to test your blood glucose level more frequently until you can establish a glycemic pattern. Even becoming more trained doing each unique activity will change your body's use of blood glucose and likely result in smaller drops in your glucose than before you trained. For additional exercise guidelines and regimen-change advice, please consult my book, *The Diabetic Athlete: Prescriptions for Exercise and Sports* (Human Kinetics Publishers, 2001). It covers diabetic-regimen changes and gives real-life athlete examples for more than 85 recreational physical activities and sports.

Maintaining Exercise for Life

The inspiration to make a change in your daily routine can come in many forms. If motivation is your biggest problem, make a game out of trying to count your daily steps. Even instructing sedentary, overweight women to walk 10,000 steps per day (monitored by a pedometer, or step counter) is more effective in increasing their daily exercise than asking them to walk 30 minutes on most days of the week. If nothing else, keeping track of your steps should at least help you become more conscious of how active you are (or aren't) and remind you to add in more steps and movement whenever and wherever you can.

Many people also complain all of the time about being too tired to exercise. What you may not realize, though, is that your lack of exercise is probably most responsible for making you feel tired. Even normally active individuals who take a few weeks off from their usual activities begin to feel more sluggish, lethargic, and unmotivated to exercise. The best thing to do is to start moving more, and you will likely begin to feel more energized and motivated to continue exercising.

If you still need more motivation to keep going, try any of the following: Put your more structured activities down on your calendar, keep track of your progress, and reward yourself for meeting your goals; recruit an exercise buddy or two to join in the fun; find ways to distract yourself during workouts to make the time pass more quickly; and keep your physical activities convenient, enjoyable, and varied to prevent excuses to avoid doing it. More importantly, don't start out working too hard, or you will likely either decide to quit or injure yourself. If you do fall off the exercise wagon, get back on it as soon as you can, but start back slowly.

Conclusions

Undoubtedly, exercise conveys certain risks and challenges for diabetic individuals, such as the risk of exercise-induced hypoglycemia. However, physical activity is an integral part of taking control of your diabetes, whether you're a beginning exerciser or an elite athlete. Anyone with diabetes can follow some basic exercise strategies to best control blood glucose levels and to exercise safely and effectively. Just keep in mind that you do not have to be an exercise fanatic to reap the benefits of increased physical activity. Adding just a little activity to your daily routine can have major health benefits. Experts suggest that even 15 to 30 minutes of walking each day is probably enough to gain substantial health benefits. Get up and get moving in every way that you can every day. If you're already a regular exerciser, then you are likely reaping maximal health benefits from your activities and should continue to do so by staying active.

For more information on getting and staying more physically active and living well with diabetes, please read *The 7 Step Diabetes Fitness Plan: Living Well and Being Fit with Diabetes, No Matter Your Weight* (Marlowe & Company, 2005). If you're already an exercise enthusiast, and particularly if you are an insulin user, consult *The Diabetic Athlete: Prescriptions for Exercise and Sports* (Human Kinetics Publishers, 2001) for regimen changes and real athlete examples for over 85 sports and recreational physical activities. For additional inspiration about living long and well with diabetes—and how physical activity plays a key role—check out our new book, *50 Secrets of the Longest Living People With Diabetes* (Marlowe & Company, 2007) by myself and Dr. Edelman. Most of all, just get up and get moving to secure your good health for the rest of your life.

6

Type 2 Diabetes Oral Medications

New Incretin Hormones and Combination Therapy

Introduction

Until 1994, there was only one type of oral medication for people with type 2 diabetes: the sulfonylureas (SFUs). This meant that people with type 2 diabetes had the option of either SFUs or insulin, or both, to control their blood glucose levels. Sulfonylureas lose their effectiveness over time, and since no one likes to take injections and it was easier for the caregivers to prescribe pills instead of an insulin regimen, many people with type 2 diabetes lived with poor glucose control for many years. Commonly, it was only when the blood glucose level becomes extremely high, into the 300- to 400-mg/dL range, that insulin therapy was initiated to finally bring down the toxic and harming glucose levels. With the advent of new oral medications, this situation is gradually improving. It is improving only gradually because some caregivers do not know about the advances made in this area, and the public is ignorant as well, which is why patient education and self-advocacy are so important. The bottom line is that if you have type 2 diabetes or know someone with type 2 diabetes, you need to know what new therapeutic advances have been made and are available right now. If you think that any of the medications you read about in this chapter may be good for you, please discuss it with your caregiver.

We now have lots of choices! Since 1994, several new types of oral medications for people with type 2 diabetes are available, with many more under development. These new oral agents can be given together and/or with insulin to more effectively control the glucose level throughout the day. Since many of these new oral agents have not been on the market for an extended period of time, it is of utmost importance that you become knowledgeable about all of them and determine if one or more of them would be helpful to you. Oral diabetes medications are generally not intended for people with type 1 diabetes or for women who are pregnant and/or are breastfeeding.

Oral Agents for Type 2 Diabetes

There are now six major classes or types of oral medications for people with type 2 diabetes:

1. Sulfonylureas (insulin secretagogues)—stimulate pancreatic insulin production
2. Nonsulfonylurea insulin secretagogues—same as SFUs
3. Biguanides—shut off excess glucose production by the liver
4. Carbohydrate absorption inhibitors—retard carbohydrate absorption in the intestine
5. Insulin sensitizers (chemical name: thiazolidinediones)—increase the body's sensitivity to insulin action
6. DPP-4 inhibitors or incretin enhancers—enhance action of incretins (explained in detail later in this chapter)

As you will learn, these six types of diabetes medications work in different ways and many can be used in combination to attain desirable glycemic control. In fact, many of them now come together in one combination pill, which will be discussed.

Sulfonylureas (Insulin Secretagogues)

Sulfonylureas, or SFUs, have been around for a long time. For decades, these were the only oral medications available for people with type 2 diabetes. They were the workhorses of the 70s, 80s, and early 90s. There are many different SFUs on the market today, and they all work primarily by stimulating the pancreas to secrete more insulin. As discussed in Chapter 1, type 2 diabetes is a condition in which the insulin secreted from the pancreas does not work well (insulin resistance). However, if the insulin level becomes high enough in the blood from taking SFUs, the glucose levels will eventually start to fall. The various SFUs on the market are listed in **Table 6-1** along with the recommended dosage range, including how often they should be taken per day (depending on the duration of action). The only SFU that requires extra caution, especially if you are elderly, is Diabinese (chlorpropamide), because it tends to stay in your system for up to 3 days even after it is discontinued. If you become ill and cannot eat, you will have the tendency to have low blood glucose for a prolonged period of time despite stopping the medication.

The SFUs are effective in bringing down the blood glucose values and are generally well tolerated by people with diabetes. However, they do have some shortfalls, but these are more of an issue with the older SFUs (**Table 6-2**). One of the main problems with the SFUs is that they lose effectiveness over time, on average after about 5 years of use; the response is different from individual to individual. The results of the long-awaited ADOPT (A Diabetes Outcome Progression Trial) pub-

Table 6-1

Prescribing Information for Sulfonylureas

Generic Name	Trade Name	Daily Dose Range (mg)	Recommended Frequency
Older Sulfonylureas			
Acetohexamide	Dymelor	250 to 3000	Twice
Chlorpropamide	Diabinese	100 to 800	Once or twice
Tolazamide	Tolinase	100 to 1000	Once or twice
Tolbutamide	Orinase	500 to 3000	Once to three times
Newer Sulfonylureas			
Glipizide	Glucotrol	2.5 to 40	Once or twice
Glipizide (extended release)	Glucotrol XL	5 to 20	Once
Glyburide	DiaBeta	1.25 to 20	Once or twice
	Glynase PresTab	0.75 to 12	Once or twice
	Micronase	1.25 to 20	Once or twice
Glimepiride	Amaryl	1 to 8	Once

lished in 2007 clearly demonstrates that SFUs fail to maintain control over time compared with other oral medications (**Figure 6-1**). Some researchers believe it is because the SFUs work by continuing to make the pancreas work overtime, eventually leading to exhaustion and reduced insulin secretion capacity over time. If the pancreas is exhausted, it cannot put out any more insulin, and you will not be responsive to SFUs anymore. Thus blood glucose goes out of control. When a person's blood glucose value starts rising while being treated with an SFU, it is usually necessary to add another oral medication or initiate insulin therapy to get the diabetes under control.

A second shortfall is that SFUs commonly cause

Table 6-2

Benefits and Shortfalls of Sulfonylureas

Benefits

- Effective at lowering the blood glucose levels (at least initially)
- Well tolerated by people with diabetes (few side effects)

Disadvantages

- Lose effectiveness over time, requiring combination therapy with other pills, incretins, and/or insulin
- Weight gain (normally just a few pounds) after the sulfonylurea is initiated
- Hypoglycemia, especially with strenuous exercise or a missed meal(s)

Figure 6-1
ADOPT: First to Fail Study

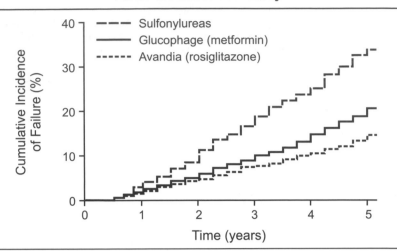

Failure defined when the morning blood glucose is consistently over 180 mg/dL. Avandia had a much lower failure rate compared with sulfonylureas as well as with Glucophage.

DREAM Investigators. *Lancet.* 2006;368:1096-1105.

5 to 10 pounds of weight gain, most likely because of the way they work. When insulin levels go up, either due to insulin secretagogues or insulin injections, the body weight also has a tendency to go up.

A third shortfall is that SFUs can cause low blood glucose (hypoglycemia), especially after strenuous exercise, if you miss a meal, or if you lose weight. It must be remembered that hypoglycemia is not a severe problem in the majority of cases and is normally recognized early and easily treated. If you are a person whose diabetes has been recently diagnosed (less than a few years ago) or if you have near normal blood glucose levels, you might be at a higher risk for hypoglycemia on SFUs than someone who has had diabetes much longer with poor control.

Hypoglycemia is discussed in Chapter 11; however, the main symptoms of hypoglycemia are shaking, sweating, palpitations (feeling your heart beating over your chest area), and confusion. If you think your blood glucose is getting too low, you should drink or eat something sweet, such as 4 to 8 ounces of fruit juice, regular soda, four to six Lifesavers, or one of the many forms of glucose tablets that are sold over the counter in pharmacies. You should always carry something sweet, such as 3 to 4 glucose tablets, and keep similar items in your car and at work or school. It may also be important to tell your family members and coworkers about helping you (if necessary) during a low blood glucose episode.

It is also important to test your blood glucose level before treating yourself with sugar to make sure that your symptoms are in fact due to hypoglycemia. This helps you and your caregiver to properly adjust your medication. You should call your doctor if you have low blood glucose reactions frequently, especially if it happens without a ready explanation, such as a missed meal or strenuous activity.

Nonsulfonylurea Insulin Secretagogues

Prandin (repaglinide) and Starlix (nateglinide) work in a fashion similar to the sulfonylureas; namely, by stimulating the pancreas to secrete more insulin. The difference is that they work faster than SFUs and must be taken before each meal. Prandin and Starlix have a completely different chemical structure than the SFUs and have been described as non-SFU insulin secretagogues. The word secretagogue is used because it explains how the SFUs, Prandin, and Starlix work by stimulating the pancreas to secrete insulin. Since Prandin and Starlix cause rapid bursts of insulin secretion when taken, it may be helpful to people with irregular eating habits (take it only when you eat). Because both Prandin and Starlix cause an elevation of the insulin levels, they can cause hypoglycemia and weight gain. These side effects are minimized by the fact that the effect of stimulating insulin secretion wears off quickly after the meal. This rapid-on and rapid-off action results in better blood glucose levels after eating and less delayed hypoglycemia or low blood sugar several hours after your meal or during exercise. In general, Prandin and Starlix should not be used with other SFUs, but they can be used safely with other oral agents. See **Table 6-3** for dosing information.

Biguanides

Glucophage (metformin) is the only biguanide on the US market and has been available since 1994. However, Glucophage has been used around the world for over 32 years. Glucophage is now recommended as the first drug of choice for people with newly diagnosed type 2 diabetes unless there is a contraindication to it. In fact, it is also recommended to be started immediately upon diagnosis along with lifestyle modification.

Glucophage is an effective medication that works mainly by preventing the liver from producing too much glucose. In the normal nondiabetic state, one of the important jobs of the liver is to produce

Table 6-3

Prescribing Information for Nonsulfonylurea Insulin Secretagogues

Generic Name	Trade Name	Daily Dose Range (mg)	Recommended Frequency
Nateglinide	Starlix	120 to 360	Two to four times a day with each meal
Repaglinide	Prandin	0.5 to 16	Two to four times a day with each meal

just enough glucose to keep the body functioning normally. However, in people with diabetes, the liver inappropriately overproduces glucose, mainly at night. This overproduction of glucose at night leads to elevated blood glucose levels, especially in the morning. This is one reason Glucophage especially improves the fasting or prebreakfast blood glucose value. Glucophage is now available in an extended-release formula (Glucophage XR) and in combination with other oral medications (see the section later in this chapter on combination medications). Both the extended-release and combination pills make your daily medication regimen a little easier and simpler (**Table 6-4**).

The benefits and shortfalls of Glucophage are listed in **Table 6-5**. Glucophage is effective in lowering glucose values and has made a major impact in this country as the first new oral drug for diabetes to become available in over 40 years after the introduction of the SFUs in the 1950s. Glucophage does not stimulate the pancreas to secrete insulin, and this is probably why there is no weight gain or problems with hypoglycemia. Weight gain and hypoglycemia are observed with SFUs, Prandin, Starlix, and insulin. In addition, Glucophage may also improve your cholesterol and triglyceride levels as well as other cardiovascular risk factors, which is an important advantage since heart disease is such a severe problem in people with type 2 diabetes.

Shortfalls of Biguanides

Glucophage is generally well accepted by patients, although it may cause mild stomach upset or loose stools when initiating therapy. If any symptoms occur, they usually do so in the first few weeks after starting the medication. In order to avoid stomach problems, I recommend starting with the lowest dose 500 mg (1 tablet) with dinner for 1 week. If no problems are present after the first week, you may increase the dose to 500 mg two times a day with breakfast and dinner, only with the advice of your caregiver. Your physician will adjust your dose further according to the level of improvement seen in your blood glucose values.

Table 6-4
Prescribing Information for Biguanides

Generic Name	Trade Name	Daily Dose Range (mg)	Recommended Frequency
Metformin	Fortamet	500 to 2500	Once
	Glucophage	1000 to 2550	Twice to three times
	Glucophage XR	500 to 2000	Once
	Glumetza	1000 to 2000	Once

Glucophage generally is a safe medication. However, it is important to have your kidney function tested before you begin taking Glucophage in order to avoid an uncommon but serious and potentially fatal problem called lactic acidosis. Testing your kidneys involves a nonfasting blood test called the serum creatinine, which must be 1.5 mg/dL or lower in men and 1.4 mg/dL or lower in women in order to take Glucophage safely. If you are older than 80 years or if your serum creatinine is borderline high, it is recommended that you perform a urine collection so that your doctor can get a more sensitive measurement of your kidney function called the creatinine clearance or GFR (glomerular filtration rate). Creatinine is a substance that comes from the kidney; levels of creatinine increase in the blood and urine when there is kidney disease present. If your kidney function is borderline, you should have repeat kidney tests at least every 6 to 12 months while being treated with Glucophage. I would also encourage you to track and keep good records of your kidney function. It is important to understand that metformin or Glucophage is not harmful in any way to your kidneys. However, metformin is metabolized (cleared from the body) by the kidney and if the kidneys are not working well, the levels of metformin in your blood can

Table 6-5
Benefits and Shortfalls of Biguanides

Benefits
- Effective in lowering glucose levels, especially in the morning
- Does not cause weight gain
- Does not cause hypoglycemia or low blood glucose
- Improves cholesterol levels

Shortfalls
- May cause stomach upset, especially when starting therapy (usually not a big problem)
- Must be cautious if kidney disease is present
- Must be cautious if congestive heart failure is present
- Must temporarily stop treatment with Glucophage if you become seriously ill or require an x-ray study using dye (see text)

elevate and cause lactic acidosis. I have been seeing patients since 1982 and I have only seen this rare problem once!

In addition, if you have a condition called congestive heart failure, you may not be an appropriate candidate for Glucophage, especially if you are taking a drug called Lanoxin (digoxin) and/or a strong diuretic such as Lasix (furosemide) or Bumex (bumetanide). (Congestive heart failure is when the blood-pumping action of your heart is not up to speed and body fluids back up into the lungs, legs, and other places.) If you have any questions about these concerns, please discuss them with your caregiver.

It is also important to remind your doctor(s) that you are taking Glucophage if you become severely ill at home, are hospitalized, or if you are going to have a radiographic (x-ray) test for which you will be receiving a dye (colored fluid). Glucophage should be temporarily halted in these situations and restarted when the acute illness or test is over and normal kidney function resumes.

Carbohydrate Absorption Inhibitors

Precose (acarbose) and Glyset (miglitol) are the two drugs in this class currently available in the United States (**Table 6-6**). They work mainly by delaying the absorption of carbohydrates after meals, thus blunting the rapid rise in blood glucose that is usually observed after eating. In a similar fashion to Starlix and Prandin, Precose and Glyset are postprandial drugs (prandial = meal). Postmeal hyperglycemia contributes to the absolute level of the glycosylated hemoglobin (or A1C) value and, over the long term, the prevalence of diabetic complications.

Precose and Glyset are safe medications that one may take with no concerns about kidney or liver disease. Precose and Glyset do not stimulate the pancreas to secrete insulin, so there is no weight gain and no problem with hypoglycemia. Their benefits and shortfalls are listed in **Table 6-7**.

Table 6-6
Prescribing Information for Carbohydrate Absorption Inhibitors

Generic Name	Trade Name	Daily Dose Range (mg)	Recommended Frequency
Acarbose	Precose	50 to 300	First bite of each meal
Miglitol	Glyset	50 to 150	First bite of each meal

Shortfalls of Carbohydrate Absorption Inhibitors

Precose and Glyset may cause excess gas (flatulence) or mild stomach upset. These side effects tend to occur when you first begin therapy. The side effects can be minimized by starting with a low dose and increasing the dose very slowly ("start low and go slow"). Instructions for initiating therapy with Precose and Glyset are listed in **Table 6-8.**

Insulin Sensitizers (Thiazolidinediones)

Insulin sensitizers (Avandia [rosiglitazone] and Actos [pioglitazone]) represent an important class of oral medications for the treatment of type 2 diabetes. They are also called TZDs, which is short for... are you ready for this... thiazolidinediones (thia-zo-la-deen-dions)! It took me 2 years to get the pronunciation of this word correct. The United States was the first country to approve the first TZD, Rezulin (troglitazone), in 1996; however, it was removed from the market due to a low incidence of severe liver damage. TZDs, or insulin sensitizers, work mainly by reducing insulin resistance. One of the earliest and main defects observed in type 2 diabetes is insulin resistance. Basically, the problem is that the body is resistant to the normal glucose-lowering effects of insulin. The end result is that the blood glucose rises because the insulin cannot do its job of getting the glucose out of the bloodstream and into the cells of the body for energy. TZDs allow the insulin that is present in the body, either secreted by the pancreas or injected by a needle, to work more effectively to lower the blood glucose levels. Avandia and Actos are the two available insulin sensitizers. The TZDs have been around for about 10 years and are available worldwide.

Avandia and Actos are easy to take because they may be taken only once a day at any time that is convenient (**Table 6-9**). In addition, TZDs are well tolerated with few side effects. In a similar fashion to

Table 6-7

Benefits and Shortfalls of Carbohydrate Absorption Inhibitors

Benefits

- Very safe medications
- Do not cause weight gain
- Do not cause hypoglycemia or low blood glucose
- Can be used with all other oral agents and/or insulin currently available

Shortfalls

- May not lower glucose levels and glycosylated hemoglobin (or A1C) as much as other medications
- May cause stomach upset and/or gas, especially when starting the drug; must titrate the dose slowly (start with a small dose and slowly increase it over time)

Table 6-8

Instructions on How to Start Precose or Glyset: Start Low and Go Slow!*†

Step 1: Start with 25 mg at breakfast only for 1 to 2 weeks

Step 2: Take 25 mg with breakfast and dinner for 1 to 2 weeks

Step 3: Take 25 mg with breakfast, lunch, and dinner for 1 to 2 weeks

Step 4: Take 50 mg with breakfast and 25 mg with lunch and dinner for 1 to 2 weeks

Step 5: Take 50 mg with breakfast and dinner and 25 mg with lunch for 1 to 2 weeks

Step 6: Take 50 mg with breakfast, lunch, and dinner

---

* Do not increase the dose further unless you have discussed this with your caregiver. If, at any step, you have bothersome gas or stomach pain, do not go to the next step; stay at the current step or revert to a previous step until your symptoms improve. Then continue with the steps as listed. Last, it is extremely important to take Precose and Glyset at the beginning of your meal(s). They will not work to lower your blood glucose if you take them more than 10 minutes before you eat. The maximum dosage of Precose is 100 mg 3 times a day, which is equivalent in efficacy or effectiveness to Glyset 50 mg 3 times a day.

† Take Precose and Glyset with the first bite of each meal.

Table 6-9

Prescribing Information for Insulin Sensitizers (Thiazolidinediones)

Generic Name	Trade Name	Daily Dosage Range (mg/day)	Recommended Frequency
Pioglitazone	Actos	15 to 45	Once a day
Rosiglitazone	Avandia	2 to 8	Once a day

Glucophage, Glyset, and Precose, TZDs do not stimulate the pancreas; therefore, hypoglycemia is not a problem and there is better long-term effectiveness, by resting the pancreas, compared with the SFUs and Glucophage (see previous discussion on the ADOPT and **Figure 6-1**). TZDs have also been shown to improve abnormal cholesterol and triglyceride levels and blood pressure. TZDs have additional effects that may help keep the heart and cardiovascular system healthy (such as reducing inflammation and the tendency of the blood to be too thick), thus reducing the risk of blood clots. The benefits and shortfalls of Avandia and Actos are listed in **Table 6-10**.

Shortfalls of the Insulin Sensitizers

The TZDs in general are very safe and well-tolerated medications. However, because of the liver problems seen with Rezulin (troglitazone), it is still required by the FDA that you have a liver function test done before you start a TZD and periodically afterward. It turns out that despite careful monitoring of the side effects of Avandia and Actos, there have been few serious problems reported relating to damage of the liver. It is a side effect that is not a big concern anymore now that these drugs have been used by millions of people with type 2 diabetes worldwide. In fact, insulin sensitizers may improve a condition called "fatty liver."

The most common side effects of the TZDs are fluid retention, commonly presenting as edema or swelling of your ankles, and weight gain. The vast majority of people who take Avandia or Actos do perfectly fine with no problems whatsoever; however, a small percentage (4% to 8%) will have some fluid retention.

Table 6-10

Benefits and Shortfalls of Insulin Sensitizers (Thiazolidinediones)

Benefits

- Easy to take (only once a day) at any time that is convenient
- Well tolerated by people with diabetes
- Do not cause hypoglycemia or low blood glucose
- Improve the abnormal cholesterol and triglyceride levels
- May improve the blood pressure and other cardiovascular risk factors
- Slows down the progressive nature of type 2 diabetes

Shortfalls

- May cause fluid retention or swelling (ankle edema)
- Can cause weight gain
- May take several weeks to see the full benefit
- May precipitate a condition called congestive heart failure if you already have a weak heart
- May increase the risk of osteoporosis in women

For some, the ankle edema is very mild and the benefits of improved glucose control far outweigh this side effect. However, some individuals may have significant swelling and the medication must be discontinued (the swelling goes away after stopping or reducing the medication). If you have a condition called congestive heart failure, discussed earlier, you may not be a candidate for an insulin sensitizer since the fluid retention may make your heart failure worse, and this is especially true if you are also on SFUs and/or insulin. Please discuss this with your caregiver if you have concerns.

The typical weight gain that is observed with Actos and Avandia in clinical studies is about 5 to 10 pounds; however, there are many variables that may affect potential weight gain. Some individuals do not gain any weight at all and others, who are on insulin and/or SFUs, may gain more weight. Once again, in my opinion, this is a small price to pay for improving blood glucose control and in turn reducing the complications of diabetes. It is important to know that because of the way the insulin sensitizers work (mechanism of action), it may take several weeks for you to observe any improvement in your blood glucose level. Your caregiver will decide the correct dose for you according to your glucose values.

DPP-4 Inhibitors or Incretin Enhancers

Januvia (sitagliptin) and Galvus (vildagliptin) are members of a new class of oral medications for type 2 diabetes called the DPP-4 inhibitors. Januvia has received FDA approval for use, and Galvus is currently under review. In order to understand how these new drugs work, I need to review how our bodies regulate glucose control. In addition to insulin, our bodies release a relatively newly discovered group of hormones called incretins, such as GLP-1 and GIP. These are abbreviations for long medical words. In any case, these hormones called incretin are normally released from the gut in response to the ingestion of food, and they work to lower glucose levels by stimulating insulin release. They also work by inhibiting glucagon, which is a good thing since glucagon works in an opposing manner to insulin and raises glucose levels. In people with type 2 diabetes, the GLP-1 and GIP incretin hormone levels are below normal. In addition, once these incretin hormones are released, they are rapidly inactivated in the gut by an enzyme called DPP-4. Here is where both Januvia and Galvus come in.

Januvia and Galvus work by inhibiting the enzyme (DPP-4) that rapidly breaks down GLP-1 and GIP, hence delaying these hormones from being degraded and prolonging their action so they can continue work to keep the blood glucose from going up, especially after eating. This is why they are called DPP-4 inhibitors. Januvia and Galvus can also automatically sense when your blood glucose level is getting near the normal range so that they can shut off their own actions to avoid hypoglycemia. In addition, neither Januvia nor Galvus causes weight gain or fluid retention. In general, the DPP-4s can be used with other oral agents; however, it is important to discuss the potential of adding this medication to your regimen with your caregiver. The prescribing guidelines are shown in **Table 6-11**.

Combination Oral Medications for Type 2 Diabetes

Combination oral medications for type 2 diabetes are becoming very popular for several reasons. Swallowing one pill that contains two effec-

Table 6-11
Prescribing Information for DPP-4 Inhibitors or Incretin Enhancers

Generic Name	Trade Name	Daily Dosage Range (mg)	Recommended Frequency
Sitagliptin	Januvia	100	Once
Vildagliptin	Galvus	—	Currently under review by the FDA

Abbreviation: FDA, Food and Drug Administration.

tive medications that work well together is simpler than taking two different pills separately. Combo pills also allow for a single copay, which may be helpful to folks on a limited income. At the current time, there are a number of combinations of oral medications and they are listed in Table 6-12.

The New Incretin Hormones: GLP-1 and Byetta (Exenatide)

What the heck is an incretin hormone? In medical school, when I was training to be a diabetes specialist, the only hormone responsible for glucose control was thought to be insulin, which comes from the

Table 6-12
Prescribing Information for Combination Drugs

Generic Name	Trade Name	Daily Dosage Range (mg)	Recommended Frequency
Glipizide/ metformin	Metaglip	2.5/250 to 20/2000	Twice with meals
Glyburide/ metformin	Glucovance	1.25/250 to 20/2000	Twice with meals
Pioglitazone/ glimepiride	Duetact	30/2 to 30/4	Once
Pioglitazone/ metformin	Actoplus Met	15/500 to 45/2550	Twice with meals
Rosiglitazone/ glimepiride	Avandaryl	4/1 to 8/4	Once
Rosiglitazone/ metformin	Avandamet	2/500 to 8/2000	Twice with meals
Sitagliptin/ metformin	Janumet	50/500 to 50/1000	Twice with meals

pancreas. In fact, most endocrinologists like myself believed that the world revolved around the pancreas and that it was the most important organ in the human body (if you are a guy, the second most important organ!). Well, a whole new class of hormones called the incretins was recently discovered to be super important in controlling blood glucose and that they come not from the pancreas but rather from the gut or small intestine.

There are a whole bunch of incretin hormones; however, one of the more important ones is called GLP-1 (glucagonlike peptide-1). GLP-1 is normally released from the gut upon ingestion of food and its main action is to prevent the abnormal rise in glucose levels after eating. GLP-1 performs many important functions in the body, which are listed below and shown in **Figure 6-2**.

1. GLP-1, when released from the gut after eating, causes the pancreas to secrete insulin, which helps to prevent blood glucose levels from rising excessively after eating.

Figure 6-2

GLP-1 Effects in Humans

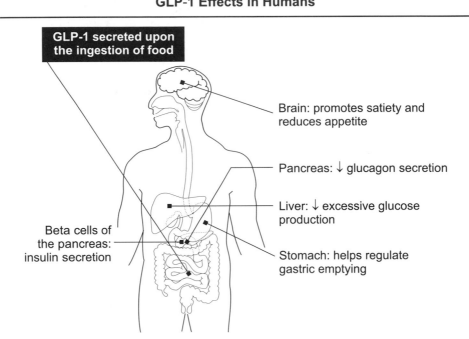

Adapted from: Flint A, et al. *J Clin Invest*. 1998;101:515-520; Larsson H, et al. *Acta Physiol Scand*. 1997;160:413-422; Nauck MA, et al. *Diabetologia*. 1996;39;1546-1553; and Drucker DJ. *Diabetes*. 1998;47:159-169.

2. GLP-1, when released from the gut after eating, causes the pancreas to decrease the secretion of glucagon, which is a good thing because glucagon leads to glucose production and elevation of glucose values. In people who do not have type 2 diabetes, glucagon goes down after eating; in people with type 2 diabetes, it inappropriately goes up.

3. GLP-1 helps to regulate the peristaltic contractions of the stomach, which turns out to be pretty important in regulating glucose values throughout the day and especially after meals. When food goes into the stomach, it is broken down by digestive enzymes but the nutrients are not absorbed and thus do not raise the glucose levels. It is only when the broken-down nutrients leave the stomach and enter the small intestine or gut do they get absorbed and contribute to postmeal hyperglycemia. In people who do not have diabetes, the peristaltic contractions of the stomach slow down when the blood glucose level is approaching the upper limit of normal (about 140 mg/dL) in an attempt to prevent the glucose level from rising above normal. Conversely, when the glucose level approaches the lower limit of normal (about 60 mg/dL), the peristaltic contractions of the stomach speed up, dumping nutrients faster into the gut for absorption, in an effort to prevent hypoglycemia. It turns out that in people with diabetes, the peristaltic contractions of the stomach are too fast and that by replacing GLP-1, the stomach motility is slowed down to the normal rate.

4. GLP-1 also has a significant effect to induce satiety, reduce the appetite, and lead to weight loss. This last effect of significant weight loss in addition to improving the glucose control is a unique combination of effects not seen with other medications for type 2 diabetes. GLP-1, when released into the circulation after eating, travels to the appetite and satiety centers in the brain, and weight loss has been a consistent finding in every clinical study conducted in people with type 2 diabetes. By the way, satiety is a term to describe the feeling of being satisfied when eating. It turns out that when people with type 2 diabetes take synthetic human GLP-1 before sitting down to a meal, they eat approximately 20% to 24% fewer calories since they experience satiety and reduced hunger.

Byetta: The First Incretin Mimetic

With all these great effects, why not give GLP-1 to people with type 2 diabetes? GLP-1 is a peptide hormonelike insulin and needs to be injected, which is not the problem. The problem is that GLP-1 is rapidly deactivated by an enzyme called DPP-4, which is found throughout the body. Once GLP-1 is released from the gut upon ingestion of food, it is deactivated by DPP-4 within 90 seconds. Hence the only way to give GLP-1 and take advantage of its benefits is to give it continuously intravenously or via some type of pump. This makes giving GLP-1 impractical. However, believe it or not, a substance called exenatide was accidentally discovered in the saliva of the Gila monster, a lizard found in Arizona, that mimics the action of GLP-1 almost exactly but it is different in one important way. Exenatide (chemical name), also called Byetta (trade name), was different enough that it did not get rapidly inactivated like GLP-1. Byetta can be given twice a day and has all of the beneficial effects of GLP-1

Byetta, which became available in 2005, is officially approved to be used in people who have type 2 diabetes and have not achieved glucose control with SFUs, Glucophage, and/or TZDs, such as Actos and Avandia. The majority of people who are started on Byetta have no side effects at all. The side effect that occurs in a minority of patients is nausea. The nausea is usually mild, mainly occurs when Byetta is first started, and typically improves over time. In rare cases, the nausea precludes the continued use of Byetta. Byetta does not cause hypoglycemia, but if used with medications that can cause hypoglycemia such as SFUs, then of course hypoglycemia is possible. The educational material given to the prescribers says that the SFU dose may need to be reduced or stopped when using Byetta concomitantly. It is not uncommon that hypoglycemia may occur as the patient loses weight on Byetta and becomes more sensitive to his or her other diabetes medications. The benefits and shortfalls of Byetta are listed in **Table 6-13**.

Byetta comes in a disposable pen that has a 1-month supply (approximately 65 doses). There are two strengths of Byetta (5-microgram

Table 6-13

Benefits and Shortfalls of Byetta (Exenatide)

Benefits
- Significant and sustained weight loss while the blood glucose level is improving
- Reduced appetite
- Does not cause hypoglycemia
- No need to change home glucose monitoring frequency

Shortfalls
- Can cause mild nausea when intiating therapy

[mcg] and 10-mcg dose pens). The prescribing guidelines recommend that the patient start on the low-dose pen for the first month and if no adverse effects occur, then go up to the 10-mcg pen thereafter (**Table 6-14**). Byetta should be taken before the two main meals of the day. If you are a light breakfast eater and your two main meals are at lunch and dinner, those are the times you should take your Byetta. Don't forget that your caregiver should prescribe the BD ultrafine 31-gauge short insulin needles that are used with the Byetta pen. They are super comfortable and there is no question that it is painless most of the time.

Byetta LAR (long-acting release) is currently being developed so that only a weekly injection will be needed rather than twice daily.

Table 6-14

Prescribing Information for Byetta

Generic Name	Trade Name	Daily Dosage Range (mcg)	Recommended Frequency
Exenatide	Byetta	5 for first month, followed by 10 thereafter	Twice with two largest meals of the day

FDA Guidelines on Using Combinations of Oral Medications, Incretin Hormones, and Insulin Together

It is important to be aware that some of the combinations of medications discussed in this chapter are not FDA approved yet. The FDA will officially approve a drug or combination of medications to be used together once an official study has been done, usually conducted by the drug company that makes one of the medications to be combined, and the data submitted to the FDA for review. It is impossible for new drugs to immediately be approved with indications for use in combination with all other diabetes medications because there are too many combinations now and it would take too long. Eventually, most effective combinations are studied and formally approved by the FDA. It is not unusual for practicing physicians with lots of clinical experience to use medications in combination "off label" before the FDA formally approves their use in this way.

General Guidelines for Taking Diabetes Medications Alone or Together

There are many variables that should be considered before any diabetes medication is chosen. There is no one perfect regimen that should be used for everyone. **Table 6-15** lists some of the variables that should be considered when choosing a medication to help control your diabetes.

Now that there are six different types of oral medication, incretin hormones, plus insulin (discussed in Chapter 6) for treating type 2 diabetes, and because we can mix and match them safely, there are many different regimens that are now possible. You have many options to choose from for the agent(s) that best fits your personal needs. There are many ways to design a successful treatment regimen for people with type 2 diabetes. A perfect regimen is one that helps you achieve normal or near-normal glucose levels, avoiding bothersome side effects, and does not disrupt your lifestyle to a significant degree. General guidelines for a successful treatment program are listed in **Table 6-16** and discussed below.

First and foremost, there is no oral agent(s), incretin hormone, or insulin that will control your blood glucose level if you are not following some type of dietary program. You can't just eat anything you want at anytime and expect a good blood glucose level. I don't expect a perfect diet from anyone, but there has to be some regularity in the types and amounts of food that you ingest.

Attaining blood glucose control with only one oral medication (monotherapy) is most successful when the diagnosis of diabetes has been made recently (within the past few years). Because of the natural history of diabetes, as discussed in Chapter 1, when the pancreas becomes exhausted, the likelihood that any single oral agent will control blood glucose values is slim to none. As times goes on, the chances increase that you will need more than one oral medication, incretin hormone, and/or insulin to control your blood glucose level.

Another rule of thumb that I promote to caregivers is that when one oral medication (no matter which type) is not controlling the glucose value, it is recommended that another oral agent or incretin hormone be added to, and not substituted for, the initial drug.

Finally, it is important not to wait too long before initiating insulin if the pills and/or an incretin hormone is not working to control

Table 6-15

Variables to Consider When Choosing an Oral Medication

- Are you overweight?
- Do you have abnormal cholesterol levels?
- How is your kidney function?
- How is your liver function?
- How good are you about taking pills regularly?
- Are you prone to having hypoglycemia?
- Do you already have a sensitive stomach?
- What does your health care plan provide for?

glucose levels. The longer you have diabetes and the higher your blood glucose value, the greater the likelihood that the oral medications will not work well enough and that you will require insulin therapy to achieve control. In certain situations, adding a single bedtime injection of a long-acting insulin to the daytime oral medication(s) and/or an incretin hormone may be quite effective and will be discussed next.

Combination Therapy: Bedtime Insulin Added to Daytime Medications

Combining medication(s) taken during the day with a single injection of a long-acting insulin at bedtime can be an effective way to achieve 24-hour glucose control. Combination therapy is important because the use of insulin plus daytime medications is a natural extension of daytime medications alone. This regimen was especially attractive when the

Table 6-16

General Guidelines for a Successful Treatment Program

- A minimal amount of dietary discretion is required
- The earlier the treatment, the better
- The chance of good glucose control on one oral medication (monotherapy) in part depends on how long the diabetes has been present
- When one oral medication alone is not controlling the blood glucose level, addition (not substitution) of another oral agent is the rule rather than the exception
- Consider the addition of bedtime insulin to your regimen if the fasting or prebreakfast glucose value remains excessively high on the oral agent(s)
- Do not hesitate, or wait too long, to switch to an insulin regimen if the oral medication(s) is not controlling your blood glucose level. Insulin is a natural hormone and the needle is nothing to fear

SFUs were the only oral medications available in the United States and incretin hormones were not yet developed; however, this type of combination should work with any of the oral agents on the market today as well as with Byetta.

This combination therapy is effective in many individuals because the evening insulin works mainly during the night and early morning to improve the fasting or prebreakfast glucose level to normal. When you start off the day with a good blood sugar value, the daytime medications work much better to control the blood glucose value during waking hours.

There are a number of practical reasons why combination therapy can be beneficial. You do not need to learn how to mix different types of insulin, and it is more desirable to be on a single injection of insulin rather than a multiple-injection regimen. In addition, you do not have to carry the insulin with you during the day since you take it only at bedtime. You can also estimate the initial dose and safely start 5 to 10 units of Lantus, Levemir, or NPH insulin if you are not overweight, or 10 to 15 units if you are overweight, at bedtime (about 10 PM ± 1 to 2 hours). Obviously, you will need to discuss the details of your regimen with your caregiver.

In either case, the dose is increased in 2- to 5-unit increments every 3 to 4 days until the fasting or prebreakfast blood glucose levels are consistently within the 80 to 130 mg/dL range. It is recommended that you remain on your current dose of oral medication(s); however, if the daytime blood glucose level starts to become excessively low, the dose(s) of the daytime medications must be adjusted downward. If this occurs, it is a good indication that combination therapy is successful. Your physician may also instruct you to make your own insulin adjustments using home glucose monitoring (**Table 6-17**). An even simpler method is to increase the dose of insulin by 2 units if the average of the previous 3 morning values was not under 120 mg/dL.

Daytime Oral Agents and Predinner Premixed Insulin

Another great clinical tool is to take a premixed insulin before dinner instead of bedtime insulin. A premixed insulin such as Humalog mix 75/25 or Novolog Mix 70/30 has 70% to 75% intermediate-acting insulin, similar to NPH, and 25% to 30% rapid-acting insulin (Humalog or Novolog). Humalog Mix 50/50 is now available as well. In this manner, the premixed insulin will help to control blood glucose immediately after dinner and help with overnight control. I usually try this regimen when the postdinner

---

Table 6-17

Instructions for Adding Bedtime Insulin to Daytime Oral Medication(s)*

- Start with a dose of __1∅__ units of NPH/Lantus/Levemir insulin given just before bedtime
- If your morning blood glucose level is higher than 130 mg/dL for more than 3 days in a row, increase the dose of bedtime NPH insulin by __3__ units
- If your morning blood glucose level is less than 80 mg/dL for 2 days in a row, decrease your bedtime NPH dose by __3__ units
- It is extremely important that you not increase your dose of insulin more frequently than every 3 days
- If you have any questions, call your caregiver who prescribed this regimen.

* This type of regimen must be prescribed by your caregiver. Do not change or start therapy on your own.

and morning blood glucose levels are both consistently too high (**Table 6-18**).

When the fasting blood glucose in the morning is brought under control, the success of combination therapy is dependent upon the ability of the daytime medication(s) to maintain glucose control throughout the day. If this cannot be achieved, some or all of the pills should be stopped and an insulin regimen started (discussed in Chapter 7).

Treatment Algorithm

Figure 6-3 is a treatment algorithm that I developed with my good friend and colleague, Dr. Robert Henry. It was originally printed in a book written for caregivers and has been modified for this book. It is a general treatment plan designed to help guide practicing physicians, nurse practitioners, and physician assistants in making therapeutic decisions for their patients. It is important to remember that these are simply guidelines and that every patient's care must be approached on an individual basis.

Case Presentations
Case #1: Monotherapy

David is a 56-year-old business executive who was told he had "a touch of diabetes" during a yearly routine physical. David felt good and had no symptoms of diabetes such as excessive thirst or urination. His mother and one brother have type 2 diabetes and weight problems, just as David does. The only other major medical condition that David has is high blood pressure (hypertension), which is being treated with an ACE

Table 6-18

Instructions for Adding Predinner Premixed Insulin to Daytime Oral Medication(s)*

- Start with a dose of __1Ø__ units of Humalog Mix 75/25, Humalog Mix 50/50, or Novolog Mix 70/30 given just before dinner
- If your morning blood glucose level is higher than 130 mg/dL for more than 3 days in a row, increase the dose of predinner Humalog Mix 75/25, Humalog Mix 50/50, or Novolog Mix 70/30 by __3__ units
- If your morning blood glucose level is less than 80 mg/dL for 2 days in a row, decrease your predinner Humalog Mix 75/25, Humalog Mix 50/50, or Novolog Mix 70/30 dose by __3__ units
- It is extremely important that you not increase your dose of insulin more frequently than every 3 days
- If you have any questions, call your caregiver who prescribed this regimen

* This type of regimen must be prescribed by your caregiver. Do not change or start therapy on your own.

Figure 6-3

Treatment Algorithm for Type 2 Diabetes

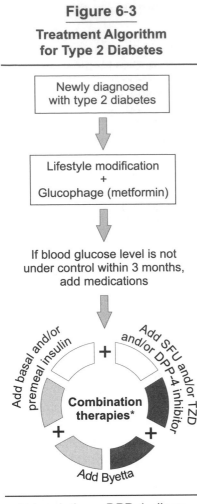

Abbreviations: DPP-4, dipeptidyl peptidase 4 [inhibitor], SFU, sulfonylurea; TZD, thiazolidinedione.

* If the combination of several oral and/or injectable medications does not control your blood glucose level, you may need a more intensive insulin regimen. See your diabetes specialist.

inhibitor (see Chapters 12 and 14). The only abnormal lab results were a fasting (first test in the morning) glucose value of 134 mg/dL and an elevated triglyceride level of 247 mg/dL. His A1C was 7.4% (normal 4% to 6%). According to the most recent American Diabetes Association recommendations, David was started immediately on Glucophage as well as lifestyle modifications.

Discussion—David was lucky to have his diabetes diagnosed early before his condition deteriorated to the point of having symptoms. The early diagnosis increases the chance that his diabetes can be controlled with diet and exercise alone and/or with only one medication. David now needs to be educated about diabetes (he should already have been knowledgeable since both his mother and his brother have the same kind of diabetes), as well as getting on a realistic diet and exercise regimen that he can follow. He should also be educated in home glucose monitoring periodically before breakfast and after a large meal. If after 3 months his blood glucose value is not in the desired range (premeal level below 120 mg/dL and postmeal value below 160 mg/dL), starting a second oral medication or Byetta is indicated. Byetta would be a good choice because of the weight loss that occurs with this incretin hormone in addition to glucose control. TZDs such as Avandia or Actos and a DPP-4 inhibitor such as Januvia would also be appropriate choices.

The choice of the medication should depend on David and his caregiver's preferences. Some factors that should go into the decision of which drug to choose are the presence of liver or kidney dysfunction, abnormal cholesterol levels, and obesity. In this particular situation, I would be cautious with an SFU, because David already has a weight problem and I do not want to expose him to the risk of hypoglycemia or low blood glucose. I agree with the choice of an ACE inhibitor for his blood pressure, and would suggest that David get a home blood pressure measuring device. His cholesterol levels should be checked after his blood glucose value has improved. Sometimes, this is all that is needed to control the cholesterol levels; however, a cholesterol-lowering medication is often needed to aggressively lower the values to normal.

Case #2: Combination Therapy

Mary is a 64-year-old obese (220 pounds) woman who has had type 2 diabetes for the past 14 years. She has been treated with an SFU for the past 10 years. Her glucose control for the past 3 or 4 years has not been good. Her most recent A1C is over 9.5% (normal range is 4% to 6%, with a goal of 7% or less). In addition, both her premeal and postmeal glucose values are excessively high (above 200 mg/dL). She is afraid of "the needle" and does not want to start insulin. In addition, Mary was recently diagnosed with early diabetic eye disease (retinopathy) and nerve disease (neuropathy).

Discussion—Unfortunately, Mary's story is a common one. The SFU has lost its effectiveness over time and her blood glucose has been excessively high for years. As a result, she is developing the classic complications of diabetes. She has several different therapeutic options at this point in time because of the availability of the newer oral medications. Even though Mary's glucose value is not under control, the SFU is probably working to some degree to keep her blood glucose from really going through the roof. This is why I would now add a second oral medication to her regimen. The choice of the second medication could be Glucophage, Avandia or Actos, Glyset, Precose, or Januvia. Once again, the choice would depend on the many different variables that go into making a decision as mentioned in Case #1 and outlined in **Table 6-10**. Byetta would also be an excellent option because of her need to improve her glucose control and to lose weight. The only two that I would not use are Starlix and Prandin since the SFUs that she is already taking work in a similar fashion.

Other options for Mary include adding an injection of Lantus, Levemir, or NPH insulin at night or adding an injection of Humalog Mix 75/25, Humalog Mix 50/50, or Novolog Mix 70/30 before dinner. Stopping the SFU and going to a full insulin regimen is a viable and effective option.

Case #3: Oral Medications

Mike is a 52-year-old very obese (270 pounds) male with the diagnosis of type 2 diabetes for the past 12 years. Seven years ago, he was taken off of SFUs and started on a full insulin regimen because of poor glucose control. Mike is now taking 55 units of premixed insulin twice a day, before breakfast and dinner. His A1C is 11%. He is frustrated with his diabetes control and his weight problem.

Discussion—Mike's exasperating situation is also very common. There are many people with insulin-requiring type 2 diabetes with inadequate control despite being on large doses of insulin (over 100 units per day). In this scenario, I would recommend adding an oral agent to his insulin regimen, with the main goal being to reduce his A1C and blood glucose value. One choice would be an insulin sensitizer such as Avandia or Actos, since these drugs work to lower insulin resistance and will allow the insulin that is present to do its job better. However, caution must be used when using TZDs and insulin together. Glucophage and a DPP-4 inhibitor would also be beneficial in this situation. Symlin is also a consideration (discussed in Chapter 7). Don't forget that he may also need a higher dose of insulin. Your choice will be determined by the variables listed in **Table 6-15**.

When the blood glucose value starts to fall after an oral medication is added, you will need to eventually lower your insulin dose by 20% to 25% if your premeal level is consistently below 120 mg/dL and/or your postmeal level drops well below 140 mg/dL. Do not make these changes on your own.

Summary

There are now six different classes of oral medications and a new category of important hormones called incretins for the treatment of type 2 diabetes. All people with type 2 diabetes should be knowledgeable about the old and new diabetes medications now available. Whether you are newly diagnosed and only on a diet and exercise program or have had diabetes for a long time and are now taking insulin, you may be a good candidate for a newer oral medication and/or Byetta now or in the near future. Each medication has it benefits and shortfalls and there are many different variables that should determine the best one for your situation.

Early diagnosis and aggressive treatment are important for long-term success. In addition, when one oral agent is not effective in controlling your blood glucose, addition and not substitution of another medication is the rule rather than the exception. The addition of evening insulin to daytime medication(s) is an easy and valuable tool for achieving glucose control in certain individuals, and there should be no delay in proceeding to a full insulin regimen when the oral medications alone cannot control the glucose levels.

There is no one perfect treatment plan for everybody. You need to work with your doctor to design the best regimen that fits your needs and your lifestyle. Having a good knowledge base regarding the available medications is crucial for you to take control of your diabetes.

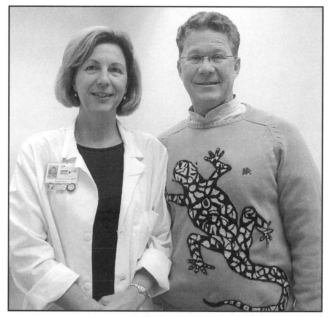

Steven Edelman displays his Gila Monster Pride by wearing a sweater that was created for him by his mother-in-law. He poses here with his wife, Ingrid.

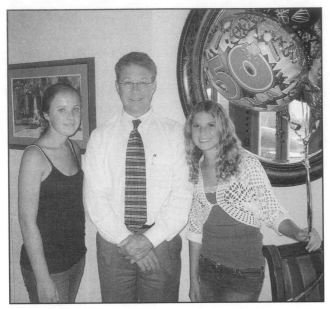

My daughters, Talia and Carina, try to cheer me up on my 50th!

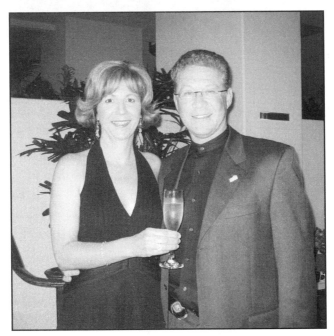

My wife, Ingrid, turns 50.

7

Insulin Therapy Must Be Custom Fit for You

Newer Designer Insulins, Inhaled Insulin, and Symlin

Introduction

Every single person you know uses insulin, whether it comes from their own pancreas, from an injection, or from an inhalation. Insulin therapy needs to be individualized to custom-fit the lifestyle of each and every individual who uses insulin to control their diabetes. It is unrealistic to drastically change lifelong daily habits to conform to a rigid and inflexible insulin regimen. Most medical textbooks usually discuss only two or three of the most commonly used insulin regimens, and this is what most physicians prescribe for their patients. However, there are many ways to design an insulin regimen that will successfully control your blood glucose throughout the day without disrupting your lifestyle. The information in this chapter will help you design or modify your insulin regimen, working with your caregiver, to better fit your personal needs and daily habits.

Important General Considerations

The sophistication of the normal human pancreas, including the way it keeps the glucose level in the normal range throughout the day, is incredible. The pancreas of a nondiabetic individual can detect minute changes in blood glucose on a second-to-second basis and respond immediately. This is why a nondiabetic person will have a blood glucose level between 70 and 100 mg/dL at all times no matter if he/she eats five hot fudge sundaes in a 2-hour period or fasts for 48 hours. It is no wonder that blood glucose levels bounce around all over the place in diabetics who must take insulin, even when we try to do "all the right things" at correct times. I like to compare our current state-of-the-art insulin injection regimens with the normal physiologic state as an old slide ruler is to the computer on the NASA space shuttle. We are trying to replace the intricate function of the normal pancreas with a few injections or inhalations of insulin per day. In addition, the way we give insulin to ourselves is very nonphysiologic and contributes to the wide swings in blood glucose levels that commonly occur on a daily basis.

When we give ourselves insulin, it is injected into the subcutaneous tissue, which is the layer of fat just below the skin. The insulin then has to travel through this fatty tissue in order to be absorbed into the bloodstream and this can take a very long time. The insulin that is released from a normally functioning pancreas of a nondiabetic individual goes directly into the bloodstream (intravenous), and that is why it works within seconds to minutes. It is imperative that one be familiar with the pharmacokinetics (time course of action) of the various types of insulin.

The time course of action (pharmacokinetics) of the various types of insulin is listed in **Table 7-1** and shown graphically in **Figure 7-1**. It is important to know when a particular insulin starts to work, has its peak action, and how long it stays in your system. This information is not only needed to design an individualized insulin regimen, but it is also crucial to determine the best times to perform home glucose monitoring. In addition, it is important to know the time course of action of the insulin you are taking to help avoid hypoglycemia or low blood glucose, especially during exercise. The last important issue is that the time course of action of the various insulins can vary from person to person and from day to day in the same person. It has been estimated that the variation in response to injected insulin on a day-to-day basis can account for up to 50% of the variability in glucose readings throughout the day.

The Different Types of Insulin
The New Rapid-Acting Insulin Analogues

It is my strong belief that in addition to the availability of home glucose monitoring, the new rapid-acting insulin analogues are one of the more important advances in diabetes therapy since the discovery of insulin in the 1920s. There are currently three rapid-acting analogues available: Apidra (glulisine), Humalog (lispro), and Novolog (aspart).

As mentioned earlier, the route of delivery of injected insulin is different from the route of delivery of insulin by the pancreas in the nondiabetic individual and, as a result, injected insulin works slowly. The older Regular insulin, when given subcutaneously, peaks much later than the actual peaking of glucose in your blood after meals, leading to wide swings in the blood glucose values throughout the day. In other words, there is not enough insulin around when you need it (just after meals) and too much insulin around later when you do not need it (3 to 6 hours after eating). The new rapid-acting insulin analogues have one structural change on the insulin molecule (for you chemists out there... an amino acid substitution). This change allows the insulin analogue to be absorbed much more quickly into the bloodstream compared with the older Regular insulin. The end result is a much better match between the peak action of insulin and the peak rise in blood glucose after eating (**Figure 7-1**). When the peak action of insulin better coincides with the absorption of food, not

Table 7-1
Time Course of Action of Insulin Preparations*

Insulin Preparation	Starts to Work	Peak Effect	Stays in Your System
Mealtime Insulins			
Short-Acting			
Regular	30 min	2-3 hr	6-8 hr
Rapid-Acting			
Apidra (glulisine)† Humalog (lispro)† Novolog (aspart)†	Minutes	1-3 hr	3-5 hr
Basal Insulins			
Intermediate-Acting			
NPH (isophane)	2-3 hr	6-8 hr	16-20 hr
Long-Acting			
Lantus (glargine)†	1-2 hr	Peakless	24 hr
Levemir (detemir)†	0.8-2 hr	Relatively flat	Up to 24 hr
Biphasic Insulin: Fixed Mixtures‡			
Humalog Mix 75/25, 50/50† 75% (50%) lispro suspension/ 25% (50%) lispro injection	Minutes	2 peaks: ~1 hr and 6-8 hr	16-20 hr
Humulin 70/30, 50/50 70% (50%) human insulin sus-pension/30% (50%) human insulin injection	30 min	2 peaks: 2-3 hr and 6-8 hr	16-20 hr
Novolin 70/30 70% NPH suspension/ 30% regular insulin injection	0.5 hr	2 peaks: 2 hr and 12 hr	Up to 24 hr
Novolog Mix 70/30† 70% aspart suspension/ 30% aspart injection	10-20 min	2 peaks: 1 hr and 4 hr	Up to 24 hr

Abbreviation: NPH, neutral protamine Hagedorn [insulin].

* This table summarizes the typical time course of action (pharmacokinetics) of various insulin preparations. Values are highly variable among individuals, depending on the site and depth of injection, local tissue blood flow, skin temperature, and exercise.

† The insulin analogues more closely mimic insulin secretion in a person without diabetes, therefore they are more effective. Peak and duration of action depends on dose.

‡ Mixtures of short- and intermediate-acting insulins.

Figure 7-1

Peak Action of Insulin Compared With Peak Rise in Glucose After Eating

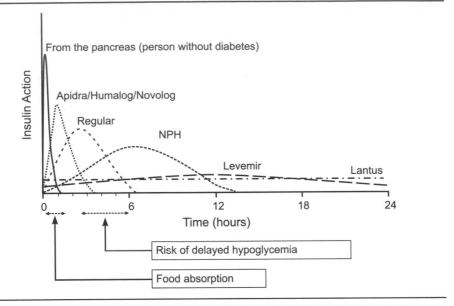

The time course of action (pharmacokinetics) for the rapid-acting insulin analogues (Apidra [glulisine], Humalog [lispro], Novolog [aspart]) is not as fast as insulin from the pancreas of a individual that does not have diabetes, but it is much more physiologic than the older Regular insulin preparation. Also shown is the time course of action of the intermediate-acting insulin (NPH [isophane]) and long-acting insulins Lantus (glargine) and Levemir (determir). Peak and duration of action depends on dose.

only are the postmeal blood glucose values lower, there is also a significant reduction in the incidence of delayed hypoglycemia. The older Regular insulin peaks long after the food is absorbed, when you are not eating anymore or when you may be exercising. Some tips for using rapid-acting insulin analogues are listed in **Table 7-2**. I do not prescribe the older Regular insulin anymore because of the benefits of rapid-acting insulin analogues. If you are on the older Regular insulin and doing fine (no problems with frequent hypoglycemic reactions, elevated glucose levels after eating, or wide swings in your values), there is no need to change. We do not have to fix what is not broken!

Long-Acting Basal Insulin Analogues

Lantus (insulin glargine) was the first long-acting peakless basal insulin analogue. By altering the structure (changing the amino acid sequences),

Lantus lasts for 24 hours without a peak. A true basal insulin ideally should not have a dramatic peak (**Figure 7-1**). Peaking of insulin should be under your control when you are able to eat or purposefully treat a high blood glucose level as with Apidra, Humalog, or Novolog. Lantus is an excellent alternative for people with diabetes who require or can benefit from a steady basal level of insulin in a very similar fashion to the basal rate of an insulin pump described in Chapter 8.

Levemir (detemir) is the newest long-acting basal insulin analogue. Levemir is made to last a long time because it is bound to albumin, a protein in our bodies that also hangs around for a long time. Levemir has been studied in people with both

Table 7-2

Tips for Using Rapid-Acting Insulin Analogues

- Take your dose about 5 minutes before your meal, unless your glucose value is excessively high
- You may need a small dose of insulin for every snack. This may not have been necessary with the older Regular insulin because it hung around in your system for 4 to 6 hours
- Make sure you have an adequate long-acting insulin dosing schedule to cover you between widely spaced meals and during the night, when the rapid-acting insulin will have left your system
- It is convenient and wise to use an insulin pen and carry it with you at all times

type 1 and insulin-requiring type 2 diabetes who require basal insulin with or without the use of rapid-acting insulin analogues (**Figure 7-1**).

The use of Lantus and Levemir has also led to a lower incidence of hypoglycemia or low blood glucose in the night, which is a great advantage to these long-acting basal insulins. Lantus and Levemir both have a more predictable time course of action compared with older basal insulins, leading to reduced unpredictable swings in blood glucose levels on a day-to-day basis. Because of their chemical properties, it is not recommended that Lantus or Levemir be mixed with other types of insulin. They must be taken alone in a syringe or via a Lantus or Levemir insulin pen. Lantus or Levemir at night or twice a day and a rapid-acting analogue at mealtimes is the "poor man's" insulin pump!

The role of a basal insulin is to keep your blood glucose in the near-normal range in between meals and overnight. If your dose of basal insulin is correct, your numbers will not drift upward or downward when you are fasting, and your blood glucose upon awakening will be normal. In fact, this is how you can test to see if your basal rate is adjusted appropriately. To test how your basal rate is working during the daytime, fast most of the day and test your glucose level every 2 hours or so. If it is hard to fast, then have an early breakfast, skip lunch, and have a late dinner, testing every few hours to see how stable your numbers are. To test how your basal

133

dose is working overnight, eat an early dinner and test your glucose level at bedtime, at 3 AM, and again upon awakening. Better yet, the use of a continuous glucose monitoring (CGM) device would be ideal to see how your basal rate is working as they measure glucose values every 5 minutes throughout the night and day (see Chapter 9). In normal individuals, the pancreas secretes a little amount of insulin all of the time, even if the person is not eating a thing all day and night. We try to mimic that normal physiologic insulin secretion with a basal insulin or an insulin pump.

Inhaled Insulin

Injectable insulin users know the challenge of injecting themselves with needles several times a day and there are many non–insulin-using folks with type 2 diabetes who are in bad control and avoiding insulin injections. Now there is another option to replace mealtime or "bolus" injectable insulin. Pulmonary inhaled insulins are currently being developed for both children and adults with type 1 diabetes and type 2 diabetes. The companies involved include Pfizer, Lilly, Novo Nordisk, and MannKind. On January 27, 2006, the Food and Drug Administration (FDA) approved the first-ever inhaled form of insulin for adults. The insulin is called Exubera and is manufactured by Pfizer. Exubera uses a novel insulin delivery inhaler developed by Nektar Therapeutics, a biotechnology company in San Carlos, California. Exubera was studied in (and is officially FDA approved for) people with type 1 diabetes and those with type 2 diabetes who are using lifestyle modification alone, oral medications, or insulin therapy. It is not yet approved for use in children. The time course of action of Exubera is very similar to rapid-acting insulin analogues such as Apidra, Humalog, and Novolog, however, the route of administration is obviously quite different. The inhaler when collapsed is the size of a small flashlight and fits easily in a pocket or purse.

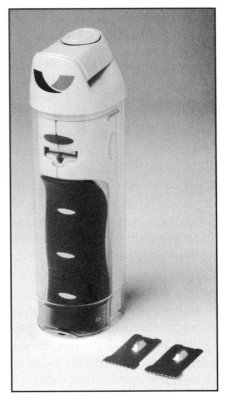

The Exubera device delivers insulin human (rDNA origin) inhalation powder.

Photo courtesy of Pfizer, Inc.

Exubera is an insulin powder that is inhaled through the mouth. The powder is stored in small "blister" doses wrapped in individual foil packets. Unlike injected insulin that is measured in units, the inhalable insulin powder is measured in milligrams (mg). The blisters of insulin are available in 1-mg and 3-mg packages. A 1-mg blister is approximately equal to 3 units of subcutaneously injected rapid-acting insulin, and a 3-mg blister is approximately equal to 8 units of insulin. The blister packets of insulin do not need to be kept in a refrigerator. People with diabetes and their health care providers will need to determine their appropriate dose requirements. If you have type 1 diabetes, you will need to continue to use a basal insulin such as Lantus or Levemir. If you have type 2 diabetes, you may or may not need a basal insulin. For example, in one of the clinical studies conducted with Exubera, patients with type 2 diabetes on oral medications alone and very poor control (A1C above 10%), were simply given Exubera with every meal and no basal insulin. The results were quite striking in that the A1C dropped about 2%, which is a very large drop compared with most other clinical study testing of diabetes drugs. In fact, many diabetes experts feel this may be the group of people in whom inhaled insulin will make the biggest impact, because many type 2 diabetics are hesitant to take insulin injections when their oral medications cannot control their diabetes.

What about the safety issues? People with diabetes have been taking inhaled insulin in clinical trials for over 7 years and there have been no serious adverse events. If you are an active smoker or have moderately severe asthma or other lung conditions, such as chronic obstructive pulmonary disease (COPD), you are not a good candidate for inhaled insulin. All candidates for inhaled insulin need to get a test of their lungs called a PFT (pulmonary function test) before starting Exubera, again after 6 months of therapy, and then once a year to make sure there is no change in lung function. A PFT is an easy and quick test in which you breathe deeply in and out into a mouthpiece hooked up to a machine that measures certain parameters. We then compare your values with the values obtained from healthy individuals. If you want to learn more about Exubera, please call 1-800-EXUBERA or visit *www.exubera.com*. It is great that we have so many choices now!

Symlin: Another Important Hormone That Partners With Insulin

At one time, insulin was thought of as the only important hormone from the pancreas that helped to control the blood glucose levels throughout the day. Well, in 1987, another hormone called amylin was discovered that came from the exact same cells in the pancreas that produced, stored, and secreted insulin. Hence, the San Diego–based company called Amylin was created by visionary Ted Greene, and what followed was a challenging 18-

year scientific trek to understand the relationship of this natural partner hormone to insulin and its role in the management of diabetes. The scientists at Amylin produced an analogue of amylin called pramlintide (sort of like Humalog is an analogue of regular insulin) and the marketing name is called Symlin. Symlin is currently approved by the FDA for people with type 1 diabetes and type 2 diabetes who use "meal-time" insulin and have not achieved glycemic control.

To make a long story short, amylin was discovered to have at least three main important functions in healthy nondiabetic humans to keep the blood glucose level in a very narrow and normal range after meals and throughout the day. When amylin is released from the pancreas at mealtimes along with insulin, its three main functions are:

1. To induce satiety (the feeling of being satisfied), reduce the appetite, and help to limit or stop overeating. (Every study to date has demonstrated significant weight loss with Symlin.)

2. To prevent the release of glucagon (another hormone from the pancreas), which is a good thing because glucagon raises blood glucose.

3. To control how fast the stomach propels food down the gastrointestinal track, limiting the rise in glucose levels after eating.

All three of these mechanisms work primarily to control how high blood glucose rises after meals (postmeal or postprandial glucose levels). Symlin has the same mechanism of action as the naturally-secreted pancreatic amylin. **Figure 7-2** shows blood glucose levels in people with type 1 and insulin-using type 2 diabetes who were on insulin alone or on both insulin and Symlin at mealtimes. As you can see, the fasting values (before breakfast) are reduced; however, the big difference is the flattening of the postmeal glucose values and the daily glucose fluctuations. In the clinical studies, many of these people lost weight compared with those who were not on Symlin, and they used less insulin to achieve the better glucose values. **Table 7-3** lists the benefits of using Symlin, and I put them in my order of importance.

Because Symlin can effectively act to reduce the amount of food ingested and the dose of insulin needed, it is important to follow the titration schedule suggested when initiating Symlin (**Figure 7-3**). In the early clinical studies, insulin was not reduced, which caused a high rate of hypoglycemia. Reducing the dose of insulin when starting Symlin has helped address this problem. The dose of premeal insulin (Apidra, Humalog, Novolog, Regular, inhaled and premixed insulins) should be reduced by about 50% in order to prevent hypoglycemia or low blood glucose. The reduction may be excessive and the dose of insulin may need

Figure 7-2

Symlin Reduces Glucose Fluctuations in Type 1 and Type 2 Diabetes

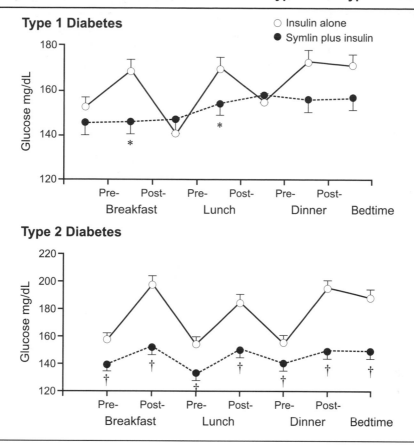

Clinical practice study of Symlin (pramlintide) 60 to 120 micrograms (mcg) before meals.

* Number in study = 265; *P* value <0.5.
† Number in study = 166; *P* value = 0.05.

Data on file at Amylin Pharmaceuticals, Inc.

to be adjusted upward according to your home or continuous glucose monitoring results.

Nausea is a side effect when initiating Symlin therapy. This is why the titration schedule shown in **Figure 7-3** starts off with a low dose and is gradually increased over time. It turns out that people with type 1 diabetes are more sensitive to Symlin in terms of nausea so the titration is slower and final dose is lower compared with those in people with type 2 diabetes. For more information please visit *www.symlin.com*. Symlin is injected at mealtime with an insulin syringe; however, a Symlin Pen should be available soon.

I have been on Symlin for over 6 years now and would not leave home without it! When I was conducting clinical studies of Symlin years ago, I was hearing positive things from the participants so I decided to try it as well. In a nutshell, it has helped me control my daily fluctuations of glucose levels and really flatten out my postmeal glucose value. I dropped 14 pounds and have kept it off and my A1C improved. My dose of rapid-acting insulin has been reduced by about 30% and after the initial adjustment period, my incidence of mild hypoglycemic reactions has diminished. Now that I have a CGM, I can really appreciate how well Symlin works to control my glucose level after meals and throughout the day.

I have personally collected a list of a few tips for successful Symlin use:

Table 7-3

Benefits of Symlin in People With Type 1 and Insulin-Using Type 2 Diabetes

1. Reduction of the frustrating daily fluctuations in blood glucose throughout the day
2. Flattening out or significant reduction of the postmeal glucose level
3. Reduction of the fasting glucose level (first thing in the morning before breakfast)
4. Lowering the A1C level
5. Help in controlling your appetite and feelings of hunger which leads to weight loss while controlling your glucose level at the same time
6. Reduction of the amount of insulin needed (especially the premeal rapid-acting insulin dose)

1. Take your dose of Symlin at the beginning of the main part of your meal.
2. Consider taking your dose of rapid-acting insulin near the end of the meal when you have seen exactly how much you have eaten.
3. If on an insulin pump, give your bolus over 2 hours (extended-wave bolus).
4. If you have not experienced the satiety and appetite effect, discuss increasing your dose of Symlin past the current recommended dose with your caregiver.

When a company such as Amylin conducts a study and presents the results to the FDA, the final recommended dose must be the dose that was used in those studies. It is not uncommon to discover better ways to use a drug once it is released for public use. Always check with your caregiver when making dose adjustments of any medication.

Although Symlin leads to weight loss, it is not officially approved by the FDA as a medication for weight control at the current time. Clinical

Figure 7-3

Initiation and Titration Schedule for Symlin (pramlintide)

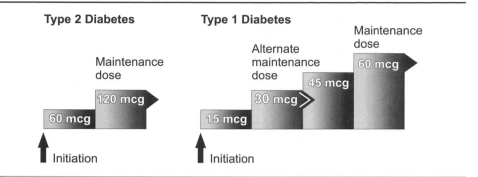

- ▪ Symlin (pramlintide) should be administered immediately before major meals or snacks
- ▪ It is recommended that mealtime insulin dose be initially reduced by 50% upon initiation of Symlin
- ▪ Symlin should be initiated at a dose of 60 micrograms (mcg) (10 units) in patients with type 2 diabetes and 15 mcg (2.5 units) in patients with type 1 diabetes
- ▪ The dose of Symlin should be increased every 3 to 7 days (as tolerated, based on nausea) until the maintenance dose is reached. Patients with type 2 diabetes require one Symlin dose titration to reach a maintenance dose of 120 mcg with major meals. Patients with type 1 diabetes require three Symlin dose titrations (in 15-mcg increments) to reach a maintenance dose of 60 mcg with major meals.
- ▪ If nausea occurs and persists at a given dose, Symlin should be reduced to the previous dose
- ▪ Once a maintenance dose of Symlin is reached, insulin adjustments should be made, based on the individual patient's self-monitoring of blood gucose and treatment goals

Symlin (pramlintide) prescribing information, 2005.

studies are currently under way to see if Symlin can be helpful as a weight loss agent in overweight people with or without diabetes.

How to "Catch Up": Insulin Algorithms, Sliding Scales, and Correction Factors

It doesn't make any sense to give the same amount of Regular or fact-acting insulin every day before every meal, no matter if the blood glucose is 80 or 350 mg/dL. It always boggles my mind to hear my patients tell me that their blood glucose was high before a meal and that they did not take any extra rapid-acting insulin to help compensate for it. Insulin algorithms, sliding scales, and correction factors are phrases to describe different methods to correct for a high glucose level between meals and at mealtimes. They are an important part of achieving glucose control on a day-to-day basis, in addition to helping make decisions about long-term adjustments. It turns out that all three terms are variations on the same theme. The problem is that many caregivers and patients may not know how to design or utilize a proper algorithm, sliding scale, or correction factor. As a result, these valuable tools are not widely used, and their use is sometimes inappropriately discouraged.

An example of an insulin algorithm or sliding scale is shown in **Figure 7-4**. As you can see, once the glucose value goes above 150 mg/dL, the dose of insulin increases one unit for every 50 mg/dL. This would also be called a correction factor of 1:50—one unit of rapid-acting insulin should be added to the total dose of rapid-acting insulin to be given for every 50 mg/dL above 150 mg/dL measured. Everyone needs to figure out what his or her correction factor is by lots of pre- and posttesting. For example, if you had breakfast at 7 AM and at 10 AM your glucose value is 276 mg/dL (damn pancakes will do it to you every time) and you would like to be close to 150 mg/dL at lunchtime in a few hours. If your correction factor is 1:50, you would take 2 to 3 units of rapid-acting insulin at 10 AM (276

Figure 7-4

Sample Algorithm of Case Presentation for "Sandy"

Name: Sandy   Date: December 15, 2006

Provider: Dr. Edelman   Phone: 858-552-8585

Time between injection and meal (minutes)	Blood glucose value (mg/dL)	Breakfast	Lunch	Dinner	Bedtime	Bedtime snack size
Humalog						
0	< 80	5	3	7	0	large
5	81 to 150	6	4	8	0	medium
5 to 15	151 to 200	7	5	9	0	small
15 to 30	201 to 250	8	6	10	3	none
30	251 to 300	9	7	11	4	none
30+	301 to 350	10	8	12	5	none
30+	351 to 400	11	9	13	6	none
30+	401 to 450	12	11	15	7	none
30+	451+	13	13	17	5	none

AM long-acting insulin dose _____

PM long-acting insulin dose 20 units Lantus   ☐ Take before dinner   ☒ Take at bedtime [current blood glucose] minus goal of 150 divided by 50 equals 2 to 3 units). You need to decide on what your goal blood glucose is and how many mg/dL your blood glucose will drop after 1 unit of rapid-acting insulin. If you are a type 1 diabetic, your correction factor will most likely be around 1:50; if you are a type 2 diabetic your correction factor may be closer to about 1:25. It is important to test before and after taking insulin to find the correct factor for you, as it is different for everyone. The dose of insulin does not matter. What does matter is your glucose value.

The 1800 rule is used if you are taking rapid-acting insulin to estimate what your correction factor may be. You take the total amount of insulin you use per day (both long- and short-acting insulin) and divide the total into 1800. For example, if you use 40 units of insulin per day (20 units of Levemir and 20 units of Novolog), an estimate of your correction factor would be 1800 divided by 40, which equals 45 or 1:45. You would then use this correction factor at meal times and between meals to correct for an elevated glucose value over what your goal is, which will be between 100 and 150 mg/dL, depending on what you and your doctor mutually decide. The 1500 rule works in the same manner if you are using the older Regular insulin instead of a rapid-acting insulin.

Figuring Out How Much Insulin You Need With Each Meal: "Guesstimating" and Carbohydrate Counting

In addition to adjusting your insulin dose according to the blood glucose level at that time using a correction factor, the amount and types of food to be eaten are important. The latest diabetic eating fashion is to count the carbohydrates and use a carbohydrate-to-insulin ratio to figure out how much rapid-acting insulin to take for the meal you are about to consume… or inhale, if you are a fast eater! A typical carbohydrate-to-insulin ratio for someone with type 1 diabetes may be 15:1 (for every 15 grams of carbohydrate consumed, 1 unit of rapid-acting insulin should be given). For example, if someone with a ratio of 15:1 is about to eat 90 grams of carbohydrate, the dose of rapid-acting insulin for that meal would be 90/15 or 6 units. This amount would be in addition to a correction dose if the pre-meal glucose level was high or above your goal range. Someone with type 2 diabetes may have a ratio of 10:1 and would take 9 units for the same meal. By pre- and postmeal testing, you can determine your appropriate ratio.

It is important to note that many people with type 1 and especially type 2 diabetes do pretty well guesstimating their dose based on past experience and trial and error. For many of us, we are creatures of habit and eat the same amounts and types of food most of the time. I suggest using an insulin algorithm based on personal experience, trying different doses with certain types and amounts of food. In a short time, with the help of premeal and postmeal home glucose monitoring, most of us will have a fairly well-defined mental "insulin menu." An insulin menu is basically how much insulin you need for a certain type of food. For example, when I eat my usual three slices of pizza, I always add an extra 8 to 10 units of my rapid-acting insulin to my usual dose in order to avoid excessively high postmeal glucose values (**Table 7-4**). In summary, it is important to figure out your dose of insulin at mealtime for the amount of food you are going to eat and correct for a high blood glucose level if you have one.

Insulin Pens

Insulin pens not only allow for an easier and more convenient way to take insulin, but they also help protect the insulin from light and heat (both of which can lead to reduced activity of the insulin). Insulin pens are used by 90% to 95% of insulin-treated patients in Europe, Asia, and Scandinavia with excellent results. Insulin pens are severely underutilized in the United States (used by only about 12% of insulin users), mainly because of ignorance by caregivers and people with diabetes. They just do not know about them and have never seen one. In addition, many health care systems do not offer them because they are slightly more expensive than using a vial and syringe.

Insulin pens are small, pen-size devices that contain a reservoir and needle for the accurate and convenient delivery of the various types of insulin (**Figure 7-5**). They are either totally disposable or reusable, replacing only the cartridge of insulin. Normally insulin pens are used for the premeal injections of rapid-acting insulin; however, insulin pens can also deliver the long-acting and premixed insulins. Don't forget that the needle of an insulin pen does not get dull because it is not shoved through the thick rubber stopper of an insulin bottle. One can unofficially use insulin needles multiple times before discarding them. I find that the injection from an insulin pen is much less painful than injecting with a syringe that I have shoved into a vial several times or than pricking my finger to test my blood glucose level.

The Role of Home or Continuous Glucose Monitoring

It is important to emphasize that there is no way to achieve glycemic control without the proper use of home or continuous glucose monitoring (CGM), no matter what type of insulin regimen you are using. Home monitoring or CGM is essential to determine how much rapid-acting insulin to give yourself before each meal and how long to wait between the injection of insulin and consumption of the meal. Glucose monitoring after meals will also help to figure out if you gave yourself too much or too little insulin. Home monitoring or CGM will also help with avoiding

Table 7-4

Example of an "Insulin Menu" Using Steve Edelman's Eating Habits

Usual Meals	Usual Humalog Dose*

Breakfast

Just coffee with milk (no food)	3 units
Bagel with cream cheese	10 units
Bowl of cold cereal with milk	12 units
Bowl of hot cereal (no milk)	7 units
Pancakes or French toast	15 units
Scrambled eggs (2) with buttered toast (1 slice)	6 units

Lunch

Tuna, turkey, or veggie sandwich	10 units
Veggie burger	12 units
Soup and salad	8 units

Dinner

My wife's usual pasta dinner	14 units
Large salad with fresh bread	10 units
Chicken, fish, or meat dinner	12 units
3 Large slices of pizza	18 units

Unusual Meals

Restaurants

Usually add 5 to 10 units to my normal dose because I always find myself eating more in a restaurant than I do at home

Desserts (Yes, I do eat desserts once in awhile!)

Small scoop of ice cream	3 units
Cookies (2 or 3)	5 to 7 units
Small piece of chocolate cake	6 to 8 units
Pudding (I love butterscotch)	4 to 5 units

* These doses are my usual normal premeal dose of Apidra, Humalog, or Novolog.

hypoglycemia, planning exercise, and making long-term adjustments in your insulin regimen (**Table 7-5**). Please see Chapters 9 and 10 to help analyze your own glucose results.

Adjusting for Exercise

If you are lucky, you can fit exercise into your daily schedule on a regular basis at the time most desirable for you. If you are like me and most other people, it is a constant battle to find any time to exercise, let alone a

Figure 7-5

Examples of Insulin Pens

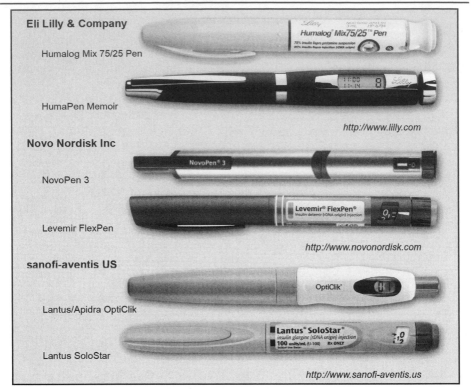

Device Name	Insulin Delivered	Consumables
Humalog Mix 75/25	Humalog (lispro)	Disposable pen (15 mL)
HumaPen Memoir	Humalog (lispro)	3-mL cartridge refill
Novo Pen 3	Novolog Mix 70/30 (aspart) Novolin 70/30 (NPH/Regular)	3-mL cartridge refill
Levemir FlexPen	Detemir (rDNA origin)	Disposable pen (3 mL)
OptiClik	Lantus (glargine) Apidra (glulisine)	3-mL cartridge refill 3-mL cartridge refill
SoloStar	Lantus (glargine)	Disposable pen

All images provided as a courtesy from Eli Lilly & Company, Novo Nordisk Inc, and sanofi-aventis US.

Table 7-5

Importance of Home Glucose Monitoring in Achieving Glycemic Control

- *Determining the premeal dose of Regular or rapid-acting insulin:* It is important to adjust the premeal dose of insulin, depending on the premeal glucose value as well as the size of the meal and anticipated exercise.

- *Timing of the insulin injection in relation to consuming the meal:* You should wait at least 30 minutes after you inject before eating if you are using the older Regular insulin and only 5 minutes if you are using the new rapid-acting analogues (Apidra, Humalog, and Novolog). This time period is appropriate only if your premeal blood glucose value is within the normal range. However, if your premeal glucose value is higher than normal, you should wait longer to give the insulin a chance to bring down your abnormally high value before you consume more calories. The timing of your insulin dose in relation to your meals is of utmost importance and is usually ignored by most patients and physicians.

- *Determining if you gave yourself too much or too little premeal insulin:* Testing your blood glucose value 1 to 2 hours after eating is important to determine whether you gave yourself too little or too much rapid-acting insulin. This postmeal testing is especially important if your premeal glucose was high or if you ate an unusual amount or type of food. If your blood glucose is too high after eating, a small extra dose of rapid-acting insulin is usually warranted. If your postmeal glucose is too low, consumption of extra calories may be appropriate to avoid a severe low blood glucose, especially if you are planning on exercising

- *Avoidance of hypoglycemia:* Home glucose monitoring is an important tool to help you avoid serious hypoglycemia. By knowing when your insulin will be peaking, you can use home glucose monitoring to detect a low blood glucose before a severe low blood glucose reaction occurs..

- *Exercise planning:* Home glucose monitoring before, after, and sometimes during prolonged exercise can give you important information for a safe and effective workout. Glucose testing before exercise is important, not only to avoid hypoglycemia but also to detect and treat severe hyperglycemia, which will definitely affect your workout. In addition, sometimes prolonged and strenuous exercise can cause delayed and severe hypoglycemia that needs to be monitored.

- *Make long-term adjustments in your insulin regimen:* Using home glucose monitoring or continuous glucose monitoring is not only important for making short-term daily adjustments in your insulin dose, it is crucial that appropriate long-term changes be made as well. For example, if the prebreakfast glucose value is consistently high, requiring the need for extra Regular or rapid-acting insulin every morning, then more evening or bedtime long-acting insulin is needed in order to avoid the morning high glucose value in the first place.

desirable time. My idea of a marathon is a swim in the Jacuzzi, a jog from the couch to the refrigerator, and a bike ride to the ice cream store (just kidding about the Jacuzzi). It is important to know how exercise affects your glucose control. Much of the information will come from pre- and postexercise home glucose monitoring or CGM and a mental diary of how certain types of exercise (including the length and degree of intensity) bring down your blood glucose level and by how much. There are no shortcuts or fancy formulas to predict how you will respond to certain types of exercise. You must test a lot and learn from experience. The best prediction of what will happen to your blood glucose is what has happened in the past during similar types of exercise. See Chapter 5 for much more on exercise.

In general, if you know you are going to exercise within 2 to 4 hours of your last dose of a rapid-acting insulin, you should reduce that premeal dose by 20% to 50%, depending on the intensity and duration of the exercise (**Table 7-6**). My usual exercise is either 45 to 60 minutes on an elliptical stepper that I have at home or on a treadmill machine at my club. I reduce my premeal rapid-acting insulin dose by approximately 25% if I exercise fairly soon after eating. You may not need to reduce your dose as much if you are using a rapid-acting insulin such as Apidra, Humalog, or Novolog, since they leave your system much more quickly than the older Regular. In order to avoid problems, it is best to exercise when your Regular or rapid-acting insulin is not peaking. If you are one of those exercise freaks who run marathons in your spare time, you obviously need to reduce your long-acting basal insulin as well by 20% to 50%.

Table 7-6

General Recommendations for Exercise and Insulin Regimens

- For anticipated mild-to-moderate exercise 1 to 3 hours after eating, reduce your premeal dose of Regular or rapid-acting insulin by approximately 20% to 50%
- For anticipated strenuous exercise over an extended period of time, not only reduce your premeal dose of Regular or rapid-acting insulin by 30% to 50%, but also reduce your long-acting insulin by 20% to 50%
- Always test your blood glucose before exercising. Consider testing your blood glucose after exercising, especially if you are developing your mental diary on how exercise affects your diabetes. Testing every 1 to 2 hours during prolonged exercise may be helpful in avoiding severe hypoglycemia
- Always carry something with you to treat a low blood glucose reaction. The day you forget will be the day you get low... Murphy's law!
- If you are a hard-core athlete, definitely join the International Diabetes Athletes Association. This nonprofit organization is also for the novice athlete

Always test your blood glucose value before and after exercising, and every 1 to 2 hours during prolonged strenuous routines. If your blood glucose is over 250 mg/dL, you should consider giving yourself a small amount of rapid-acting insulin, depending on the time of your last dose and how sensitive you are to insulin. If your last dose was within 1 or 2 hours, it might be safer to not take any extra insulin. If your blood glucose level is in the low or normal range (less than 120 mg/dL), you should consider taking in some carbohydrates before exercising. Once again, if your last injection was within 1 or 2 hours, it is more likely that your blood glucose level will become low during exercise than if your last injection was given over 5 hours prior to the activity.

Case Presentations of Commonly Used Insulin Regimens

For people with type 1 diabetes, there are two main effective regimens, which include the basal/bolus or basal/prandial regimen and insulin pump therapy, discussed in detail in Chapter 8.

The regimens most commonly used in people with type 2 diabetes are combination therapy (oral agents during the day plus a basal insulin), the split-mixed and premixed regimens, and the basal/prandial approach. I will describe an example of each one to give you an idea of what they entail.

The Basal/Bolus or Basal/Prandial Regimen

Case #1: Type 1 Diabetes

Kirk is a 45-year old man who has had type 1 diabetes for 22 years. He is a construction worker and sometimes has a problem with consistent meal times and doing regular exercise. Many years ago, he was switched from NPH twice a day to Lantus 25 units at bedtime and he is also on the rapid-acting analogue Apidra, given before meals. He learned to count his carbohydrates and his ratio is 15:1 (for every 15 grams of carbohydrates consumed he takes 1 unit of Apidra) and his correction factor is 1:50 (for every 50 mg/dL he is above his goal of 120 mg/dL, he will take an extra 1 unit of Apidra). He adjusts his Lantus dose based on his morning glucose value and his Apidra dose is based on his postmeal glucose value. He is also on Symlin 10 units with each major meal. His A1C has been in the low 7% range with 1 to 2 hypoglycemic reactions a week. He recently got a Dexcom STS continuous glucose monitor (see Chapter 9), which has allowed him to fine-tune his regimen and reduce his A1C to 6.7% in addition to almost eliminating completely his low blood glucose reactions.

The basal/prandial regimen is the most physiologic regimen, in addition to insulin pump therapy. The basic concept is to try and mimic the normal insulin secretory pattern of a nondiabetic. The pancreas of a normal nondiabetic secretes a little bit of insulin all the time (basal rate), even in the fasting state, and puts out little squirts or boluses for every meal. The normal pancreas only secretes rapid-acting insulin directly into the bloodstream, where it works almost instantaneously. Lantus, Levemir, and NPH are basal insulins that have been chemically altered to be longer acting, similar to any sustained-release medication.

Insulin Pump Therapy

Case #2: Type 1 Diabetes

Mary is a 22-year-old female with type 1 diabetes since the age of 5. She has been on insulin pump therapy using Humalog for the past several years and loves the freedom it gives her in terms of the ease of boluses and controlling her blood glucose values overnight. Her basal rate is set at 0.7 units an hour except between the hours of 3 AM to 8 AM, when it automatically goes up to 1.0 units per hour. This increase in her basal rate of insulin is to counteract the dawn phenomenon (see Chapters 8 and 9 on pump therapy and CGM for more details of pump therapy and the dawn phenomenon). Her carbohydrate-to-insulin ratio is 20:1, and her correction factor is 1:60. She is obviously more sensitive to insulin than Kirk. She also uses a CGM which helps her prevent her blood glucose level from going too low at night, especially important since she lives alone.

Combination Therapy: Oral Medications During the Day and a Basal Insulin

Case #3: Type 2 Diabetes

John is a 65-year-old Hispanic male with type 2 diabetes for 12 years. When he was first diagnosed, he was on diet and exercise alone but soon after, both glyburide and Glucophage were added to get his glucose level under control. This worked for a few years. Later, Actos was added to his regimen, which helped, but his A1C was still above goal at 7.4%. John's home glucose monitoring data showed that his fasting glucose level in the morning was in the mid 200-mg/dL range. His caregiver prescribed 10 units of long-acting basal insulin Levemir at bedtime and slowly increased the dose to 55 units over the next few weeks to get his morning blood glucose level in the 80- to 130-mg/dL range. His dose of oral medications was not changed and his A1C eventually came down to 6.5% with no episodes of hypoglycemia.

Combination therapy is an effective and efficient way to get the A1C to goal. While John and his caregiver chose Levemir for his basal insulin, the other available long-acting insulin is Lantus. There are differences between these insulins so it wise to discuss them with your caregiver. If combination therapy does not get the A1C to goal, it may be necessary to advance the insulin regimen to a split-mixed or basal/bolus strategy.

The Split-Mixed/Premixed Regimen

Case #4: Type 2 Diabetes

Brenda is a 47-year-old overweight woman who has had type 2 diabetes since the age of 39. She did not respond well to oral agents and is currently treated with 25 units of NPH and 15 units of Regular before breakfast and 20 units of NPH and 12 units of Regular units before dinner. Her overall glycemic control is poor with an A1C of 8.2%. Her home glucose monitoring records show that her blood glucose is bouncing all over the place from high (over 200 mg/dL) to low (below 60 mg/dL); however, there are two consistent trends: The trends show that her postbreakfast and postdinner blood glucose levels are too high, commonly in the 300 mg/dL range.

She is currently being treated with a split-mixed insulin regimen. This regimen consists of an injection of a combination of NPH and Regular insulin prior to breakfast and dinner. Although this regimen is used quite frequently in type 2 diabetes and much less commonly in type 1 diabetes, it may have limitations especially in type 1 diabetes, including:

1. There is no Regular or rapid-acting insulin given for lunch. Hyperglycemia is not uncommon in the early afternoon.
2. The morning NPH peaks 6 to 8 hours after injection, leading to hypoglycemia in the late afternoon, especially if the midday meal is light or is missed.
3. The NPH given before dinner usually peaks in the early morning, leading to hypoglycemia during the night (1 AM to 3 AM).
4. Since the evening NPH is given before dinner (around 6 PM to 7 PM), it loses effectiveness by the next morning, and it is not uncommon to have persistent prebreakfast hyperglycemia or high blood glucose.

Brenda's main problem was high postmeal glucose values. She was switched to the rapid-acting analogue Novolog to help improve her postbreakfast and postdinner blood glucose level. She also reduced the calorie content of her midday meal so that her postlunch blood glucose value was improved.

1. Her postmeal glucose level improved tremendously
2. She enjoyed a little more flexibility in the timing of her insulin dose since the rapid-acting insulin analogue given before or soon after the meal have the same results in glucose control.

Brenda's A1C value came down to 7.1% 5 months after making the changes. A few months later, Brenda switched to the premixed insulin,

Novolog Mix 70/30, in a pen since her ratio of NPH to Novolog was about 70/30. She loved the convenience of the pen. Her A1C drifted below 7.0% over the next 6 months.

The Basal/Bolus or Basal/Prandial Regimen

Case #5: Type 2 Diabetes

Sandy is a 50-year-old, obese woman who has had type 2 diabetes for the past 5 years. She originally was treated with a split-mixed regimen, but was changed to a basal/prandial regimen several years ago when she started to work the graveyard shift (11 PM to 7 AM) as a surgical nurse. Her daily schedule consists of going home after work and going straight to bed until 1 PM or 2 PM without eating anything. She then has a regular type of lunch consisting of a sandwich or salad. Her dinner is normally at 8 PM every night with her husband. She has breakfast at the hospital during one of her breaks between 4 AM and 6 AM, although this eating time is variable since emergency surgeries are not predictable.

Sandy's regimen has changed through the years but currently consists of 25 units of the basal insulin Levemir given at around 8 AM before she goes to sleep, with a few units of Novolog only if her glucose level is high (above 180 mg/dL). She also takes 15 units of Levemir at dinner (8 PM) along with her Novolog dose, according to her premeal blood glucose value (insulin algorithm). She gives herself small boluses (about 8 to 15 units) of Novolog before breakfast, lunch, dinner, and other small snacks. She does pretty well adjusting her dose and does not use carbohydrate counting. She loves the Novolog and Levemir Flex pens, which make her daily life with diabetes easier. One year ago, Sandy started Symlin as her postmeal value was difficult to get below 200 mg/dL and she was well over her ideal body weight. She eventually got her A1C below 7% and lost a significant amount of weight at the same time.

Sandy's regimen is a great example of a custom-fit insulin regimen. Her basal/prandial regimen was designed to fit her schedule. She has a good baseline insulin dose with the new long-acting Levemir given about 12 hours apart and the rapid-acting insulin analogue Novolog given before each meal. She has the freedom to eat her meals at any time that is convenient for her. She also has the freedom to skip meals, provided she checks her blood glucose value to make sure it is not too low or too high. A good baseline insulin dose should not allow your value to get too low or too high, even if you do not eat. If your blood glucose level gets too low in the fasting state, your long-acting insulin dose is too high and must be adjusted. On the other hand, if your glucose value goes too high in the fasting state, your long-acting insulin dose needs to be increased.

Summary

Designing an insulin regimen that fits your lifestyle is important for achieving and maintaining glycemic control (**Table** 7-7). To do this successfully, you must have a basic understanding of the time course of action of the different insulins as well as know the benefits of Symlin. You must also not only perform home glucose monitoring at the appropriate times and strongly consider CGM, but you must also be well informed on how to respond to your glucose values. The use of an insulin algorithm or correction factor is vital to make the day-to-day decisions in your treatment plan as well as making long-term adjustments. Every dose of premeal insulin must be guesstimated, keeping several facts in mind, including the premeal glucose value, amounts and types of food (carbohydrates) to be ingested, and anticipated exercise. With experience and time, you will develop mental diaries and insulin menus of how certain types of meals and exercise routines affect your diabetes. You will be able to use this information in addition to carbohydrate counting to come up with the best guesstimate of what insulin dose should be given at any particular time or in any situation. Eventually, adjusting your daily insulin regimen will be as easy and routine as brushing your teeth. You have the ability to have a flexible lifestyle while achieving excellent glycemic control on insulin. Being educated and motivated to work with your caregiver to design the perfect insulin regimen for you is the key. We now have many new insulins and Symlin to choose from, and with the advent of continuous glucose monitoring, excellent control with minimal hypoglycemia is easily possible.

Table 7-7

Insulin Regimens Commonly Utilized

Type 1 Diabetes
- Basal/bolus regimen (also called basal/prandial)
- Insulin pump therapy

Type 2 Diabetes
- Combination therapy (oral agents during the day in addition to a basal insulin)
- Premixed or free-mixed regimen (intermediate-acting and rapid-acting insulin given 2 or 3 times a day)
- Basal/bolus regimen
- Insulin pump therapy

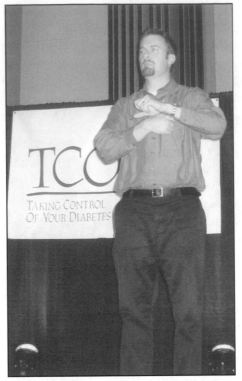

A volunteer signing for the hearing impaired at a TCOYD conference.

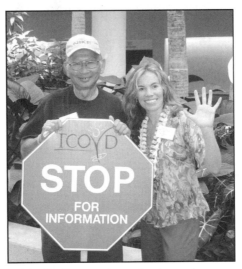

Michelle Day and a volunteer at a TCOYD conference held in Hawaii.

8

Today's Insulin Pumps With Smart Features

*by John Walsh, PA, CDE
and Ruth Roberts, MA*

Copyright © 2007, Diabetes Services, Inc.

Introduction

The number of people using insulin pumps has grown rapidly since their introduction nearly 30 years ago to well over 400,000 worldwide. Much of this growth has come from pump wearers enthusiastically sharing their experience. When used well, an insulin pump helps the wearer feel better, live more freely, and have fewer diabetes-related health problems.

The decision to go on a pump is often a turning point in diabetes care. Those who use pumps say things like, "For the first time in years, I can eat when I want to" or "I can really control my blood glucose now, and I feel better, too."

Why Consider a Pump?

Keeping the blood glucose as close to normal as possible is the primary goal in diabetes, whether using injections or a pump. Today's smart pumps have helpful features (see section *Smart Pump Features and Their Use* within this chapter) that offer the best choice for many people in reaching this goal. Many health professionals who have diabetes them-selves prefer pumps because they provide a convenient and effective way to mimic the pancreas. In 1998, when only 6% of people with type 1 diabetes were wearing a pump, 60% of diabetes nurse educators and 52% of physicians who had type 1 diabetes were on an insulin pump.

Pumps benefit people of all ages, from infants to those in their 80s and 90s. They have been shown to help people who have peripheral or autonomic neuropathy, early kidney disease (microalbuminuria), and reti-nopathy. Pumps also benefit those who have a dawn phenomenon, erratic control, or insulin resistance. The improved control possible with a pump may even reverse some health damage associated with complications.

How a Pump Works

Powered by common AA or AAA batteries, an insulin pump uses a rapid-acting insulin that is programmed for delivery as basals and

153

boluses to better mimic normal insulin delivery. Basal rates replace the background release of insulin from a normal pancreas. These can be programmed to change every 30 minutes in increments as small as 0.025 or 0.05 unit per hour to balance the increased insulin need that many people experience before dawn or the decreased insulin need during long periods of exercise or activity (**Table 8-1**). Basal rates can be temporarily increased or decreased in 5% increments over 30 minutes for up to 72 hours in most pumps as needed for illness, exercise, or other situations.

Boluses cover the carbs in meals or snacks, and can be used to lower any high readings that may occur. Once a pump is programmed with a carb factor and a correction factor by the user and health care provider, the user simply enters how many carbs will be eaten and the user's current blood glucose. Their smart pump can recommend an appropriate carb or correction bolus. Entry of the blood glucose also allows the pump to accurately reduce this bolus for any bolus onboard (BOB) or insulin still active from recent boluses.

Table 8-1
Insulin Delivery Using an Insulin Pump

Basal—a continuous 24-hour delivery that matches background insulin need. The basal is given as units per hour, ranges between 0.4 and 1.6 units per hour for most adult pumpers, and usually makes up about half of the total daily dose (TDD) of insulin.

Carb Bolus—a spurt of insulin delivered quickly to match the carbohydrates in a meal or snack. Most adult pumpers use 1 unit per 5 to 25 grams of carb.

Correction Bolus—a spurt of insulin designed to bring a high blood glucose back to target. For most adult pumpers, 1 unit lowers the blood glucose between 20 and 120 mg/dL (1 to 6.7 mmol).

Basal Insulin and Basal Rates

Basal delivery from a pump mimics nature with a steady delivery of small amounts of insulin around the clock. Basal rates are set to balance normal daily changes in counter-regulatory hormones and activity. Many teens and adults require a higher basal rate in the predawn hours to counteract a dawn phenomenon that starts about 3 AM daily. It is caused by a natural increase in growth hormone production at this time. If no extra insulin is provided, the blood glucose would rise and be high when the person awakens. As a person approaches middle age, the dawn phenomenon along with the increased need for insulin often declines or disappears entirely.

154

Accurate basal rates make the blood glucose stay level overnight or when meals are skipped during the day. When someone has their basal rates set correctly, their blood glucose will rise or fall no more than 30 mg/dL (1.7 mmol) during 8 hours of sleep or during any 5-hour period of fasting while awake.

Basal rates usually make up about 50% of the total daily dose (TDD) of insulin. Considering individual variations, effective basal rates rarely fall below 40% and only occasionally rise above 60% of the TDD. Carb boluses make up most of the remainder, with a small percentage of the TDD, usually less than 8%, used for correction boluses.

Pumps offer temporary basal rates and alternate basal profiles. Temporary rates can be increased to handle occasional illnesses or decreased during and after long periods of exercise or activity. A user can also switch between alternate basal profiles if insulin requirements differ on weekends versus weekdays, or during menses for women. Some pumps now offer a weekly schedule that allows unique basal profiles and missed-meal bolus alerts to be set up and started automatically on different days of the week. This can be especially helpful for those whose activities vary from day to day.

Boluses

Boluses are short spurts of insulin given to cover carbs or correct high blood glucose levels. Unlike basal rates, boluses are not programmed ahead of time but are given when they are needed.

Carb Boluses

The amount of carbohydrate in a snack or meal determines the size of the carb bolus required to cover it. The more carbs, the larger a bolus will need to be, so accurate carb counting or a very consistent diet is critical for accurate insulin dosing.

A personal carb factor is used to determine the size of the bolus that is needed for each meal and snack. A carb factor is an insulin-to-carb ratio worked out by the user and health care provider. It is how many grams of carb 1 unit of insulin will cover for an individual pumper. Like the basal rates, the carb factor can be adjusted as needed to improve control, and different carb factors can be entered for different times of the day if needed. A smart pump divides the total carbs in a meal or snack by the carb factor to determine an accurate carb bolus for each meal and snack.

Boluses from a pump are not delivered directly into the blood like the insulin delivery from a pancreas. Instead, the pump infuses insulin into fat below the skin, from where it is gradually absorbed into the bloodstream. This delay in uptake means that carb boluses have to be given well before a meal begins to have their best effect. Although a meal bolus given right before eating may occasionally provide reasonable control, whenever possible boluses are given at least 15 to 20 minutes before eating to get the best postmeal blood glucose level possible, except, of course, when the blood glucose is low at the beginning of the meal. When carbs are accurately counted and matched with a premeal bolus using an accurate carb factor, the glucose will rise no more than 40 to 80 mg/dL (2.2 to 4.4 mmol) and return to the target range 4 to 5 hours later.

Correction Boluses

The normal pancreas and counter-regulatory system work so well that a healthy person has no high or low blood glucose, but insulin delivery as basals and boluses from a pump cannot be as effective. A high blood glucose can occur whenever too little insulin is given for basal or bolus coverage, although other causes may contribute. When a high blood glucose occurs, a correction bolus is given to bring it down safely. The higher the blood glucose, the more bolus insulin is needed to bring it down.

The correction factor indicates how far the blood glucose will fall per unit of insulin. It is used to determine how much bolus insulin to take to bring a high reading down to target without going too low. Once the correction factor is programmed into a pump, correction boluses will be automatically calculated, with reductions made as needed for any active BOB (**Table 8-2**).

Keep in mind that a pump must be thoroughly checked if a high blood glucose is unusual or unexplained. When infusion site or mechanical problems occur, a correction dose must be given by syringe or insulin pen to ensure

Table 8-2

Today's Smart Pumps Excel at Control

- Precise insulin delivery allows most pumpers to achieve blood glucose within an acceptable target range most of the time. If you use a smart pump and your blood glucose often goes too high or too low, your basal rates, carb factor, correction factor, or duration of insulin action can be changed to better fit your needs
- Never accept having a high A1C or experiencing erratic control if you use a smart pump. A smart pump should deliver excellent overall results. If it does not, modify your lifestyle or tweak your insulin settings until it does

delivery. Take action to lower the blood glucose before getting involved in troubleshooting the pump.

Testing and setting basal rates, carb factor, and correction factor should be completed within 4 to 6 weeks after a pump start. Once blood glucose is well controlled, occasional adjustments will be needed as weight, activity, or seasons change, or when blood glucose control is no longer optimal.

Is a Pump Better Than Multiple Injections?

Better Insulin Delivery

Healthy beta cells in the pancreas release precise amounts of insulin to cover two basic needs: a steady background flow to orchestrate the release and uptake of glucose and fat for fuel and a burst for carbs when eaten. To mimic the normal pancreas, multiple daily injections (MDIs) or a pump provides background insulin and boluses of insulin for carb coverage. In addition, correction boluses are taken to lower a high blood glucose, a state that does not occur in a nondiabetic person.

A pump has an advantage over MDI because it uses a rapid-acting insulin to provide the basal or background infusion that the body needs around the clock to keep the blood glucose from rising when no food is eaten. Faster and more precise insulin adjustments can be made for things like a dawn phenomenon or a change in activity. The same rapid-acting insulin is delivered as a bolus or quick release of insulin when carbs are eaten. If a high blood glucose occurs, a correction bolus can lower it without needing to take an additional injection.

A pump allows the wearer to more easily tailor their insulin to life's events, such as exercise, a change in schedule, or an illness. Because the same insulin is used for both basals and boluses, these doses can be interchanged when more or less insulin is needed. For instance, when a pump is disconnected for water sports, a "disconnect" bolus can be given to replace the basal delivery that will be lost during this time. This bolus-for-basal replacement allows the blood glucose to be maintained for at least 3 to 4 hours off the pump. One pump already offers an estimate for how much bolus insulin will be needed for a selected time off the pump.

More Convenience and Flexibility

In life, work hours vary, meetings and events occur randomly, meals may be delayed or missed, and eating is often done on the run. On weekends, you may want to rise early or sleep late, and exercise more or less than usual and at different times of the day. Eating may change to accommodate larger family or holiday meals or be delayed to allow dining after a movie. As meals, activity, stress, and sleep change, so must insulin levels.

Greater Precision

Dose calculations with today's pumps are simpler and more accurate than MDIs or classic pumps. Once an appropriate carb factor and a correction factor are entered into a pump, it can recommend an accurate bolus anytime the user enters how many carbs they will eat and their current blood glucose. The pump keeps track of any BOB and adjusts carb and correction boluses to prevent insulin stacking when active bolus insulin remains from recent boluses.

The precise insulin delivery of a pump can better match the demands of an active lifestyle. Basal insulin flow is adjusted to keep the blood glucose in a normal range overnight or when meals are skipped. Basal settings that work well do not change until the wearer needs to change them, such as for longer periods of exercise or activity. Exclusive use of rapid-acting insulin allows both bolus doses and basal rates to be tailored quickly for spontaneous eating and exercise.

People who are sensitive to insulin and require small doses especially benefit from the precision of a pump. Those who need less than 30 to 35 units a day love a pump with which doses are delivered in increments as small as 0.025 (twenty-five thousandths) of a unit. If a single unit of insulin will lower the glucose by 100 mg/dL (5.6 mmol) or more, even a small miscalculation spells disaster. A pump's precision, along with carefully calculated doses that account for any BOB, can save the patient from the low readings that often plague them when using a syringe.

More Reliable Insulin Action

With injections, one or more doses of a long-acting insulin are required each day. In contrast to older long-acting insulins, newer ones like Lantus (glargine) and Levemir (detemir) display less peaking and have more consistent activity. Yet even with a more consistent insulin, variation in insulin activity will occur whenever the time of an injection varies, such as when sleeping late on a weekend, or when sweaty in hot weather when absorption of the large pool of insulin may occur faster. In contrast to the variable action of a long-acting insulin, a pump uses only rapid-acting insulin delivered in small amounts throughout the day. This reduces variable insulin delivery from as much as 25% with injections to only 3% on a pump.

Some users may find that the newer injected long-acting insulins have a greater peak in activity along with a shorter than 24-hour action time compared with other users. Many diabetes clinics find that over a third of their patients require two injections a day to offset the shorter action time seen in these individuals or to accommodate changes in the time of injection. Often the flatter action of these new long-acting insulins may not match a person's true basal insulin need, and, unlike with a pump, doses cannot be quickly adjusted to accommodate a spontaneous change in activity.

Compared with using MDIs with Lantus or Levemir, pumps provide more stable glucose readings. Basal delivery from a pump can be more easily matched to the variable background needs of those who have a dawn phenomenon, those whose waking or work hours vary, and those who engage in strenuous exercise at different times of the day. Over 75% of pumpers use more than 2 basal rates a day and most use 3, 4, or 5 daily rates to match their background insulin need. Basal rates on a pump can be programmed to adjust every 30 minutes to match the body's need at different times of the day.

Easier Problem Solving

A pump allows the effects of basal rates and boluses to be separated and tested. This helps to clarify which insulin dose is likely responsible for a control problem. Basal delivery is tested and adjusted first because this allows the blood glucose to stay flat overnight and when a meal is skipped. Then the pump user selects a carb factor that keeps the post-meal blood glucose from rising too high with a minimum of lows and highs before the next meal. If the carb count for a meal is inaccurate or the carb factor is incorrect, the blood glucose 2 hours later will show an unwanted rise or fall. Because the basal rate has already been tested, the bolus for that particular meal will likely be the problem.

If a blood glucose is high, a correction bolus should safely bring it back to a desired target range. The correction factor and bolus can be tested by whether they bring the blood glucose to the target range sometime between 4 hours, when 70% to 75% of the bolus activity has occurred, and as much as 5 to 6 hours later when that bolus activity ends.

Less Hypoglycemia With a Lower A1C

Several research studies have shown lower A1C values and less hypoglycemia with pumps versus MDIs, meaning that less time is spent in both the low and the high blood glucose ranges. As experience on a pump grows, low blood glucose generally becomes less frequent and less severe. Today's smart pumps and continuous glucose monitors are more likely to prevent hypoglycemia through use of smart features.

Prevention of lows becomes possible when reminders are set to test after boluses, bolus doses are based on a meal's carb count and the current blood glucose, and adjustments are made by the BOB. Tracking of the BOB allows a pump to determine how much additional bolus insulin is needed to lower a high reading or how many carbs will be needed to prevent an upcoming low blood glucose once a blood glucose test is done.

Less Hypoglycemia Unawareness

Hypoglycemia unawareness happens when someone's awareness of low blood glucose is reduced. This occurs after the person's internal stores of stress hormones are depleted following a series of frequent lows. Lower stress hormones cause fewer symptoms to occur. Thinking becomes severely impaired before symptoms are noticed. (See Chapter 11 for more on hypoglyemia.)

Once basal rates, carb and correction factors, and duration of insulin action are properly set, the wearer has fewer lows, as well as more time to recognize symptoms and correct a low blood glucose. Most long episodes of hypoglycemia occur during sleep. Basal rates on a pump can be precisely programmed to match small changes in insulin needed to prevent night lows.

Fewer Morning Highs

"If I wake up high, my whole day is shot!" is a typical complaint from people with diabetes. Morning highs are difficult to bring down and often require several correction boluses, less food, or more exercise throughout the day to return the blood glucose to target. A precisely timed increase in the early morning basal rate lessens glucose production by the liver, improves uptake of glucose by muscle cells, and reduces excess fat release. This allows a person with type 1 diabetes and a strong dawn phenomenon or someone with type 2 diabetes and insulin resistance to wake up with normal fasting blood glucose.

Smart Pump Features and Their Use

The newer pumps have added features that help improve glucose control compared with older classic pumps. First appearing in late 2002, these smart features include built-in math calculations that provide more accurate bolus measurements, as well as helpful alarms and reminders and comprehensive memory recall. Today's pumps simplify management of complex interactions between insulin levels, blood glucose, and carb intake. This allows users to achieve desirable glucose levels with less effort.

In addition to the benefits of accuracy, precision, and convenience, the history contained in pumps can quickly reveal how insulin is being used and identify where control problems may arise. Forgotten or skipped boluses can be quickly spotted. Basal/bolus imbalances are easy to identify. Insulin doses, blood glucoses, and carb intake can be tracked to make troubleshooting easier.

These innovations require the pump user to learn and apply rules and judge situations well to improve their control. Many pump wearers do not use all the new features. This decreases the benefits derived from today's smart pumps that simplify dose decisions and improve dose accuracy, resulting in improved A1C levels, glucose stability, and overall health. Better training is often needed to benefit from these advanced features.

Carb Factor

A personal carb factor programmed into the pump makes carb coverage easier and more accurate. One carb factor may be programmed for the entire day or different ones for specific meals of the day. When the number of carbs to be eaten is entered in the pump, it calculates the bolus needed to cover them, while compensating for any BOB (see also *Bolus Onboard*). Some pumps offer a built-in carb database that simplifies carb counting. Users can create their own list of favorite foods along with the exact carb count for them.

Carb Bolus Types

Besides standard carb boluses, there are two additional carb bolus types. One is called an extended or square-wave bolus, and the other a combination or dual-wave bolus. These are used to match carbs with a low glycemic index or combination foods that digest slowly, to cover a time of prolonged snacking and grazing, or with medications like Symlin (pramlintide) or GLP-1 inhibitors like Byetta (exenatide). These drugs slow food digestion and are extremely helpful for lowering postmeal glucose values to stabilize control. Extended and combination boluses are also helpful when digestion has been slowed by gastroparesis. For instance, a combo bolus may best match the digestion of specific foods with part of the bolus given immediately and the rest over the next 90 or 120 minutes.

Correction Factor

A personal correction factor (called insulin sensitivity factor or ISF in some pumps) programmed into the pump along with glucose targets for different times of the day makes it easier to correct high readings. When a high reading is entered in the pump, it will determine the precise bolus required to bring the blood glucose to target.

Blood Glucose Target

A personal blood glucose target or target range can be entered into the pump for each meal and at bedtime. This range is *not* the same as similar personal ranges that signify acceptable clinical goals. In contrast, the target range on a pump is the glucose the pump is attempting to achieve on a future blood glucose test, usually 3 to 5 hours later. The pump will calculate the current insulin dose based on data previously input by the user in order to aim for this target at a later time. For example, if a reading of 140 mg/dL (7.8 mmol) is desired for bedtime at 10 PM, this target should be set into the pump by 6 PM to allow time for the pump to attempt to achieve this goal.

Duration of Insulin Action

One unanticipated challenge that faces those on smart pumps is how to select a duration of insulin action (DIA or how long a bolus lowers the blood glucose) that works for them and does not cause problems. An accurate DIA helps prevent insulin stacking when boluses are given close together. Stacking occurs because insulin from previous carb and correction boluses is still active in the body. The time for your DIA must be accurate to allow BOB to properly calculate subsequent carb and correction boluses once the first bolus of the day has been given.

It takes a minimum of 4 to 6 hours for all of the insulin action from a recent bolus of rapid insulin to stop lowering the blood glucose. Insulin has little effect on the glucose for the first 15 to 20 minutes, reaches a halfway point in activity at just over 2 hours, and has the other half of activity tail off over about 5 to 6 hours or more after the bolus is given.

Today's pumps allow a wide range of times to be selected for the DIA, from 1.5 to 8 hours. This range is designed to handle faster genetically-engineered insulins that may appear in the future, as well as older Regular insulin. This range is far wider than the action time for the insulin currently used. Every pump comes with a default setting for DIA. This default setting can often be changed to a more effective and sometimes safer setting.

An appropriate DIA setting for today's insulins (Novolog [aspart], Apidra [glulisine], and Humalog [lispro]) is between 4 and 6 hours. A DIA time shorter than this will hide true bolus insulin activity.

Bolus OnBoard (BOB)

Frequent boluses are easy to give on a pump. This convenience can benefit the user by lowering the A1C and reducing glucose variability, but frequent boluses can also lead to insulin stacking. When a carb bolus is given for dinner, another for an unplanned dessert, and then a correction bolus is needed for the high reading that follows, the resulting insulin pileup can be confusing when the amount of bolus insulin remaining in the body needs to be determined. This is important because it helps you decide whether you need more insulin to cover a high, whether you need to eat more carbs to raise your blood glucose and avoid an impending low, or whether you need to cover additional carbs you are about to eat.

When a blood glucose test has been entered into the pump and a correction bolus is to be given, today's smart pumps automatically take into account bolus onboard or BOB, also known as insulin on board and active insulin. This prevents hypoglycemia caused by insulin stacking. It is especially helpful for those who live alone and those who have hypoglycemia unawareness or a history of frequent lows. Knowing the amount of BOB can prevent someone from giving too much insulin. For instance, a high bedtime reading may require no correction bolus if enough residual bolus insulin remains to bring the blood glucose down, while a blood glucose already at target at bedtime may be dangerous if excess BOB is still active.

Reminders and Alerts

Reminders and alerts on smart pumps can be customized for safety and to improve control. For instance, a postmeal reminder can be set to recheck your blood glucose 90 minutes or 2 hours after a bolus has been given. Testing at this time allows the meal bolus to be evaluated as to whether extra carbs are needed to prevent a low or a correction bolus is needed because the meal bolus was too small. This helps prevent lows and speeds correction of highs.

Reminders can also be set to ensure that boluses are given at specific times of the day. Some pumps can be set to sound an alarm if no bolus is given at the usual time, such as between 11:45 AM and 12:30 PM for lunch. If a bolus is started but not completed because a user gets distracted, a smart pump can sound an alert that the bolus was not finalized. Another reminder can be set to notify when the next infusion site change is due. Others will automatically remind the user to retest the glucose 15 or 20 minutes after a low blood glucose to ensure the treatment has corrected the low, or 90 minutes to 2 hours after a high reading to ensure a correction bolus is working. Helpful reminders like these minimize human error and improve control.

An auto-off feature can be a lifesaver for those who travel or live alone. When auto-off is activated, the pump turns itself off if one of the pump buttons has not been pressed within a certain amount of time, such as 8 or 9 hours overnight. This protects against the continuation of basal insulin delivery if the wearer becomes incapacitated due to hypoglycemia.

Alternate Basal Insulin Profiles and Weekly Schedules

Current pumps allow for different basal profiles to be entered into a pump, such as a weekend profile to accommodate an increase or decrease in activity at this time or a profile for women during menses. These alternate basal profiles currently adjust only basal rates, not the carb and correction factors that accompany them. Future pumps will allow these factors to be adjusted along with the alternate basal profile.

Some pumps now offer weekly schedules that enable routine basal profile changes, such as weekday to weekend, to be automatically done at the same time each week so they are not forgotten. Reminders and alerts can be set up to start automatically on different days of the week. This can be especially helpful for those whose activity or schedule varies from day to day. Schedule changes can even be adjusted for missed-meal bolus alerts when meal timing varies from day to day.

Basal/Bolus Balance and Correction-Bolus Tracking

Basal and bolus doses have to be balanced for optimum control. The pump wearer's basal/bolus balance can be calculated from the average insulin doses per day or provided directly by the pump. This helps check insulin usage and spot the cause of any problems that may arise. For adults with type 1 diabetes, glucose control is usually best when basal insulin delivery makes up 40% to 65% of the TDD. If control problems occur, the pump's memory can be quickly checked to determine the percentage of the TDD currently used for basal rates, carb boluses, and correction boluses. Many diabetes clinicians check basal/bolus balance at each clinic visit because it is so helpful for improving control.

Many smart pumps separately perform correction-bolus tracking to determine how much correction-bolus insulin was used over the last 2 to 30 days to bring down high blood glucose readings. Normally, correction boluses should make up less than 8% of the TDD. When more than 8% of the TDD is being used to bring down high readings, some of this insulin needs to be shifted into basal or carb bolus doses to reduce the number of high readings.

Pump-Meter Combos

Some pumps have an associated meter that sends blood glucose readings directly into the pump for convenient calculations. This means that your pump can calculate an accurate correction bolus to prevent insulin stacking. Direct entry of glucose values ensures accurate data entry, reduces human error, speeds bolus calculations, and ensures that every blood glucose reading is used to suggest appropriate boluses after accounting for BOB. If your meter does not automatically enter readings into your pump, be sure to do this yourself each time a test is taken. Only by entering your blood glucose into your pump can you benefit from your pump using BOB for bolus calculations.

Disposable Adhesive Pumps

A new pump, the Omnipod (**Figure 8-1**), is the first wearable pump on the market. It is a small disposable pump in the shape of a pod that attaches directly to the skin. This eliminates the need for an infusion line and an infusion set, which are the most likely parts of a typical pump system to fail. Automated insertion of a small cannula from the pod itself creates an easy and consistent application. Each pod with batteries, motor, and electronics is entirely discarded after 48 to 72 hours of use. A personal data manager, completely separate from the pump pod, must be available at all times to communicate with the pod.

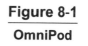

Figure 8-1

OmniPod

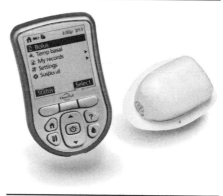

Choosing a Pump and Infusion Set

When choosing a pump, take the time you need to make a good choice. You will depend on this pump for 4 to 5 years, so discuss different pumps and pump options with your doctor and health care team to select the features that will be most helpful.

Ask local pump representatives to demonstrate their pumps. Ask lots of questions and discuss the advantages of each pump and assess the support provided. Look for a pump support group or go to a diabetes conference where pumpers are talking about pumping and pump vendors are showing their products. This may take some time, but you will be better informed and able to make a better decision.

The pump company will prepare the paperwork to submit to your insurance carrier or Medicare to cover their share of the pump and supplies and can help you deal with any insurance questions.

Choosing an Insulin Pump

Insulin pumps differ in their features and ease of use. Your needs may make one pump a better choice than another. When selecting a pump, consider the following:

1. What appeals to you about the pump? Look, feel, and color, features, accessories?
2. How easy is the pump to program and use?
3. How easy are the buttons to push? A bolus should be easy to deliver, but giving a bolus accidentally while gesturing, reaching into a pocket, or displaying the pump to inquisitive friends should not.
4. What type of reminders and alarms does the pump have?
5. How finely can basal rates be programmed for children and insulin-sensitive adults who require low basal rates? How often does basal delivery occur?

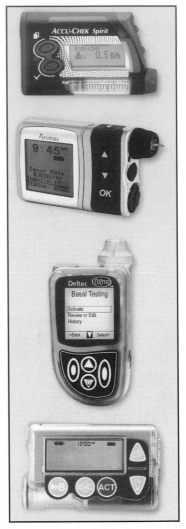

Research available features and capabilities of different insulin pumps before purchasing. Pictured here are *(from top to bottom)* the Accu-Chek Spirit (Disetronic), the Animas 1250 (Animas), the Deltec CozMo (Smiths Medical), and the MiniMed Paradigm (Medtronic).

6. How easy is it to stop a bolus? If the pump is for a child, can a caregiver easily learn to stop the pump in an emergency?

7. Can you hear or feel the alarms? Will you know if your insulin delivery has stopped?

8. How much information is stored in the pump's memory? How easy is it to access? This is important if you get distracted and forget to give a bolus, or if you want to check on your current BOB or active insulin, or if a parent wants to verify bolus delivery by a child.

9. If required, can the pump survive rough use? Is the pump waterproof? Is it easy to disconnect before showering or swimming?

10. What level of customer service is provided by the manufacturer? 24-hour telephone support? Assistance with insurance coverage? Warranty? Ease of upgrading to a newer pump? Trial period? Shipment of temporary supplies to different addresses? How soon will a replacement arrive if needed?

Choosing an Infusion Set

Using an infusion set that works well is one of the more important steps in making your pump experience successful. The infusion set and site are the weakest link in pumping. If a particular set causes skin irritation, falls off when swimming or sweating, or is easily dislodged, problems with your control will occur. For success with a pump, the infusion set must be reliable and comfortable. When selecting a pump, consider:

1. How much body fat do you have?

2. Which sites on your body are best to use?

3. Do your belt or clothing choices limit wearing a set near the waist?

4. Does your activity level limit you to certain sites?

5. Which type and size infusion set will work best for the body locations you prefer?

6. Can you easily detach from your pump for showering, etc? Some sets disconnect right at the infusion site, while others have a separate connector located a few inches away.

7. Will you need a device to aid with insertion of the infusion set?

8. Straight-in metal sets are reliable and easiest to insert, even using only one hand. Slanted Teflon sets may be more reliable for some users than straight-in Teflon sets. Inserters tend to work best with straight-in sets.

9. Suggested set sizes: for children under 12 and very lean adults with a body mass index (BMI) less than 24 or 25, try 6-mm straight or 13-mm slanted sets. For a BMI less than 27 or so, use

8-mm straight or 17-mm slanted sets. For a BMI over 27, try 10-mm straight or 17-mm slanted sets. See **Table 4-1** to determine your BMI.

Most infusion sets are reliable and work well. However, problems with a particular set, like a tendency to detach, crimping of the Teflon during insertion, or a series of unexplained high blood glucose readings caused by set failure will not be apparent until a set is worn for some time. A particular infusion set may cause a skin rash or irritation while another one will not. A trial run with various sets is likely to pick up most of these problems. Finding the right infusion set can have a major impact on the satisfaction you get out of pumping, and there are many good choices.

Summary

Pumps have some drawbacks. If site-preparation techniques are poor, an infection may occur at the infusion site. Infusion sets can come loose and lead to ketoacidosis if testing is infrequent. Attachment to a pump can be perceived as a drawback or be a real one that needs to be dealt with by those who swim or play contact sports. A pump can never be more successful than the ability and effort of the person responsible for its use.

When a pump is used well, the wearer feels better, lives more freely, and is far less likely to have diabetes-related health problems. Confidence about good diabetes management enables the wearer to feel more in control of daily living. "My friends (family, co-workers) say that I look healthier and more alert" is a frequently heard comment. The improved sense of well-being and the better quality of life that come from improved control motivate many people to do even better as time goes on.

Pump wearers find that less effort is required to achieve control and that there is less impact from diabetes on their life. Although the prevention of long-range problems is always a goal, most people find that the day-to-day convenience and flexibility of a pump are better personal motivators. They like the immediate sense of security and the better quality of life, along with the added benefit of knowing they are preventing future health problems through improved control. When the pros and cons are carefully weighed, a pump clearly offers significant advantages for people who want a healthy and enjoyable life.

9

Continuous Glucose Monitoring

Technology That Will Improve the Life of People With Diabetes

by Steven V. Edelman, M.D.
and Timothy S. Bailey, MD, FACP,
FACE, CPI

Introduction

Home glucose monitoring (HGM) has been one of the more important advances in diabetes care, but it does have limitations. There are 1440 minutes in a day, and even when people are testing their blood glucose frequently during the day, it only gives a snapshot of what is happening. Continuous glucose monitoring (CGM) can now fill those wide and potentially dangerous gaps. We do not lack the knowledge about how to treat the disease, but rather do not currently have the tools to do it safely and effectively.

For the past 36 years, like millions of Americans living with diabetes, I have struggled to control my blood glucose level as best I could while avoiding the lows. I personally have avoided unconsciousness from hypoglycemia, but at a price. I have diabetic retinopathy, kidney dysfunction, and neuropathy. The best way to describe how I felt when I went on my first CGM was like I finally got my eyesight and hearing back after being partially blind and deaf since June of 1970!

The challenge now is to get this technology into the hands of the people who could benefit the most. This will take a concerted effort to educate the people living with diabetes, the professional community, and the insurers. This chapter is an excerpt from a full CGM guide that can be downloaded from the TCOYD web site and was sponsored by an unrestricted educational grant from Dexcom.

What Is a Continuous Glucose Monitor and Who Should Use It?

A CGM system is a device that measures glucose levels throughout the day and night. Some of these devices provide measurements every 5 minutes or up to 288 values every 24 hours. The device works by having a sensor inserted under the skin (which you can do easily at home). The sensor takes glucose measurements at frequent intervals. It then transmits these values wirelessly to a handheld, cell phone–sized device, which enables you to see glucose values and trends. CGM is primarily for people with type 1 diabetes, insulin-requiring type 2 diabetes, gestational diabetes, and anyone with hypoglycemia unawareness.

At the current time, CGMs are not meant to replace traditional blood glucose meters—they work together with fingerstick readings to give you a more complete understanding of what is happening to your glucose level. You should always confirm your CGM readings with a fingerstick before you take any action such as taking an insulin dose. **Figure 9-1** shows two CGMs currently available and one that is under development.

Benefits of Continuous Glucose Monitoring

The continuous readings that are provided every 5 minutes create a trend line, which you can use to help understand how insulin, food, exercise, and other variables affect your glucose values. Traditional fingersticks provide a point-in-time glucose value, but do not tell you whether your glucose levels are rising or falling, or how fast these changes are happening.

Continuous monitoring allows you to see these trends in glucose and, after confirming with a fingerstick, to make adjustments to your insulin or take other appropriate action. Alert levels can be individually set for both high and low glucose levels, helping you better detect and manage hyper- and hypoglycemia. CGM can help you respond more quickly to changing glucose levels and take control of your diabetes management by using the information provided from continuous monitoring (**Figure 9-2 A** and **B**).

Stay in Target—Avoid Highs and Lows

Clinical research shows that using CGMs can help you spend less time hypoglycemic, less time hyperglycemic, and more time in your target zone. CGMs allow you to set a range of target control, including the high and low levels that are recommended by your caregiver or diabetes management team. You can customize these levels at your doctor's office or at home. CGM uses three zones: target, high, and low (**Figure 9-3**).

Always Use Your Trend Information With Your Glucose Value

Glucose trends show your glucose levels over a period of time. Both your glucose value and the direction in which your glucose level is headed are important. From the glucose-trend graphs below, you can see that the same glucose value of 220 mg/dL can mean different things, depending on the trend.

Figure 9-1

CGM Systems Currently Available and Under Development

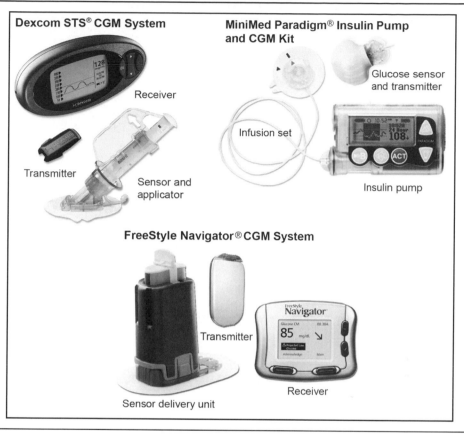

Dexcom STS® CGM System

Receiver

Transmitter

Sensor and applicator

MiniMed Paradigm® Insulin Pump and CGM Kit

Glucose sensor and transmitter

Infusion set

Insulin pump

FreeStyle Navigator® CGM System

Transmitter

Sensor delivery unit

Receiver

Abbreviation: CGM, continuous glucose monitoring.

The value of a CGM system over point-in-time finger sticks is that glucose values are determined on a minute-to-minute basis while the system is attached to the body. An insulin pump delivers insulin via an infusion set inserted into the abdominal region based upon glucose values as reported by a transmitter using radio frequency (RF) wireless technology. The transmitter is linked to a sensor attached to the abdomen by a tiny wire through the skin that measures glucose levels in the cellular fluid. The Dexcom STS (*www.dexcom.com*) and MiniMed Paradigm (*www.minimed.com*) are currently available. The MiniMed Guardian (not shown) is also available. It is essentially the same system as the MiniMed Paradigm but without the insulin pump, functioning only as a CGM. The FreeStyle Navigator (*www. abbottdiabetescare.com*) is still under development in the United States, although it has received approval in Europe.

Photos courtesy of Dexcom, Medtronic Diabetes, and Abbott Diabetes Care.

Figure 9-2

Examples of Four Fingersticks Taken and Values From CGM During 24 Hours

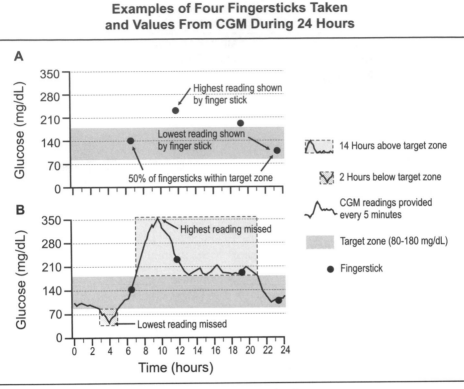

Abbreviation: CGM, continuous glucose monitoring.

A) These fingerstick point-in-time readings show that half of the values throughout the day were within the target zone (80-180 mg/dL) and half were outside. None of the four readings fell below the target zone (potentially dangerous glucose levels). The highest reading shown was 230 mg/dL. *B)* CGM readings of the same patient in the same day reveal substantially more information. Higher glucose readings (over 330 mg/dL) on this same day as well as lower glucose readings (under 60 mg/dL) are recorded, both of which were missed by fingerstick readings alone. About 16 hours were spent outside of the target zone. A portion of this time outside the target zone was unknown to the person, because fingerstick readings did not show glucose values or trends between these points.

Rising Trend

In **Figure 9-4**, the glucose value is above the target zone and is continuing to rise. After confirming the reading of 220 mg/dL with a fingerstick, a rising trend may prompt you to take additional insulin or begin exercising.

Falling Trend

In **Figure 9-5**, the glucose value is falling and headed back into the target zone. After confirming the reading of 220 mg/dL with a fingerstick, a falling trend may prompt you to watch and wait. If the trend continues to fall rapidly, even if the glucose reading is still within the target zone, it may prompt you to eat some fast-acting carbohydrates.

Constant Trend

In **Figure 9-6**, the glucose value is above the target zone and is constant. After confirming the reading of 220 mg/dL with a fingerstick, a constant trend may prompt you to take additional insulin or begin exercising.

Don't Overreact—Understand "Turnaround Time"

Turnaround time is the time it takes to reverse a trend. There is a delay that it takes for insulin to take effect once it is administered, even with rapid-acting insulin such as Novolog or Humalog. When your glucose trend is going up, it may still rise for a while before it comes down if you take insulin. When your glucose trend is going down, you may still go down for a while before it comes up if you take glucose or other carbohydrates. In some cases, it is best to watch and wait before you react to a slowly rising or slowly falling glucose level.

Figure 9-3

Three Zones of CGM:
High, Target, and Low

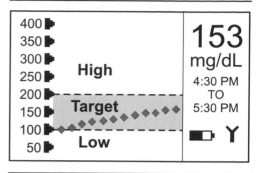

Abbreviation: CGM, continuous glucose monitoring.

The dashed lines in this graph show a sample target glucose zone of 100 mg/dL (low) to 200 mg/dL (high). When glucose goes above the high target level or below the low target level, the CGM will alert you to let you know that you are outside of your target zone. Once you are alerted, you have the option to take action early in order to avoid wide swings in glucose values.

Figure 9-4

Rising Trend

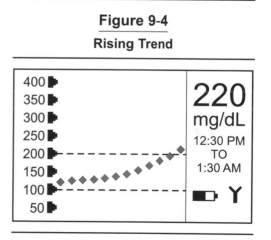

Three Views of the Same Trend at 3 PM

These charts in **Figure** 9-7 are the same trend line shown over different periods of time: 1 hour, 3 hour, and 9 hour. This person ate a meal and took insulin at noon, and soon after you can see the glucose trend starting to rise. Although glucose initially went up, the 3-hour trend graph shows that it began to level off and then went back into the target range (as insulin began to take effect and brought the glucose level back down). The 1-hour and 3-hour glucose-trend graphs are the best graphs to show that the rise in glucose is leveling off, indicating that a watch-and-wait approach may be appropriate. This turnaround time needed to reverse the trend is shown in the shaded area of each of the three graphs. The 3-hour and 9-hour glucose-trend graphs show that the total turnaround time in this example was about 2 hours.

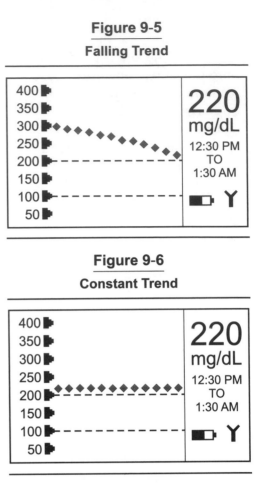

Figure 9-5

Falling Trend

Figure 9-6

Constant Trend

CGM Considerations

When evaluating CGM devices, it's important to recognize that CGM is a relatively new technology that may not work consistently all the time.

Sensor Irregularity

There may be occasions when the CGM device does not provide glucose data, alerts, or trend information. Most often this is because the sensor is experiencing an irregularity in its signal and the receiver has determined that it cannot display an accurate reading.

Start-Up Period

When the sensor is first inserted beneath the skin, it requires a start-up period (2 to 10 hours), plus calibration (entering blood glucose

Figure 9-7
Three Views of the Same Trend at 3:00 PM

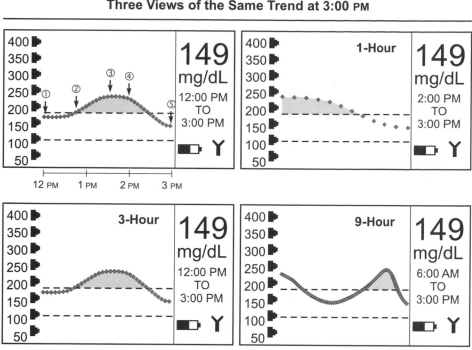

1) 12:00 PM—ate and took insulin; 2) 12:45 PM—glucose starts to rise; 3) 1:30 PM—insulin peaks; 4) 2:00 PM—glucose levels off and starts to fall; 5) 3:00 PM—current glucose reading is 149 mg/dL; no action required at this time as glucose is within target zone.

values obtained from your blood glucose meter into the CGM system) before it can begin providing continuous glucose information.

Calibration Required

Most CGM devices require 2 to 4 fingersticks in addition to the software processing (performed by the receiver) in order to calibrate the system each day.

Supplement to Fingersticks

Continuous glucose monitoring devices are FDA-approved for adjunctive use and are intended to complement, not replace, the glucose values you receive from your blood meter. Diabetes management decisions should not be based solely on CGM readings.

Margins of Difference

Even with calibration, the CGM device will generally not provide the exact same glucose value as your blood glucose meter. On average, most CGM device readings are about 5% to 20% different from those of your blood glucose meter. As the technology improves, the CGM devices will achieve better accuracy.

Reimbursement

Health insurance companies do not currently reimburse for CGM. At this point, insurance plans may or may not be paying for the device on an individual basis.

How to Get the Most Out of This Chapter

Following are three clinical situations that you may encounter while using a CGM. Several more cases are described in the full CGM Guide posted on the TCOYD web site (*www.tcoyd.org*). Each example will begin with a real-life situation and the corresponding 1-hour glucose-trend graph and, in many cases, the 3-hour glucose-trend graph as well. In cases that involve overnight glucose control problems, the 9-hour glucose-trend graph will also be shown. After you read the case history, you will be asked questions. You should try to answer each question as best you can and then read the explanation that follows each question. If you select an incorrect answer, please read the explanation very carefully before you go on to the next question.

This chapter is meant to illustrate how to interpret the information provided by your CGM device. Our hope is that by the time you review the case scenarios, you will be able to make more effective and safe decisions regarding your diabetes care.

Section 1: Blood Glucose Levels on the Rise
Scenario #1

John is a 32-year-old male who has had type 1 diabetes for 20 years. He is currently on 25 units of Lantus at bedtime as his basal insulin and a rapid-acting insulin (Apidra [glulisine]), which he takes before meals and for correction boluses. His correction factor is 1:50, which means that 1 unit of a rapid-acting insulin like Apidra, Novolog (aspart), or Humalog (lispro) will lower his glucose level about 50 mg/dL. His carbohydrate-to-insulin ratio is 15 to 1, which means that for every 15 grams of carbohydrates consumed, he will take 1 unit of Apidra. John's blood glucose upon awaking was 72 mg/dL, and he ate breakfast at 8 AM (60 grams of carbohydrates). He took 4 units of Apidra, calculated this way:

60 grams carbohydrates in meal ÷ 15 grams/unit (insulin ratio)
= 4 units for meal dosage

At 9:20 AM, the high alert (set at 180 mg/dL and shown by the upper dashed lines in the graphs below) went off. John did a fingerstick to confirm his glucose level, reviewing the 1-hour (**Figure 9-8**) and 3-hour (**Figure 9-9**) glucose-trend graphs.

Question 1a. Options for Treating High Glucose Levels

Which of the option(s) below is the best suggestion for John to follow at 9:20 AM when his high alert went off? (There may be more than one correct answer.)

  A. Watch and wait (give no additional insulin)
  B. Walk for an hour at a brisk pace
  C. Give a correction dose of 2 to 3 units
  D. Adjust the carbohydrate-to-insulin ratio to 12:1 at breakfast if this scenario repeats itself every morning

Explanation

The correct answers are B, C, and D, depending on the situation. Watching and waiting when the glucose level is rising fairly steeply after a meal usually

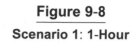

Figure 9-8

Scenario 1: 1-Hour

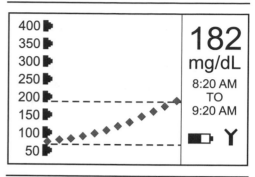

Figure 9-9

Scenario 1: 3-Hour

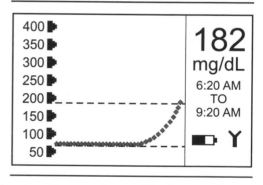

means that not enough rapid-acting insulin was given with that meal. Blood glucose levels are not always the same after meals, even if we have had that same meal numerous times before. There are so many variables that affect the glucose readings, including stress, exercise, medications, etc. This is why it is important to be able to use a correction dose to account for unexpected elevations in your glucose values. Normally, if you just tested your blood glucose with your blood glucose meter 2 hours after a meal and got a 182-mg/dL reading, you might have been perfectly satisfied. However, the CGM data clearly show that if nothing is done, the blood glucose level may continue to rise and stay elevated for hours.

One question you might ask is: Given that the correction factor is 1:50 and that 2 to 3 units of Apidra (answer C) would drop the blood glucose level 100 to 150 points, if John is only at 182 mg/dL, shouldn't this amount of insulin cause hypoglycemia? The big difference in this situation is that you have important trend information that tells you not only that the blood glucose level is 182 mg/dL, but also that it is rising steeply. This really helps you give a more appropriate correction dose and limit the amount of time spent in the hyperglycemic range.

Aerobic exercise for an hour (answer B), especially within 1 to 2 hours after your last injection of a rapid-acting insulin such as Apidra, will help to lower your glucose level. If you have an opportunity to exercise, you would not give any insulin and would watch to see what happens to your number while you exercise. If it does not come down, you can give a correction dose later (with an amount determined by your blood glucose level and trend over time as well).

Answer D is also correct—if you find that your blood glucose level is above 180 mg/dL morning after morning, you need to make the long-term adjustment by changing your breakfast carbohydrate-to-insulin ratio. It is usually recommended to make small changes slowly and wait several days to see how your adjustment affects your glucose levels.

Question 1b. Avoiding Postmeal Highs

John gave himself a correction dose of 3 units of Apidra at 9:20 am. Over the next 90 minutes, his glucose level peaked at 232 mg/dL, but started to trend downward. By noon, it was 122 mg/dL with a flat or level trend (**Figures 9-10** and **9-11**).

What could John do differently in the future in order to avoid the same situation of high postmeal glucose values in scenario 1? (More than one answer may be correct.)

A. Take 2 to 3 extra units on top of his usual 4 units when he eats the same

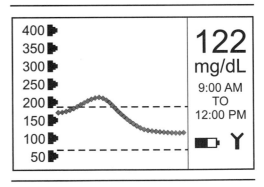

Figure 9-10

Scenario 1/Question 1b: **1-Hour**

Figure 9-11

Scenario 1/Question 1b: **3-Hour**

type of breakfast that he ate that day (eg, only when he eats 60 grams carbohydrates such as Cheerios with milk)

B. Change the carbohydrate-to-insulin ratio from 15:1 to 12:1 for the breakfast meal
C. Eat only two thirds of his normal breakfast
D. Change the composition of the breakfast to include fewer refined carbohydrates and more protein and fat

Explanation

Answers A, B, C and D could all be correct, depending on the situation. Taking 2 to 3 extra units of a rapid-acting insulin (answer A) is a viable option. The correction dose of 2 to 3 units that John gave himself at 9:20 AM worked well. Thus the same correction dose could be given at the beginning of the meal, in addition to his calculated initial dose, in order to avoid the high postbreakfast blood glucose level in the first place. If this scenario happens most of the time, answer B would be appropriate. Changing the carbohydrate-to-insulin ratio is an excellent option if John is going to eat the same type of breakfast on most days. This would work since his postmeal values are typically high when he uses the 15 grams of carbohydrates to 1 unit of rapid-acting insulin ratio. Reducing the carbohydrate-to-insulin ratio allows for a higher dose of rapid-acting insulin per serving and in this scenario would indicate that John should take 5 units for breakfast instead of 4 units:

$$60 \text{ grams carbohydrates in meal} \div 12 \text{ grams/unit (insulin ratio)}$$
$$= 5 \text{ units for meal dosage}$$

If this change does not solve the problem, he could try a 10:1 ratio for breakfast. It is important to look for trends and patterns and not make long-term changes based on one blood glucose result. Last, John's carbohydrate-to-insulin ratio of 15:1 may be perfectly adequate at lunch and dinner.

Eating two thirds of his normal breakfast (answer C) would help his postmeal glucose values. However, if that leaves John hungry after breakfast and leads to snacking and overeating at lunch, this would not be the best option. This option would improve or solve the problem, but John would have to make that decision himself. All changes really are up to the individual living with diabetes and his or her diabetes care team.

Changing the composition of the breakfast from a refined carbohydrate meal, such as cold cereal and milk, to one that has more fat and protein (answer D) would reduce postmeal glucose values. One must be aware of his or her limitations for fat if high cholesterol is a problem or of limitations for protein if kidney problems are present. Normally, a balanced breakfast of carbohydrate, fat, and protein is the best choice; however, personal preferences, living situation, budget, etc., may limit the ideal choices. Now that we have rapid-acting insulin, Symlin, and CGM, we can control postmeal glucose values regardless of the amount or type of foods eaten.

Section II: Blood Glucose Levels on the Way Down

Scenario #2

Ruth is a 76-year-old woman with insulin-requiring type 2 diabetes. She has many relatives with diabetes, and when she retired from her job as a banker at age 65, she was diagnosed with diabetes. After taking oral medications for 5 years, her average blood glucose level rose to more than 200 mg/dL, and she started taking insulin. She now takes 60 units of Lantus (long-acting basal insulin) at bedtime, 20 units of Apidra (rapid-acting insulin) with breakfast, 10 units of Apidra with lunch, and 25 units of Apidra with dinner. She also takes 1000 mg of oral metformin (Glucophage) twice daily. She weighs 169 pounds and is 5'4" tall.

She is meticulous with her diabetes treatment. Last month, she purchased a CGM and has been using it every day. She set her low blood glucose alert to 60 mg/dL and high glucose alert to 200 mg/dL. Her last A1C value was 6.2%, and she has been able to avoid many complications of diabetes. However, she has macular degeneration (damage to the macula or the eye), and her vision is not as good as it once was.

Ruth went to Napa, California, to spend a week tasting wine with her husband. She went to bed at 11:15 PM with a glucose level of 128 mg/dL and took her usual 60 units of Lantus. Within 45 minutes of injection, she was awakened by a low-glucose alarm. Her monitor read 53 and showed a sharp decline in blood glucose (**Figures 9-12** and **9-13**).

Question 2a. Using Different Insulins

What answer do you think is most likely to have caused Ruth's blood glucose level to drop? (Only one answer is correct.)

A. Ruth forgot to have her bedtime snack
B. Ruth mistakenly took 60 units of Apidra at bedtime (instead of Lantus)
C. The batteries were low in the receiver, which led to a falsely low reading
D. The insulin went bad and was working too quickly

Explanation

The correct answer is B. While this may seem improbable for a woman as careful as Ruth, it happens not infrequently. It may be due in part to all of the newer insulins being clear or colorless and, therefore, difficult to distinguish from one another.

Prior to the introduction of Lantus and Levemir, all clear insulins were faster-acting products. NPH is cloudy and easy to distinguish from clear, short-acting insulin. Currently, there is no consistent way to distinguish commonly used insulins other than by reading the labels, which is difficult for people with limited vision. To minimize the potential for confusion, some doctors suggest using insulin pens for meal therapy and a vial and syringe for long-acting insulin therapy.

Missing a bedtime snack (answer A) can cause problems for people who are taking excessive basal insulin. However, it usually results in a much slower decrease than that seen here, so answer A is incorrect. However, if Ruth drank a great deal of alcohol during her wine tours, it could have made her more vulnerable to hypoglycemia, as drinking alcohol can lower glucose levels.

Figure 9-12

Scenario 2: 1-Hour

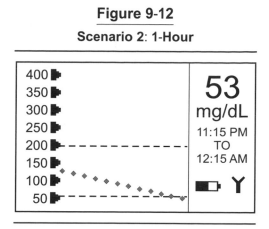

Figure 9-13

Scenario 2: 3-Hour

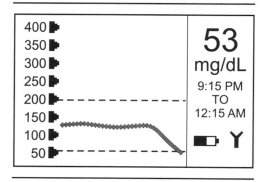

Answer C is also incorrect. When the monitor's batteries are low, there is a low-battery indicator. The low-battery state does not lead to false readings. The monitor is designed to shut off the display of readings in case of suspected inaccuracy of the device.

When insulin is exposed to extreme temperatures or used beyond its expiration date, there is generally a reduced potency. An increased insulin effect has not been seen, so answer D is incorrect.

Question 2b. Options for Treating Low-Glucose Levels

Ruth took four glucose tablets and woke her husband. What should she do next? (Only one answer is correct.)

A. Call her doctor and ask for further advice

B. Call room service to order some desserts

C. Confirm that her glucose level is really low by a fingerstick test and continue to take glucose tablets and any other available carbohydrates until the CGM shows a glucose level greater than 100 mg/dL and a rising trend

D. Inject herself with 1 mg of Glucagon and call the paramedics immediately

Explanation

The correct answer is C. Treatment of her accidental mistake is urgent, and quick action is required to avoid severe hypoglycemia. The insulin she took will keep her at risk for hypoglycemia for at least 4 hours, so she should not go back to sleep. Having a CGM will allow her to closely watch her blood glucose level.

Answer D would be correct if she was unable to take anything by mouth. If she had type 1 diabetes and took this amount of rapid-acting insulin and was not very close to a hospital, taking Glucagon and calling the paramedics would not be an unreasonable choice.

Calling the doctor (answer A) would be a good idea if Ruth didn't know what to do or if she didn't realize her mistake. However, patients using CGMs tend to be among those most informed about diabetes.

Answer B is unwise for short-term treatment, due to the unpredictable time it may take to get the food. In addition, answer B has the potential for overtreatment (depending on the type and amount of desserts eaten) and could lead to high blood glucose levels. However, ordering a small snack from room service may make all of those glucose tablets more palatable.

Ruth has had a rough night so far. Her initial glucose level when she confirmed it by fingerstick with her blood glucose meter was 68 mg/dL. It has been 2 hours since her low glucose alarm went off. She has not only exhausted her supply of glucose tablets, but she also ate a bagel leftover from lunch and drank the only 2 bottles of regular soda that were in her minibar. Her husband has finally come back with dessert. Look at her 1-hour and 3-hour glucose-trend graphs in **Figures 9-14** and **9-15** and decide what she should do next.

Question 2c. Treatment Following a Low Glucose Value

What should Ruth do now? (Choose the one best answer.)

A. Decide not to eat the desserts and go to sleep, as she was confident her glucose was not going to drop further

B. Have a decaf cappuccino and watch the monitor closely for another hour before doing anything else

C. Continue eating, but more slowly

D. Give 10 units of Apidra to prevent rebound hyperglycemia

Explanation

Answer B is the best option, since she has reversed the falling glucose trend and has a glucose level high enough to be reasonably safe. Remember, she has type 2 diabetes, and because of the associated insulin resistance, overdoses of insulin are less catastrophic (as compared with such a high dose of Apidra in a thin person with type 1 diabetes).

Answer A is incorrect. Although Apidra is a rapid-acting insulin, it remains active for 4 to 5 hours, and she is not out of the woods yet with regard to hypoglycemia risk.

Answer C might be an option if glucose levels begin to trend downward again.

Answer D would be unwise as the time frame during which she is at risk for hypoglycemia has not passed. Most likely, Ruth's glucose level will not be in the normal range in the morning due to overtreatment of her lows with food. However, this is preferable to hypoglycemia. With the use of CGMs, both overtreatment of hypoglycemia and risk of hypoglycemia can be safely reduced.

Figure 9-14

Scenario 2/Question 2b: 1-Hour

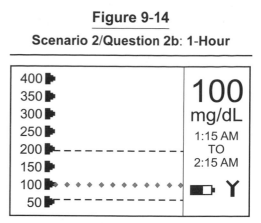

Figure 9-15

Scenario 2/Question 2b: 3-Hour

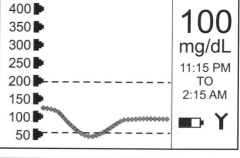

Question 2d. Adjusting Your Target Range

Which setting change on her CGM receiver should Ruth consider? (Choose the one best answer.)

A. Raise the high-glucose alert to 250 mg/dL
B. Raise the low-glucose alert to 100 mg/dL
C. Call the manufacturer of the company to change the fixed low warning of 55 mg/dL
D. Turn off the audible alarms

Explanation

Answer B is the correct answer. Raising the threshold for a low alarm can improve safety, as it gives you more time to anticipate a potential low. Although the alarm on the device may annoy you, the increase in safety from hypoglycemia can be worth it (particularly if you have hypoglycemia unawareness).

Raising the high-glucose alert in Ruth would offer no benefit (it is already somewhat high at 200 mg/dL), so answer A is incorrect.

Answer C is incorrect because the low-glucose alarm warning (set at 55 mg/dL) cannot be altered. This option would also be unwise because of safety concerns.

Answer D would be unwise as the audible alerts might be very helpful to Ruth, particularly during the night.

Section III: Blood Glucose Levels During the Night
Scenario #3
Mary is a 19-year-old college student who has been living with diabetes for less than a year. She uses an insulin pump with the basal rate set at 0.6 units per hour for 24 hours (a basal rate is a constant amount of insulin delivered throughout the day and night by an insulin pump in very small increments). The basal rate maintains blood glucose values in the normal range between meals, overnight, and during periods of fasting. Mary's correction factor is 1:50 and her carbohydrate-to-rapid-acting insulin ratio is 15:1. She commonly goes to bed with a good blood glucose level, but it is high upon awakening in the morning. She has dinner at 6 PM on most nights and does not snack after dinner. She usually goes to bed around 11:00 PM. Please see her 9-hour glucose-trend graphs in **Figures 9-16, 9-17,** and **9-18** from the previous 3 nights.

Question 3a. Nocturnal Hyperglycemia –Second Culprit
Which option below best explains what is happening with Mary overnight? (Only one answer is correct.)
  A. Mary is experiencing the Somogyi reaction (rebound hyperglycemia as a result of a hypoglycemic reaction)
  B. Mary's insulin pump is malfunctioning
  C. Mary is experiencing the dawn phenomenon, which is early morning resistance to insulin
  D. Mary has gastroparesis

Explanation
Option C is the correct answer. The dawn phenomenon is a well-characterized problem that is common in people with diabetes. People without diabetes commonly need more insulin in the early hours of the morning to keep the blood glucose levels from rising. This need for more insulin is thought to be due to natural circadian (natural biologic cycle of the body) elevations in anti-insulin hormones such as the growth

hormone. If you do not have diabetes, the pancreas merely secretes a little more insulin during this time period, which is normally between the hours of 3 AM and 7 AM. However, if your pancreas does not secrete enough insulin because you have diabetes, your glucose level will go up during this time unless you compensate for it.

Answer A is not correct. The Somogyi reaction is a situation where there is rebound hyperglycemia after one has a hypoglycemic reaction. When one has a hypoglycemic reaction, there is sometimes a natural physiologic response to protect one from extremely low glucose values by secreting hormones such as epinephrine (also called adrenalin) and glucagon that raise the glucose levels. As you can see from the 9-hour displays, Mary is not getting into the hypoglycemic range, so this option is not correct.

There is no reason why the pump would malfunction at such a specific time period, so answer B is not correct.

Gastroparesis, delayed absorption of food after it enters the stomach, which is further described in Chapter 17, would not take 9 hours to cause hyperglycemia, so answer D is not correct. Mary eats dinner at 6 PM and the glucose values do not go up until around 3 AM. Gastroparesis usually causes a delay in postmeal glucose elevations of about 2 to 4 hours.

Figure 9-16
Scenario 3: 9-Hour

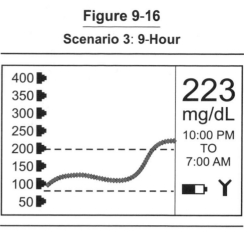

Figure 9-17
Scenario 3: 9-Hour

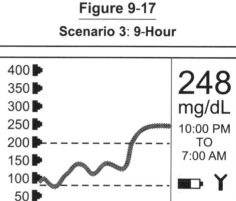

Figure 9-18
Scenario 3: 9-Hour

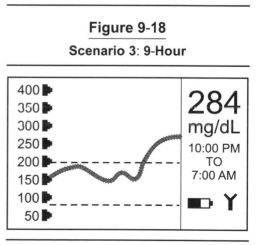

Which of the options below might help to prevent this situation causing elevated glucose level in the early morning? (There is one best answer.)

A. Have Mary take an injection of NPH insulin at bedtime
B. Program a second basal rate into Mary's pump where the rate is increased by 30% to 0.8 units/hour, starting at 3 AM until 7 AM
C. Have Mary do 30 to 45 minutes of aerobic exercise starting at 3 AM
D. Have Mary change her normal sleep hours, so that she goes to bed much later than 11 PM

Explanation

Option B is the best answer. One advantage of insulin pump therapy is that you can have more than one basal rate throughout the day and night. You can adjust your basal rate according to your activities, including exercise and whether you experience the dawn phenomenon. Having an increased basal rate during the time of the dawn phenomenon is normally very effective at preventing the rise in glucose in the early morning hours. CGM is really ideal for making the diagnosis quickly and accurately. It can also help you make the correct insulin adjustment.

Giving NPH at bedtime (answer A) would also help the situation; however, the timing of NPH insulin is not as precise as increasing the basal rate on an insulin pump. In addition, adding intermediate-acting insulin such as NPH at night to a patient on a pump adds unnecessary complexity to the insulin regimen. Changing Mary's sleep habits (answer D) and exercising in the middle of the night (answer C) are unreasonable options.

Summary

For people on insulin and with hypoglycemia unawareness, CGM is one of the more important advances in the past several decades. Home glucose monitoring only captures a snapshot of what is happening throughout the day and night, while CGM provides much more information on trends and patterns. CGM allows many people with diabetes (including me) to achieve a better A1C in a safe manner with less hypoglycemia. Please go to the TCOYD web site (*www.tcoyd.org*) to watch the TCOYD-TV episode on continuous glucose monitoring and to download the full version of the CGM guide with more case scenarios.

10

Know Your Numbers

You need to know your numbers because it is your diabetes, your life, your blood, and your results! Know Your Numbers is a regular part of the widely-recognized TCOYD newsletter. I have chosen just a few of the many scenarios that have appeared in the newsletter over the past several years for inclusion in this chapter. Testing your blood glucose level and recording it in a logbook is not enough. You need to know what your goals of control are, both before and after meals, and then be able to interpret your own numbers. You also need to know what actions to take to achieve your goals... whether it is adjusting your own medication (if cleared with your caregiver) or just recognizing that you need to make a phone call well before your next scheduled appointment because you are having a consistent problem. Read each case history and examine each logbook carefully. Try to figure out what the problem is before you read the explanation. *Know Your Numbers* is a great example of what TCOYD is all about: education, motivation, and self advocacy. Please see the TCOYD TV episode on home glucose monitoring on the Web site (*www.tcoyd.org*). If you are not a member of TCOYD, please go online or call to join so that you can receive our newsletter on a regular basis.

Type 1 Diabetes and Carbohydrates

Case #1

Logbook CS-1 is from a 15-year-old boy who has had type 1 diabetes since the age of 6. He is treated with Lantus (glargine) at night (24-hour basal insulin) with rapid-acting Novolog (aspart) before meals. He carefully and accurately figures out how much Novolog he needs to take before each meal by counting the carbohydrates in that meal. His ratio is 1 unit of rapid-acting insulin (Novolog in this case, but Humalog [lispro] and Apidra [glulisine] are also rapid-acting insulins) for every 10 grams of carbohydrate consumed. As you can see, his post-breakfast numbers are through the roof almost every day, commonly above 300 mg/dL.

After a thorough dietary history, I discovered that his typical breakfast consisted of orange juice (8 oz), a bowl of cold cereal (his favorites are Trix and Captain Crunch) with 1% milk, and two pieces of toast with diet jelly. This breakfast contains not only a ton of carbohydrates, but they are all simple or refined carbohydrates, which means they get broken down quickly once eaten. They raise the postmeal blood glucose levels extremely high, very quickly. There is no way any amount of rapid-acting insulin can handle this load of simple carbohydrates at one time.

There are several solutions, including changing the breakfast to contain less carbohydrates and more protein, eating more complex carbohydrates, and spreading out the calories over several hours. He may also consider starting Symlin (pramlintide), the new hormone recently approved for people on insulin, to flatten out postmeal glucose levels.

Logbook CS-1

Usual Target Before Meals: 70-130   **BLOOD GLUCOSE**   Usual Target 1-2 Hours After Meals: 70-180

DATE	INSULIN			BREAKFAST		LUNCH		DINNER		BED TIME	OVER NIGHT	COMMENTS
	TYPE	AM	PM	BEFORE	AFTER	BEFORE	AFTER	BEFORE	AFTER			
S				121	362	186		161	179			Dinner 6:30 pm Bedtime 9 pm
S				97	410	159		212	187			
M				116	299	At school		113				
T				159	351	At school		149	–			
W				126	320	At school		225	118			
Th				84	281	At school		261	145			
F				162	427	At school		144	197			

Prediabetes

Case #2

Peter is a 56-year-old man with a history of being overweight, along with high blood pressure and abnormal cholesterol levels. His mother, brother, sister, and two paternal uncles have type 2 diabetes. He came to my office to ask what he can do to prevent diabetes.

I gave him a loaner glucose meter and he came back with the results shown in **Logbook CS-2**. As you can see, his before-breakfast numbers range from 86 to 123 mg/dL and his after-meal values go as high as 198 mg/dL. The official ranges for the fasting (before food in the morning) and postmeal glucose values for people who are normal, prediabetic, or diabetic are shown in **Figure 1-2**.

Peter's values are not normal, but neither are they within the diabetes range. He clearly has prediabetes. I recommended a good dietitian and exercise physiologist to slowly begin practical lifestyle changes that will help him to avoid developing full-blown diabetes.

188

After we see how his blood glucose does with lifestyle modifications, I will make sure Peter is aware of medication options to see if he wants to be aggressive about attempting to prevent diabetes. It is important to state that the FDA has not officially approved any medication for the prevention of type 2 diabetes. The bottom line is that each person at risk needs to be dealt with on an individual basis.

Logbook CS-2

Usual Target Before Meals: 70-130

BLOOD GLUCOSE

Usual Target 1-2 Hours After Meals: 70-180

DATE	INSULIN			BREAKFAST		LUNCH		DINNER		BED TIME	OVER NIGHT	COMMENTS
	TYPE	AM	PM	BEFORE					AFTER			
				102					—			
	TYPE	AM	PM	86					—			
	TYPE	AM	PM	98					187			
	TYPE	AM	PM	—					145			
	TYPE	AM	PM	123					198			
	TYPE	AM	PM	—					—			
	TYPE	AM	PM	117					141			

Continuous Glucose Monitoring

Case #3

Logbook CS-3 comes from a 32-year-old woman who has been living with type 1 diabetes since she was 6 years old. Laura is on an insulin pump and her correction factor is 1 unit for every 50 mg/dL above 120 mg/dL—meaning that it takes 1 unit of fast acting insulin to lower her blood glucose level 50 mg/dL. Her insulin to carbohydrate ratio is 1:15—meaning she takes 1 unit of insulin for every 15 grams of carbohydrate. She tests her blood glucose 6 to 10 times a day and tries to eat and exercise regularly; however, she works full time, has three young boys (4, 6, and 10 years old) and has a husband who is frequently not at home due to his profession. Laura had a severe hypoglycemic reaction one night while her husband was out of town. Her oldest son heard her thrashing about in bed and called 9-1-1. Because Laura has had diabetes for over 26 years, her body does not respond to low blood glucose as it used to. Earlier in her life, she would always wake up feeling shaky and sweaty if she had a low blood glucose, but she did not experience those symptoms—and she didn't wake up on her own. Since that episode,

189

Laura is afraid of having another severe unconscious reaction when she is home alone with her kids. She now purposely runs high at night to avoid a low blood glucose level but at the cost of organ-damaging hyperglycemia. When she wakes up with a high blood glucose, she must take a large correction bolus of insulin, which on occasion leads to hypoglycemia before lunch and creates a roller coaster type of situation that is hard to control. A continuous glucose monitor (CGM), which can be programmed with predetermined high and low level alerts, would not only help Laura avoid serious lows but also help her get off the roller coaster. A device that provides continuous blood glucose readings would allow Laura to see the rising and falling blood glucose trends and would greatly improve her glucose control safely.

Logbook CS-3

				BREAKFAST		LUNCH		DINNER		BED	OVER	
DATE	INSULIN			BEFORE	AFTER	BEFORE	AFTER	BEFORE	AFTER	TIME	NIGHT	COMMENTS
Mon 5/8	TYPE	AM	PM	113		152		159		(221)		
Tues 5/9	TYPE	AM	PM	(178)		64		128		192		
Wed 5/10	TYPE	AM	PM	163		71		162		(264)		
Thurs 5/11	TYPE	AM	PM	(201)		[52]		(199)		213		
Fri 5/12	TYPE	AM	PM	121		[44]		(244)		186		
Sat 5/13	TYPE	AM	PM	125		136		257		(277)		
Sun 5/14	TYPE	AM	PM	(215)		[39]		(377)		(302)		

Usual Target Before Meals: 70-130
BLOOD GLUCOSE
Usual Target 1-2 Hours After Meals: 70-180

Disconnecting the Pump

Case #4

John is a 17-year-old teenager who was diagnosed with type 1 diabetes 5 years ago. He plays on the high school football team. He has also been extremely happy on an Animas pump using Novolog insulin for the last 2 years. During practice and the games, he removes his pump for up to 2 hours at a time. As you can see (**Logbook CS-4**), his numbers after practice are not too bad but they seem to rise extremely high after dinner even though the amount and types of food are similar to other nights without exercise. What is happening?

When you are on a pump, there is no long-acting insulin onboard. The pump is giving only rapid-acting insulin. The insulin not only gets into the system quickly, but it also leaves the body quickly. When a pump is disconnected for 2 hours, the insulin levels in the body get very low. Although his blood glucose is not super high after exercising intensely, it eventually rises excessively because of that deficit in insulin. Pump wearers really should not disconnect for more than 45 minutes. If it is necessary, then there are ways to deal with the situation, such as using long-acting insulin in combination. See *The Untethered Regimen* on the TCOYD web site in the *Article Archives* found under *Dr. Edelman's Corner.*

Logbook CS-4

DATE	INSULIN			BREAKFAST		LUNCH		DINNER		BED TIME	OVER NIGHT	COMMENTS
	TYPE	AM	PM	BEFORE	AFTER	BEFORE	AFTER	BEFORE	AFTER			
M				122		164		175	341	221			Foot ball practice (off pump) 3-5:30 pm
T				211		153		129	191	175			
W				110		146		157	433	297			Foot ball practice (off pump) 3-5:30 pm
Th				234		/		166	201	174			
Fr				97		115		134	397	251			Foot ball practice (off pump) 5-7 pm
S				190		/		126	/	191			
S												

BLOOD GLUCOSE

Usual Target Before Meals: 70-130

Usual Target 1-2 Hours After Meals: 70-180

Premixed Insulin

Case #5

Logbook CS-5 is from an overweight 63-year-old veteran with type 2 diabetes who is on the older 70/30 premixed insulin twice a day before breakfast and dinner. The main difference between the older 70/30 and the newer Novolog Mix 70/30 (70% insulin aspart protamine suspension and 30% insulin aspart [rDNA origin] injection) is that the Regular insulin is replaced by the newer rapid-acting insulin analogue Novolog Mix 70/30. The two fairly obvious trends are that the postmeal blood glucose level is consistently about 200 mg/dL and that the patient's blood glucose is getting on the low side before meals. These two problems can be improved by substituting the new Novolog Mix 70/30 for the older formulation. In fact, this is what happened with this patient and his numbers. After eating, he did not get above 200 mg/dL regularly and his premeal numbers came up to a more normal and safer range.

Logbook CS-5

| | | | | BREAKFAST | | LUNCH | | DINNER | | BED | OVER | |
| DATE | INSULIN | | | BEFORE | AFTER | BEFORE | AFTER | BEFORE | AFTER | TIME | NIGHT | COMMENTS |
	TYPE	AM	PM									
8/3				91	284	72		164	211	69		
8/4				117	222	62		141	–	87		
8/5				112	302	110		122	322	94		
8/6				87	198	–		97	–	77		
8/7				74	–	124		153	222	98		
8/8				121	–	69		–	298	121		
8/9				132	275	102		148	194	97		

Usual Target Before Meals: 70-130 — **BLOOD GLUCOSE** — *Usual Target 1-2 Hours After Meals: 70-180*

Low Blood Glucose Overnight

Case #6

These glucose readings are from a 15-year-old boy who has had type 1 diabetes for 4 years. He is currently taking NPH before he goes to bed at 9 PM (in addition to his daytime insulin). As you can see (**Logbook CS-6**), he is going to bed with a fairly good value, but his morning number is consistently high. His mother tells me that he has been having nightmares and his pajamas have been soaked with sweat in the mornings. On one occasion, he wet his bed, which is highly unusual for him.

Logbook CS-6

Usual Target Before Meals: 70-130 — **BLOOD GLUCOSE** — *Usual Target 1-2 Hours After Meals: 70-180*

| | | | | BREAKFAST | | LUNCH | | DINNER | | BED | OVER | |
| DATE | INSULIN | | | BEFORE | AFTER | BEFORE | AFTER | BEFORE | AFTER | TIME | NIGHT | COMMENTS |
	TYPE	AM	PM									
10/8				211		152		182		146		
10/9				249		/		171		162		
10/10				231		134		/		113		
10/11				197		128		120		142		
10/12				202		167		114		/		
10/13				183		/		139		171		
10/14				189		144		121		141		

What is probably happening is that he is getting too low during the middle of the night and not waking up to take something sweet. Bed-wetting, sweating, and nightmares are classic symptoms of hypoglycemia at night. He is taking NPH insulin at 9 PM, which has its peak action 6 hours later, causing him to have hypoglycemia at 3 AM.

When the blood glucose drops too low at night, many other anti-insulin hormones such as adrenalin, glucagon, and growth hormone are produced to counteract the low, commonly resulting in an elevated number in the morning. Two ways to confirm if this patient's blood glucose is getting low are to test his glucose level at 3 AM or hook up a CGM overnight. Lowering his nighttime dose or switching him to peakless insulin such as Lantus may also be helpful.

Combination Therapy

Case #7

Logbook CS-7 comes from a 59-year-old man with type 2 diabetes on combination therapy. Combination therapy refers to a regimen of oral medications taken during the day and an intermediate-acting insulin (such as NPH [isophane]) or a long-acting insulin (such as Lantus) given at bedtime. In his case, he was on Amaryl (glimepiride) and Avandia during the day and 45 units of Lantus taken at bedtime, which is normally at 10:30 PM. On some mornings, his number looks great. But why did he awaken twice over the past week with a high blood glucose and then have a higher than usual number during the rest of the day?

Logbook CS-7

Usual Target Before Meals: 70-130				BLOOD GLUCOSE							Usual Target 1-2 Hours After Meals: 70-180
DATE	INSULIN			BREAKFAST		LUNCH		DINNER		BED TIME	OVER NIGHT	COMMENTS
	TYPE	AM	PM	BEFORE	AFTER	BEFORE	AFTER	BEFORE	AFTER			
M				112				137				
T				101				—				
W				197				164				
Tn				122				146				
F				97				117				
S				213				179				
Su				115				136				

As it turns out, he sometimes fell asleep on the couch after dinner and did not take his bedtime dose of Lantus. This problem was easily fixed. Because Lantus is a 24-hour basal insulin without a peak, he was told by his doctor to take the daily injection in the morning instead of at bedtime. Lantus works well as long as it is given at roughly the same time each day, no matter what time of day it is.

Medical Stress and Glucose Control

Case #8

It does not take a rocket scientist to notice that the blood glucose levels begin looking pretty good in **Logbook CS-8**, and then all of a sudden they go downhill and stay downhill. Upon questioning this person with diabetes, there were no changes in his diet, exercise routine, stress, or medications. Larry is a 57-year-old male who has had type 2 diabetes for 13 years. He also takes medication for high blood pressure and abnormal cholesterol levels. He checked his insulin, which was not expired and has been kept in a cool place since he received it. The only things that were different were that he was feeling more tired than usual, he was having a hard time climbing up the stairs to his apartment, and his ankles were a little swollen.

It turned out that he had a silent heart attack and, because his heart muscle was permanently damaged, it was not pumping enough blood to the rest of his body, making him feel lethargic. Remember that any type of serious medical condition, such as a heart attack, can lead to elevated blood glucose levels. In fact, sometimes the unexpected and unexplained higher blood glucose values will be your only clue. Remember this and let your caregiver know!

Logbook CS-8

Usual Target Before Meals: 70-130   **BLOOD GLUCOSE**   Usual Target 1-2 Hours After Meals: 70-180

DATE	INSULIN TYPE	AM	PM	BREAKFAST BEFORE	AFTER	LUNCH BEFORE	AFTER	DINNER BEFORE	AFTER	BED TIME	OVER NIGHT	COMMENTS
12/5				88	97	89	111	79	92			
12/6				77	125	79	117	82	135			
12/7				90	131	87	126	96	148			
12/8				76	101	82	180	190	212			
12/9				188	247	191	242	197	256			
12/10				185	210	196	222	187	243			
12/11				192	237	202	241	196	248			

Fine-Tuning Your Correction Factor

Case Study #9

Joan is a 27-year-old woman who has been living with diabetes for 4 years. She takes 25 units of Levemir (detemir) at night for her long-acting basal insulin and Novolog before each meal for her rapid-acting insulin. She calculates her premeal boluses of Novolog based on how many carbohydrates she is going to eat (one unit of Novolog for every 10 grams of carbohydrate) and what her blood glucose level is at the time of the meal (correction factor). Her correction factor is 1:50, meaning that 1 unit of Novolog will bring her blood glucose level down 50 points. For example, if she is going to eat 60 grams of carbohydrates (60/10 = 6 units) and her blood glucose level is 200 mg/dL at the time of the meal (100 mg/dL over her target number of 100 mg/dL), she would take an extra 2 units to "correct her number." This then adds up to a total of 8 units of Novolog for her meal. The problem is that this system does not always work out for her (**Logbook CS-9**).

Logbook CS-9

| | | | BREAKFAST | | LUNCH | | DINNER | | BED | OVER | |
DATE	INSULIN		BEFORE	AFTER	BEFORE	AFTER	BEFORE	AFTER	TIME	NIGHT	COMMENTS
	TYPE / AM / PM		131		111		167		136		
	TYPE / AM / PM		98		82		71		201		
	TYPE / AM / PM		175		159		191		154		
	TYPE / AM / PM		(289)→		(344)→		(275)→		189		
	TYPE / AM / PM		197		213		162		180		
	TYPE / AM / PM		114		121		164		213		
	TYPE / AM / PM		(235)→		(267)→		(194)→		149		

Usual Target Before Meals: 70-130 — **BLOOD GLUCOSE** — Usual Target 1-2 Hours After Meals: 70-180

To a trained diabetes specialist who looks at glucose logbooks all day, it seems that her correction factor is not working for all situations. When her blood glucose level is 200 or less before a meal, the correction factor works well and her postmeal blood glucose level is in range (140 to 180 mg/dL). However, if her premeal blood glucose level is above 200 mg/dL, the correction seems to underestimate her insulin requirements and she ends up with her level too high after that meal. This situation is actually quite common and it relates to the fact that the body is more resistant to the insulin injected if the blood glucose level is excessively high. Many of my patients have a different correction factor depending on their blood glucose level, ie, if it is less than 200 mg/dL, the correction factor may be 1 unit per 50 mg/dL; for blood glucose levels above 200 mg/dL, it would change to 1 unit per 35 mg/dL. This is fine-tuning at its best. If you have any questions, e-mail me. I know this can be a little confusing. **Remember**: *Please, do not change your insulin dose without talking with your caregiver first!*

Going to Bed Fine, Waking Up High

Case #10

If you look at the glucose levels at lunch, dinner, and bedtime of **Logbook CS-10**, they are not too shabby. This person has type 1 diabetes and the degree of bouncing is not unusual at all, even though it bugs the heck out of us! The main problem is that the glucose upon awakening is far too high. Something is happening overnight that is leading to elevated blood glucose values in the morning.

Logbook CS-10

Usual Target Before Meals: 70-130				**BLOOD GLUCOSE**				Usual Target 1-2 Hours After Meals: 70-180	

DATE	INSULIN			BREAKFAST		LUNCH		DINNER		BED TIME	OVER NIGHT	COMMENTS
	TYPE	AM	PM	BEFORE	AFTER	BEFORE	AFTER	BEFORE	AFTER			
25				231		112		132		154		
26				210		96		141		147		
27				197		102		126		167		
28				184		117		104		131		
29				237		86		101		111		
30				224		69		123		120		
1				191		98		134		156		

There are many possibilities that could explain these numbers. The first is that there may not be enough long-acting insulin given the evening before. This person is on NPH before dinner, along with rapid-acting insulin Novolog. Since the bedtime numbers are good, the Novolog dose at dinnertime does not need to be adjusted. If one tested at 3 AM, the number should be higher than at bedtime but not quite as high as the morning value. The second possibility is that this person is having hypoglycemia in the middle of the night without waking up and then rebounding to a high glucose level because of the many hormones that are released by the body to fight off low glucose levels. The effect is called the Somogyi phenomenon, and in this situation, the blood glucose level will be on the low side if measured in the middle of the night. The third possibility is that this person could be experiencing the "dawn phenomenon": a normally occurring situation where, increased insulin requirement in the early morning. In this scenario, the blood glucose levels are okay until about 3 AM and then they rise until the morning.

There is one good way to find out what is happening... test in the middle of the night. It is a bummer but... no pain, no gain. I would also suggest getting a CGM device (see Chapter 9).

Dry Labbing It!

Case #11

This 36-year-old person with type 2 diabetes appears to be working hard to control his diabetes and it looks like it is under excellent control (**Logbook CS-11**). He is testing four times a day without missing a single time and his numbers look excellent.

Logbook CS-11

DATE	INSULIN			BREAKFAST		LUNCH		DINNER		BED TIME	OVER NIGHT	COMMENTS
	TYPE	AM	PM	BEFORE	AFTER	BEFORE	AFTER	BEFORE	AFTER			
7/19				144		115		130		120		
7/20	TYPE	AM	PM	120		105		125		144		
7/21	TYPE	AM	PM	134		94		125		124		
7/22	TYPE	AM	PM	115		124		144		94		
7/23	TYPE	AM	PM	115		105		130		134		
7/24	TYPE	AM	PM	124		144		120		140		
7/25	TYPE	AM	PM	135		125		95		110		

Usual Target Before Meals: 70-130 — **BLOOD GLUCOSE** — *Usual Target 1-2 Hours After Meals: 70-180*

However, there is something definitely wrong with this picture. The numbers do not vary much and there are too many numbers that are exactly the same or end with zero or five, which is mathematically not likely. This person had an A1C of 15%, indicating that his average blood glucose level is, in reality, 250 to 350 mg/dL!

This person was just making up these numbers because he did not test at all and/or was ashamed to tell his caregiver he was not testing. It is so important to realize that having bad blood glucose levels does not mean you are a bad person. Falsifying your glucose value only hurts you. We must all overcome the emotional barriers of dealing with "bad numbers" and realize our health care providers can only give us the best care possible if we are honest with them.

Good A1C, but on a Roller Coaster

Case #12

In this person's logbook is that the numbers jump from as low as 36 to high as 478 mg/dL on a daily basis (**Logbook CS-12**). What must be so frustrating for this person with diabetes is that there are no consistent trends, which makes it almost impossible for the caregiver to make any adjustments in the insulin or oral-agent dose. For example, if the morning prebreakfast values were always high, then increasing the nighttime dose of long-acting insulin or oral agent would be appropriate. If one third of the numbers are low, one third too high, and the last one third are just right, then any adjustment would not be appropriate and possibly dangerous. What is amazing is that the A1C was 7.1% indicating great control but it is important to remember that the A1C is just an average and does not reflect the day-to-day ups and downs. Usually, in cases like this one, the person with diabetes may first need to improve the consistency of his/her daily eating and exercise schedule to try and reduce the day-to-day fluctuations. Obtaining a CGM device would be invaluable to help get off the roller coaster.

Logbook CS-12

				BREAKFAST		LUNCH		DINNER		BED	OVER	
DATE	INSULIN			BEFORE	AFTER	BEFORE	AFTER	BEFORE	AFTER	TIME	NIGHT	COMMENTS
	TYPE	AM	PM	72		234		111		263		
	TYPE	AM	PM	144		/		94		179		
	TYPE	AM	PM	356		68		156		105		
	TYPE	AM	PM	42		115		/		39		
	TYPE	AM	PM	121		35		279		345		
	TYPE	AM	PM	225		478		315		119		
	TYPE	AM	PM	127		/		60		156		

Usual Target Before Meals: 70-130

BLOOD GLUCOSE

Usual Target 1-2 Hours After Meals: 70-180

Summary

Know your numbers!

11

Hypoglycemia

Origins, Prevention, and Management

by Patrick J. Boyle, MD

Introduction

Hypoglycemia (low blood glucose) is undoubtedly the limiting factor preventing many motivated patients with diabetes from achieving their goal of near-normal blood glucose concentrations. So, quite correctly, hypoglycemia prevents us from preventing long-term complications. If it were easier to achieve better glucose control without substantial hypoglycemia risk, then diabetes would, in part, be much less of a national health care dilemma.

Common Themes With Type 1 and Type 2 Diabetes

First, you need a bit of general background information on hypoglycemia. The body has a series of redundant hormonal responses for limiting how low of a blood glucose one can have. These systems also allow recovery from hypoglycemia. The first line of defense should be a reduction in insulin production as the blood glucose falls just below the normal range.

Insulin's primary function is to tell your liver not to make glucose. Without insulin, your body can make extraordinary amounts of glucose (even running into concentrations in the thousands of milligrams per deciliter [mg/dL]). Insulin can entirely shut off liver glucose production. In fact, we try to take advantage of this fact by having patients take their insulin before meals in order to give the liver the signal that making glucose will not be necessary while food is being absorbed. The absence of insulin-producing beta cells results in the loss of this important buffer against low blood glucose in patients with type 1 diabetes. When a person with type 1 diabetes gets a low glucose concentration from injection of relatively excessive amounts of insulin, there is no capacity to regulate the body's total insulin concentration – once it is injected beneath the skin, there is no taking it back!

Patients with type 2 diabetes are not sensitive to the insulin that they do make. Therefore, if hypoglycemia begins to occur, their insulin-producing beta cells simply shut down the production of insulin and the body runs off of what was put under the skin. So hypoglycemia in patients with type 2 diabetes is much less common compared with that in type 1 diabetes patients.

The next line of defense is release of glucagon, a hormone produced in cells adjacent to the insulin-producing beta cells in the pancreas. Glucagon goes to the liver and tells it to release stored glucose and to make new glucose. But there's a problem here, too. The alpha cells that make glucagon become dysfunctional and fail to respond to hypoglycemia the longer one lives with either type 1 or type 2 diabetes. The exact reason for this failure is not known, although it is generally believed that the alpha and beta cells communicate back and forth with one another through chemical and nerve signaling in order to cause release of glucagon when you need it. Unfortunately, when the beta cells are destroyed, the communication becomes one-sided, and appropriate glucagon release is lost in the face of low glucose concentrations. Abnormally low, but not absent, glucagon responses are also known to be part of the type 2 diabetes picture.

When glucagon is not available to correct low glucose concentrations, there is another backup plan. The adrenal glands, which sit on top of the kidneys, release the hormone adrenalin (or epinephrine), which tells the liver to break down stored glucose and make new glucose. Adrenalin is like glucagon in this sense, but it induces its effect from completely independent biochemical steps.

During hypoglycemia, rising adrenalin concentrations also tell muscles to stop using glucose and redirect the fuel to the brain. Humans can develop deficiencies in either glucagon or adrenalin and they can still have perfectly normal glucose concentrations. Coupled with diabetes and the need to inject insulin, the defect in glucagon puts adrenalin in the driver's seat as the factor preventing hypoglycemia.

Adrenalin release that occurs during a low blood glucose event has one other desirable side effect—it makes the patient nervous, shaky, and hungry. These symptoms of low blood glucose should drive you to eat and directly help correct the low. But, you guessed it, there is one more glitch in the system, particularly in patients with type 1 diabetes. The release of adrenalin can be lost in response to hypoglycemia (we will go into this more later) and so now we have a patient who cannot reduce internal insulin production, does not release glucagon due to a loss of communication between alpha and beta cells, and also does not have the backup hormone that causes some of the symptoms of hypoglycemia, plus biochemically driving the creation of new glucose production from the liver! With this critical failure, you are now extremely vulnerable to hypoglycemia, and cannot tell when you have a low glucose due to a loss of warning signals.

A couple of final hormones can help to a certain degree. Cortisol from the adrenal glands and growth hormone from the pituitary gland in the brain are released during hypoglycemia but are not important in an immediate response. Instead, they contribute to resolution of the low glucose if it persists for hours (like over the course of a night). So even though you may not be growing in height, you still make growth hormone and it has an additional function of helping you out during a prolonged period of low blood glucose.

The brain is in charge of your body's entire response to a low glucose concentration. The brain runs on glucose, but it can learn to burn breakdown products of fat during times of fasting. Without glucose, the brain stops working, and you pass out. On the way down to unconsciousness, electrical activity can become chaotic in the brain, leading to seizures. Given this near-absolute dependence on glucose for fuel, the brain directs the redundant set of backup systems described above. But there is one final trick for preserving the flow of glucose to your brain. In the face of repeated low blood glucose levels, the brain gets the signal to increase its efficiency in extracting glucose from the circulation. Small channels in the brain allow the movement of glucose into the brain. These channels increase in number if a patient is repeatedly below the normal glucose concentration. By "up-regulating" the number of these channels, the brain is able to suck more glucose out of the circulation at lower glucose levels, thereby preserving its own function.

Here is the dark side of intensified diabetes management: If you push your therapy enough so that you are frequently experiencing blood glucose levels below normal, you may end up with a great A1C, but your brain is going to change its metabolism so that it can maintain a normal "brain glucose concentration" during subsequent hypoglycemia. This may sound like a great idea except that now, in the face of what should be a glucose level that triggers all of the defense mechanisms, the brain is satisfied that it has enough energy, and it doesn't respond to the low body-glucose concentration. In and of itself, this would be no big deal, but the ability to pull this trick off is not infinite. So there is a glucose concentration at which your brain cannot compensate, and it will finally have to shut down operation. The margin of safety from the point at which you are finally made aware of the low brain-glucose level and when you pass out becomes very narrow. After a person with this problem eats something to treat the reaction, it is still going to take minutes for the absorption to occur and there may not be enough time between when they finally get the signal to eat and when they lose consciousness. This is referred to as hypoglycemia unawareness. Mostly we see this in patients with type 1 diabetes, and so we will deal with prevention and treatment of the problem in that section below.

Complications of diabetes, particularly in small blood vessels, are directly linked to A1C both for patients with type 1 and type 2 diabetes. During the Diabetes Control and Complications Trial (DCCT), we demonstrated that better overall glucose levels would prevent eye and kidney disease, as well as reduce nervous system disease. Recently, a history of good glucose control was found to reduce the risk of heart attacks 15 years after the end of the trial. So one would be hard pressed to find a reason not to achieve as near normal glucose control as possible—except for those pesky low blood glucose levels! Although your brain is probably swimming from the review of the preceding facts, be thankful that the system was put together with as much backup built in, otherwise the general public, even without diabetes medications, would be experiencing hypoglycemia all the time!

Type 1 Diabetes

Some limitations exist in your response to a low blood glucose. Let's meet the challenge head on. First of all, in trials of intensified diabetes management, like the DCCT, 60% of the severe episodes of hypoglycemia (seizures/comas/episodes requiring the help of someone else) occurred between the hours of midnight and 4 AM. Measuring your blood glucose level immediately before you go to sleep *every night* is a key way of predicting which nights you are more vulnerable. If you are less than 100 mg/dL, you know this is going to be a night that you are going to need more of a snack, or even some liquid glucose plus a snack.

Given the fact that many patients who achieve near-normal A1C values become accustomed to glucose values of 75 mg/dL to 90 mg/dL, you cannot rely on the "I feel fine" factor. You would do something completely different with a blood glucose of 75 mg/dL than you would with 175 mg/dL, right? You might even skip the snack for 175 mg/dL. I tell my patients that if their glucose is less than 80 mg/dL at bedtime, they should have 6 oz of juice or milk, plus their usual snack.

Snacks may be unnecessary for insulin pump–managed patients, since the programming can be set at the minimum amount to achieve a normal fasting value and reduce the risk of lows during sleep. If you are on a long-acting insulin, like Lantus (glargine) and Levemir (detemir), you are going to go through a period of the night when you have too much insulin in your system to meet your needs. To cover for this fact, you will need to have a small snack, in the neighborhood of 25 grams of starch (half of a peanut butter sandwich, a small container of yogurt, or one half cup of cottage cheese).

Let's say, instead, that you are at 250 mg/dL at bedtime. How long was it since your evening meal? If you eat late (within 2 hours of lying down), resist the urge to take more insulin — the dinnertime insulin is still working and you are likely to see a fall in your blood glucose in the next hours. If it has been 4 hours since you took insulin for your evening meal, then maybe you will need to do a "touch up." Realize, though, that you are not going to be awake to sense the onset of and excessive fall in glucose and so you may not want to be so aggressive.

Many patients use correction factors of 1 unit of insulin for every 50 to 75 mg/dL over a target of 150 mg/dL. So for a blood glucose of 250 mg/dL at bedtime, you might take 2 units of rapid-acting insulin to correct before morning (remember that you cannot mix any other type of insulin in the same syringe with Lantus if that is what has been prescribed for you). My advice is not to try and correct to 100 mg/dL. Shooting for this degree of tight control is asking for trouble over the night. Insulin replacement is not a perfect science and if you try to make it into that, you will eventually pay for it in the way of a major low blood glucose during the night. An occasional fasting glucose of 150 mg/dL is not going to ruin your overall A1C.

This brings up one other topic that is worth mentioning. Insulin has the power to prevent complications. Power is addictive. I have seen more than my fair share of people who come to the conclusion that if they can tolerate a glucose concentration of 65 mg/dL and not have any symptoms, then they must be safe. They conclude that lower is better. One of my great teachers coined a phrase that is still true: "Hypoglycemia begets hypoglycemia." The more lows you have, the more lows you are going to have. Remember that you lose the symptoms of low glucose concentrations the more times you experience them.

As much as we strive to help patients reduce the number of high blood glucose levels they have, we also have to work equally hard to minimize the number of lows. The A1C is just the average blood glucose level, and you can get a "great number" with a lot of lows balanced against a lot of highs. When you interact with your diabetes team, do not forget that you are more than a number every 3 months—you have to consider your day-to-day control, both highs and lows.

I Am Not Drunk, I Have Diabetes

Alcohol deserves special mention in this section, especially for the patient with type 1 diabetes. Alcohol prevents the liver from making glucose. Insulin does the same thing in a different way, and the two added together can be double trouble. Drinking is part of growing up and so in my young patients, I understand that they are going to experiment—especially when they go off to college. Everything in moderation is a good motto for liquor and diabetes. Because judgment is impaired during hypoglycemia and also with alcohol intoxication, you can imagine the effect of the two of them together. I used to give patients cards that read "I'm not drunk, I have diabetes," since hypoglycemia can be mistaken for drunken behavior. I have gotten realistic enough to understand that humans will experiment in risk-taking behaviors even after having been informed of the danger—and I do not give out those cards anymore! If you are going to drink, then take precautions to have something near you to treat a reaction during the night. If I could get you to do it, I would have you wake up in the night and check a blood glucose. At least have a small additional snack before falling asleep—alcohol-associated hypoglycemia usually occurs hours into your sleep period.

Sex Is Exercise

While we are talking about hypoglycemia in the bedroom, let's also cover the risk of hypoglycemia after sex. Sex is exercise. You use muscles for this activity just as much as though you went to the gym or for a swim. The longer the duration of sexual activity, the greater the use of glucose to fuel the muscles in your legs and arms.

Exercise involves muscles using glucose. Every time you exercise, you should know what your glucose level is going into the episode. Some of my patients prefer to have a snack before exercise or sex in order to prevent hypoglycemia. The longer the exercise period, the more monitoring you should do and the more calories that you may need to ingest. A long bike ride on a Saturday could require frequent snack intake to keep you from getting too low.

Treating Hypoglycemia

Treatment of hypoglycemia is a simple task, as long as you have your head about you. The first few times it happens, you will feel the overwhelming urge to open the refrigerator door and inhale everything in front of you. Eating or drinking more than you actually need to correct the low blood glucose is not going to make you return to normal any faster! Your best bet is to drink 6 to 8 oz of your favorite juice. The goal is to treat your glucose back up to a normal value, not to drive it into the stratosphere.

It will take at least 10 minutes for your blood glucose to start to recover. To reassure yourself that you have stayed the same or started to go back toward normal, recheck your glucose often the first few times that you experience a low.

Liquid sugar is always going to be better than a solid, and so I suggest that patients buy and carry with them small boxes of juice. They do not require refrigeration and they have about 12 to 18 grams of sugar in them—just the right amount for one reaction. Thus the temptation to overdo the treatment is partially taken out of your hands. Alternatively, you might choose to have glucose tablets with you since they are also convenient and do not spoil. But remember that you will have to eat 3 to 5 tabs to get the right amount of sugar to treat the reaction.

Milk is one of the best treatments for a low blood glucose, but you have to be near a refrigerator, so it is not practical when you are away from home. About 6 oz of milk is sufficient, and because of the protein and fat in it, carbohydrate absorption is slowed down so you get a slower but more sustained return to normal.

Solid substances, other than glucose tabs, are always going to be slower to fix the low blood glucose because they have to be broken down from their solid form. I advise against candy bars and ice cream for the treatment of insulin reactions since you get a lot of calories along with the sugar. In the long run, all patients are going to have to fight the battle of weight gain, even patients with type 1 diabetes who are slender at the time of diagnosis.

Glucagon

In an emergency, there is nothing like an injection of glucagon to save the day. Although your body may not appropriately release glucagon during a low-glucose period, an injection of 1 mg, prescribed by your physician, is very powerful. The injection can be given in muscle or fat.

Generally, the patient's parent, significant other, or an appointed person will be the one administering it, because the time to use it is when you cannot swallow. If the brain does not have enough glucose, it cannot coordinate the muscles in the throat to do the swallowing action. Giving someone sugar by mouth at that point will cause part of the treatment to go into the lungs. If the person with you assesses that you are not capable of swallowing, then they need to get out the glucagon.

Some formulations of glucagon require that the liquid be mixed with the solid prior to injecting it. Give the person most likely to administer the glucagon an opportunity to become familiar with the type of glucagon you have been prescribed. It will take 15 to 20 minutes for your glucose to recover from this treatment, but that is faster than most paramedics can come to the rescue. It is probably preferable to most people to wake up to a familiar face rather than to that of a stranger hovering above them.

Losing Consciousness

If you have gotten such a low glucose that your brain's electrical activity is not working well, you may have a seizure or convulsion. Fortunately, you will not remember most of what happens, but it can be frightening to the person helping you to watch your arms and legs jerk uncontrollably. Direct your likely helper to turn you on your side so that if you drool, it goes out of your mouth and not down into your lungs. Besides not giving you sugar by mouth, also tell him/her not to put anything in your mouth. (In the old days, people thought that they needed to keep patients from biting in their tongues when they were low. Putting a finger into someone's mouth experiencing a seizure is a great way to lose it!) Talking through this procedure ahead of an occurrence with the person most likely to treat you will prevent a great deal of chaos during an episode.

Brief periods of this severe kind of low are not likely to lead to brain damage. If glucagon is given, the effect of restoring the glucose to normal may be short-lived, and when you are able to do so, you should eat something. However, many people become nauseous after receiving glucagon, so I recommend crackers and water to keep it simple. These seem to be less likely to increase the nausea.

Hypoglycemia Unawareness

Considering all of the patient-driven tools we have discussed to protect against hypoglycemia and the redundancies in hormonal responses with which we have all been equipped, bad events still happen. Vigilance in monitoring your glucose concentrations is undoubtedly the key to knowing where you are going to be in the next hours. As cumbersome as testing frequently may be, it still represents the key method of preventing low bloods glucose levels.

After accounting for unusual exercise, missed snacks, and alcohol consumption, 90% of the severe episodes of hypoglycemia in DCCT remained unexplained. Many of the investigators believed it was the development of hypoglycemia unawareness that explained much of the excess risk.

Patients who develop hypoglycemia unawareness, who very carefully avoided subsequent low glucose concentrations for even short periods regain their symptoms of hypoglycemia. If you develop unawareness, try backing off on how tightly you are running your blood glucose levels. Set your target a little higher. You will not compromise your A1C control that much, but you will regain your ability to know when you are low and increase the safety for yourself and for those around you. Driving a car with a low blood glucose is obviously dangerous and can be substantially reduced by monitoring your blood glucose and then doing something about it!

Case #1: Type 1 Diabetes

Let's recap all of this information by reviewing the case of a patient I took care of who died tragically after living with diabetes for 26 years. This patient had rather severe diabetic gastroparesis, which means that food she ingested processed too slowly from the stomach into the small intestine where absorption should occur. This is a form of neuropathy that is fairly common in both type 2 and type 1 diabetes. When it happens, gastroparesis makes patients with type 1 diabetes particularly more vulnerable to low blood glucose levels, since insulin injected before the meal may get into the circulation more rapidly than the glucose from the food can be absorbed. Further, the recovery from hypoglycemia can be slow since even the rate of absorption of sugar from a liquid treatment is slow.

The patient in this story was a nurse who worked early morning shifts. She lived alone, and one morning she failed to come into work on time. She had experienced repeated bouts of low blood glucose levels that she had tried to prevent and treat appropriately but because she had developed hypoglycemia unawareness, she often did not know she was very low. She always measured a bedtime glucose concentration, and sometimes would take a few extra units of rapid-acting insulin at bedtime if her glucose was too high (she used 1 unit for every 60 points above 150 mg/dL).

Because of the erratic absorption of the glucose from her diet, predicting where her blood glucose value was going to be at any time of the day or night was difficult. She had eaten a typical evening meal the night before this major episode of hypoglycemia and had taken 4 units of rapid-acting insulin, infused by her pump over 2 hours beginning at the time of the meal. (One way of managing the issue of getting too much insulin in the system before the food has a chance to be absorbed in such patients is to have them take the dose at or after the time of the meal, or, if one is using an insulin infusion pump, we recommend spreading the dose out over several hours.) At bedtime, 2 and a half hours after the meal, she found she was too high and took an extra 4 units of rapid-acting insulin. (This patient was a great record keeper and had written it down in her logbook.) Her background insulin was delivered by an insulin pump. Her most recent A1C was 7.0%.

When she failed to show up for work, her colleagues called her home, and one of them eventually went over to check on her. At 10 AM, she was found lying in bed taking short, shallow breaths every now and then. She could not be aroused. After having her blood glucose treated with emergency intravenous glucose by the paramedics, her blood glucose was over 200 mg/dL. Three months later, she had still not come back from her coma, developed pneumonia, and after a difficult course, she died.

This case represents a rare but real risk of managing type 1 diabetes intensively. Admittedly she had a condition (gastroparesis) that further predisposed her to getting low, but she made one critical error: she took a large dose of insulin at bedtime. So she was heading into the most vulnerable time of the day with an already impaired ability to detect hypoglycemia, and now had a lot of insulin in her system.

Four units may not seem like much to some patients who have type 2 diabetes and who may take over 100 units of insulin per day, but the usual insulin replacement dose average in a 110-pound woman (this woman's real weight) is only about 40 units. An extra 4 units represents a 10% increase given at a time when she was not eating anything. (As it turns out, she did the math wrong with the correction factor and took 1.5 units more than she should have.)

One other important lesson is taught from this sad case: repeating or supplementing insulin doses within 4 hours of the injection of a previous rapid-acting insulin dose can lead to trouble. The final effect of the first dose is not known before the next dose is given. We walk a fine line of enough is good enough and a bit more is dangerous.

Type 2 Diabetes

Remember that all of the preceding mentioned lines of hormonal protection are available to patients with type 2 diabetes, plus they have the capacity to shut down their own body's production of insulin in the face of falling blood glucose concentration. Therefore, it is much more difficult to cause severe hypoglycemia in these patients.

Some of the oral medications for the control of type 2 diabetes can cause hypoglycemia, particularly the sulfonylurea (SFU) medications (Glucotrol [glipizide], Glibenclamide [glyburide], and Micronase [glyburide] are examples) by causing the beta cells to pump out their insulin even in the face of a normal or low blood glucose.

The leading population at risk is generally the elderly. Because many older folks tend to eat a larger meal during the middle of the day and a lighter evening meal, they can run out of fuel during the night. The SFUs work for 24 hours and therefore increase the risk of hypoglycemia during sleep.

The other main class of medications, metformin and the thiazolidinediones (TZDs), do not drive the body to make more insulin and therefore have very limited, if any, ability to cause low blood glucose levels. But when combined with an SFU, hypoglycemia can be seen with metformin and/or a TZD. The risk of hypoglycemia with these combinations is probably a function of the baseline hemoglobin A1C being much closer to normal before the second medication is added.

Generally, when hypoglycemia occurs in someone with type 2 diabetes, it is not associated with loss of consciousness. The event still needs to be treated, but the more severe episodes seen in patients with type 1 diabetes are thankfully fairly rare. The newest class of medications to become available to treat patients with type 2 diabetes, the GLP-1 agonists (Byetta [exenatide]), have no capacity to cause hypoglycemia by themselves. Given with metformin or TZD medications, exenatide does not cause an increased risk of hypoglycemia. But when an SFU is present, the addition of exenatide increases the risk of nonsevere hypoglycemia substantially during the first months of treatment. If you are on an SFU when exenatide is added to your treatment, the dose of the SFU should be reduced.

Case #2: Type 2 Diabetes

Severe hypoglycemia can and does occur when insulin treatment is added to any of the preceding therapies. To demonstrate this point, let me tell you the story of a woman with type 2 diabetes who was managed with metformin and SFUs. She was not at her target A1C, so the decision was made to add insulin to her treatment regimen. She measured her glucose every morning and then took her insulin before driving to the nursing home where she worked. Her routine was to eat breakfast after she got to work.

One morning she had a glucose concentration of 64 mg/dL at home, took her insulin, and about 40 minutes later was in a head-on accident with an 18-wheeler. The driver of the truck saw her slumped over the wheel as she swerved across the median into the front of his rig.

Her glucose concentration at the site of the accident was low, and on arrival to the emergency room it remained low. She now lives in a mentally compromised state in a long-term care facility. Some disconnect had occurred in her education about the use of insulin, eating, and driving.

Insulin is an important addition to the treatment of many patients with type 2 diabetes, and this case is a reasonably uncommon story, but nonetheless, severe hypoglycemia can also be associated with insulin use in both forms of diabetes.

Summary

While hypoglycemia can be a barrier to getting the best control over your blood glucose, most times it is a bother in your day that takes time away from being at your best. Prevention is the best strategy for managing hypoglycemia. If it cannot be prevented, then try not to overtreat it because you will set up the vicious cycle of yo-yoing up and down. Last, especially if you have type 1 diabetes, try to trust someone to be close enough to you that they can spot that your blood glucose is low, even if you are relatively unaware.

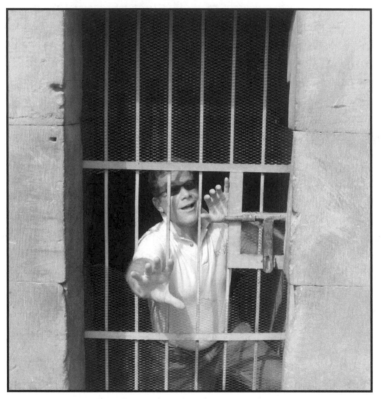

Jailed for a bad A1C value!

12

Trust Me! You Do Not Want to Have a Heart Attack or Stroke

Introduction

I lost my best friend, Ken Facter, to a sudden and unexpected heart attack at the young age of 41. Most people with diabetes do not realize that heart disease or atherosclerosis is one of the more serious and common complications in people with diabetes as well as in the general public. Atherosclerosis is the process of the buildup of fat deposits in the arteries or blood vessels, making it more difficult for blood to pass through them. The end result is total occlusion, leading to severe damage of the tissues of the heart and

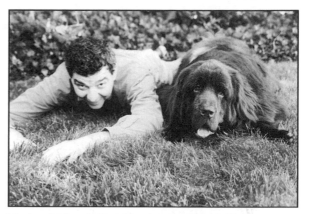

My best friend, Ken Facter, and his faithful companion, Chief.

brain. The classic microvascular complications of eye, kidney, and nerve disease are usually discussed and more often stressed in the diabetes literature. Heart attack, stroke, and clogging of the blood vessels of the legs are classified as macrovascular complications because they involve the large (macro) arteries or blood vessels of the body. We now know that preventing and aggressively treating the risk factors for macrovascular disease is equally important.

You may find it surprising that up to 80% of people with type 2 diabetes "get off the bus" because of heart attacks and strokes, and not from the classic microvascular complications. I hate to be so morbid as to use words such as mortality or death; I like to use the phrase "get off the bus" instead. I hope this more gentle term does not take away from the seriousness of the problem. Heart disease and stroke are the leading killers of Americans, diabetic or not. **Figure 12-1** demonstrates how dramatic the situation really is. This figure shows the mortality (death rate) due to coronary artery disease in men and women with type 2

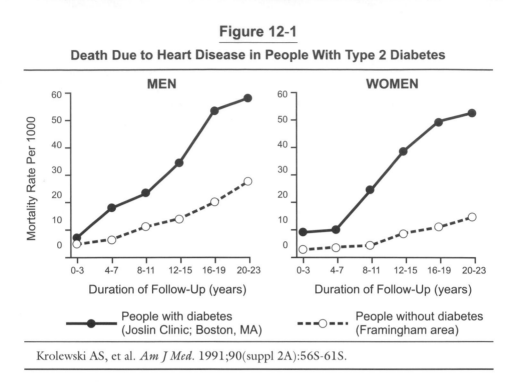

Figure 12-1

Death Due to Heart Disease in People With Type 2 Diabetes

People with diabetes (Joslin Clinic; Boston, MA)

People without diabetes (Framingham area)

Krolewski AS, et al. *Am J Med.* 1991;90(suppl 2A):56S-61S.

diabetes compared with the rate in people without diabetes over time. The mortality rate is recorded as the number of deaths per 1000 people. Time zero indicates the time of diagnosis of diabetes in these people, whose are in the neighborhood of 40 to 50 years of age. You can see that in only a few short years after the time of diagnosis, the death rate due to heart disease in people with diabetes starts to significantly accelerate and separate from that in the nondiabetics. Please notice that in nondiabetic individuals, the women have fewer heart problems compared with men. This fact is referred to as a "cardiovascular advantage" that nondiabetic women usually enjoy compared with nondiabetic men. However, now look at the death rate due to heart disease in the diabetic women compared with that in the diabetic men. It is the same, and the cardiovascular advantage is lost. The explanation for this phenomenon is unclear, but one thing is certain: Women with type 2 diabetes are at extreme risk for premature heart disease, especially after they reach menopause.

Another major problem is that people with diabetes may have a diminished sensation of the early warning signs of heart disease (for example, chest pain). This can lead to a dangerous situation since treatment can be instituted early if a person goes to the emergency room or clinic with chest pain rather than sitting at home, unaware that heart disease is present (the medical term for this condition is *silent ischemia*). The reason for this lack of awareness of cardiac symptoms is unknown, but may be related to pain fibers being damaged by diabetes just as occurs with neuropathy in the feet. In a similar fashion to retinopathy and diabetic kidney disease, serious and advanced heart disease can be present without any symptoms. Unfortunately, when the first symptom (such as chest pain) finally occurs, it may be too late to intervene. Awareness of these potential problems by you and your doctor is the key.

People with type 2 diabetes are normally diagnosed later in life and, therefore, are more likely to have heart disease just because of their advanced age in addition to the added effects of poorly controlled diabetes on the large blood vessels. High blood pressure and high cholesterol levels also contribute to the increased risk of heart disease. People with type 1 diabetes do not develop heart disease until later in life because they are usually diagnosed with diabetes at a much younger age, although the incidence is still much higher than in people of the same age without type 1 diabetes.

You must be aware of the risk factors for heart disease and stroke so that you can do everything in your power to prevent, detect, and aggressively treat them. This chapter will focus on the important information that you need to know to take control of the situation. Trust me—you do not want to be a cardiac cripple or a paralyzed stroke victim.

Risk Factors for Heart Disease and Stroke

You and your caregiver can modify several of the risk factors that contribute to heart disease. Unfortunately, you cannot change your age, gender, family history, or the fact that you are a diabetic. However, it is important that you look at each one of these risk factors carefully and decide if you can improve your own situation. The more risk factors that you have, the more aggressive you should be with modifying the changeable ones. The risk factors are listed in **Table 12-1** and discussed below.

Table 12-1

**Risk Factors for
Heart Disease and Stroke**

- Existing heart disease (atherosclerosis)
- A family history of heart disease (atherosclerosis)
- Age >45 years in men and >55 years in women
- Diabetes
- Tobacco smoking
- Severe weight problem
- High blood pressure
- Abnormal cholesterol levels

Existing Heart Disease or Atherosclerosis

If you already have had a heart attack or stroke, then your chances of having further problems are greatly increased. Now is the time to be the most aggressive to modify your risk factors. I have patients who have lived long and healthy lives after their first heart attack because they did take the situation seriously.

Family History of Atherosclerosis

Heart disease is a hereditary condition. If anyone in your immediate family has had heart problems, you may be at greater risk. Your immediate family includes your siblings, parents, uncles, aunts, and grandparents. Sorry, but your healthy spouse will not help you out here. Having a family history of heart disease is a very important risk factor, and although we cannot change our family history, we can be aggressive with our treatment plan.

Age and Gender

Age and gender play important roles in determining risk status. If you are a man and older than 45 years or a woman older than 55 years, your risk of heart disease significantly increases. These numbers were determined from large epidemiologic observational studies in nondiabetic individuals. Many experts say that the age limits should be 10 years lower for people with diabetes. If you are a female, please note what I said earlier about having diabetes and the risk of heart disease.

Existing Diabetes

Obviously, you cannot change the fact that you have diabetes, but you can work on improving control of your diabetes. It has been shown that you can reduce heart disease by improving your glucose control. The effects of aggressive blood pressure and cholesterol control most likely have greater influence over the rate of heart attacks and strokes but glucose control also plays a role. Excessive levels of glucose in your blood end up sticking to and damaging the blood vessels of your body. The arteries that deliver oxygen to your heart, brain, and lower extremities seem to be especially vulnerable. It is not just your eyes, kidneys, and nerves that are adversely affected by poor glucose control.

Cigarette Smoking

I know that cigarette smoking is a tough habit to break, but it really is a killer in terms of causing heart attack and stroke, especially in people with diabetes. It is definitely one of the worst habits to have as a diabetic and one of the more difficult to stop (other than eating those hot fudge sundaes). It has been shown that there is a powerful negative synergistic effect between smoking and diabetes. Even if you cut down your smoking by 50%, you will have done yourself a great favor. I will not dwell on this point, because I know you get grief from everyone around you if you currently smoke. Do anything you can, using any technique, to stop or reduce your cigarette consumption. Trust me—you do not want to be in need of a heart or lung transplant.

Severe Weight Problems

If you are 20% to 30% over your ideal weight, then you certainly do not need me to tell you that the excessive adiposity (fat) puts a tremendous strain on your heart. People with severe weight problems need a supportive health care team, including a clinical psychologist, to help them overcome emotional barriers and adhere to a weight-loss and maintenance program. It is not easy, and currently there is no magic pill for weight loss. We do have new drugs that may be very helpful for people with diabetes to lose weight, such as Byetta (exenatide) and Symlin (pramlintide); Acomplia (rimonabant) is currently under development.

High Blood Pressure

High blood pressure is an important modifiable risk factor. Keeping your blood pressure in the normal range will help prevent macrovascular disease (heart attack and stroke), as well as microvascular disease (kidney failure and eye disease). Controlling your blood pressure is discussed in Chapter 14 and will be discussed further in this chapter.

Abnormal Cholesterol Levels

Abnormal cholesterol levels are common in people with diabetes and are one of the main contributors to accelerating the atherosclerotic process. The cholesterol abnormalities seen in people with diabetes are complicated and deserve a detailed discussion later in this chapter.

Controlling High Blood Pressure

Aggressive blood pressure control is probably one of the more powerful interventions for reducing the incidence of heart attack and stroke. As mentioned earlier, I believe it is important that every person with high blood pressure have a home blood pressure–monitoring device, just as every person with diabetes should have a glucose-monitoring device. You should also take several readings a week at different times and record them for *you* to analyze and discuss with your caregiver. You can pick up a blood pressure–monitoring device at your local pharmacy or larger discount store. Choose one that you feel comfortable using and one that has a good return policy. It is also important to bring your blood pressure device with you on your office visit once or twice a year to have the staff check it for accuracy.

It is imperative that you know how normal blood pressure is defined. The American Diabetes Association currently recommends treatment to lower blood pressure to at least less than 130/80 mm Hg, and if you have evidence of protein in your urine (microalbuminuria), your blood pressure should be less than 120/80 mm Hg.

In general, there are some basic treatment strategies that I follow that may help you in working with your caregiver to tailor your program to effectively reach your blood pressure goals. These general treatment strategies are listed in **Table 12-2** and discussed next.

Do Not Delay Aggressive Therapy

Once high blood pressure is detected, there should be no delay in instituting aggressive therapy. Many doctors and patients wait too long before antihypertensive measures are undertaken. High blood pressure does not normally cause any pain or discomfort, and because of this fact, therapy is too often delayed. Believe it or not, for some patients, it takes several years before the appropriate treatment regimen is in place. Do not let yourself go untreated.

Table 12-2

General Treatment Strategies for Treating High Blood Pressure in People With Diabetes

- Do not delay aggressive therapy
- Know your blood pressure goals and values
- Know about the side effects of the drugs you take
- Design a regimen that is simple and easy to follow on a day-to-day basis
- Combining medications may be needed
- Avoid drugs that exacerbate your diabetes and other associated conditions

Know Your Blood Pressure Goals and Values

You need to know what your blood pressure runs on average during your daily activities. Your blood pressure at the doctor's office may not be indicative of your true values. This is why you need to get a blood pressure–monitoring device and use it at home and other places such as work. This will allow you to determine whether your blood pressure values are within the goal range most of the time. Remember that blood pressure values fluctuate during the day, so repeated measurements are important in order to get an adequate overview of your blood pressure.

Know About the Side Effects of the Drugs

It is your responsibility to know the side effects of the drugs with which you are being treated. Read and ask questions about the side effects. Some of the side effects you will be able to live with (especially because you knew about them ahead of time) and others will limit your use of a particular medication. Fortunately, we do have lots of choices.

Design a Regimen That Is Simple and Easy to Follow

Design a regimen that is simple and easy to follow on a day-to-day basis. Most people can take medications two times a day on a regular basis without forgetting. It is more difficult to take medications three times a day and almost impossible for most people to take drugs four times a day for an extended period of time. Most likely, you will be on high blood pressure medication indefinitely. Many of my patients, including myself, take several blood pressure medications in the morning and at bedtime. I use two little cups in which I put my blood pressure pills. I prepare the two cups at bedtime so that after I wake up and brush my teeth, the second morning cup of pills is ready and waiting for me to swallow. I also keep a small supply of pills at work just in case I forget to take them at home. I ask my wife and kids to call me if they find that my little pill cup is full after I leave for work. Everyone's habits and schedules are different, and you need to design a pill schedule that works easily for you. Even if you have the smartest doctor in the world and access to the best drugs, it is of no benefit to your health if your medication schedule is too complicated so that you forget to take the drugs regularly.

Combining Medications

The hypertension of diabetes is a tough condition to treat, and it is the rule, rather than the exception, that you may need more than one type of blood pressure medication. I am on three different medications that work in different ways to control my blood pressure. In addition, at least 60% of my patients with diabetes and hypertension need more than one medication to control their blood pressure. Remember that it's not how many pills you take, but rather how well your blood pressure is controlled. Most of the various antihypertensive medications can be used together safely with little or no side effects. Some of the common combinations will be discussed later.

Treatment Options

There are many different types of medications that are available to lower your blood pressure. You need to become familiar with them so that you can carry on an intelligent conversation with your caregiver and play an active role in your treatment plan. **Table 12-3** lists the various categories of blood pressure medications with a few examples of each type.

It is not really feasible or necessary to discuss in detail the pharmacologic therapy for high blood pressure. There are entire medical textbooks written on this subject alone. Conversely, I feel it is important to discuss some of the therapeutic strategies for monotherapy (using only one drug) and combination therapy that are commonly prescribed for people with hypertension and diabetes. The main goal is to get the blood pressure down to at least 130/80 mm Hg and to less than 120/80 mm Hg if there is evidence of protein in the urine that is indicative of kidney damage. If the blood pressure goals are not reached with a single drug, then a second agent is added to the first one (combination therapy). It is not uncommon for people with diabetes to need three and four different medications to control their blood pressure. It is much better to have normal blood pressure and be on four different types of medication than to have elevated blood pressure and be on only one drug. It is sometimes difficult to get over that psychological block about "taking all of those damn pills."

ACE Inhibitors and ARBs

An ACE inhibitor or an ARB is usually the drug of choice when initiating antihypertensive therapy; this is also discussed in Chapter 14. ACE inhibitors have been proven effective at preventing and slowing the progression of atherosclerosis, in addition to protecting the kidneys.

Angiotensin-converting enzyme inhibitors and ARBs have few side effects and are tolerated well. ACE inhibitors and ARBs can be taken once or twice a day and can be safely combined with other medications to reduce the blood pressure to the desired goal. There are two situations in which ACE inhibitors should be used with caution: The first is in people who have a tendency to have high potassium levels in the blood. The second is a condition called renal artery stenosis. ACE inhibitors can also cause a persistent, dry cough in a small percentage of people.

Direct Renin Inhibitor

Tekturna (aliskiren) is a new type of blood pressure–lowering agent called a direct renin inhibitor. Tekturna reduces the effect of renin (a hormone in the kidney that in high levels will cause high blood pressure) and the harmful process that narrows blood vessels. Tekturna helps blood vessels relax and widen blood vessels so blood pressure is lowered. It can be added to all other blood pressure–lowering agents

Table 12-3

Blood Pressure Medications*

Angiotensin-Converting Enzyme (ACE) Inhibitors
- Benazepril (Lotensin)
- Captopril (Capoten)
- Enalapril (Vasotec)
- Fosinopril (Monopril)
- Lisinopril (Prinivil, Zestril)
- Moexipril (Univasc)
- Perindopril (Aceon)
- Quinapril (Accupril)
- Ramipril (Altace)
- Trandolapril (Mavik)

Angiotensin Receptor Blockers (ARBs)
- Candesartan (Atacand)
- Eprosartan (Teveten)
- Irbesartan (Avapro)
- Losartan (Cozaar)
- Olmesartan (Benicar)
- Telmisartan (Micardis)
- Valsartan (Diovan)

Direct Renin Inhibitor
- Aliskiren (Tekturna)

Calcium Channel Blockers
- Amlodipine (Norvasc)
- Diltiazem (Cardizem, Cartia XT, Dilacor, Diltia XT, Tiazac)
- Felodipine (Plendil)
- Isradipine (DynaCirc)
- Nicardipine (Cardene)
- Nifedipine (Adalat)
- Nifedipine GITS (Procardia XL)
- Nimodipine (Nimotop)
- Nisoldipine (Sular)
- Verapamil LA (Calan SR, Covera-HS, Isoptin SR, Verelan)

Alpha-Blockers
- Doxazosin (Cardura)
- Prazosin (Minipress)
- Terazosin (Hytrin)

Centrally Acting Agents
- Clonidine (Catapres, Catapres-TTS)
- Guanabenz (Wytensin)
- Guanfacine (Tenex)
- Methyldopa (Aldomet)

Indoline Diuretic
- Indapamide (Lozol)

Thiazide Diuretics
- Chlorothiazide (Diuril)
- Hydrochlorothiazide (Esidrix)
- Methyclothiazide (Enduron)

Beta-Blockers
- Atenolol (Tenormin)
- Betaxolol (Kerlone)
- Bisoprolol (Zebeta)
- Carvedilol (Coreg)
- Metoprolol (Lopressor, Toprol-XL)
- Nadolol (Corgard)
- Propranolol (Inderal, Inderal LA)

Combinations
- ACE inhibitors and diuretics (Lotensin, Captozide, Vaseretic, Monopril HCT, Prinzide, Zestoretic, Uniretic, Accuretic)
- ARBs and diuretics (Atacand HCT, Teveten HCT, Avalide, Hyzaar, Benicar HCT, Micardis HCT, Diovan HCT)
- Beta-adrenergic blockers and diuretics (Tenoretic, Ziac, Lopressor HCT, Corzide, Inderide LA, Timolide)
- Calcium channel blockers and ACE inhibitors (Lotrel, Lexxel, Tarka)
- Other combinations (Moduretic, Clorpres, Aldoril, Minizide, Diupres, Hydropres, Aldactazide, Dyazide, Maxzide)

Combination to Treat Hypertension and Abnormal Cholesterol Levels
- Caduet (amlodipine/atorvastatin)

* Not all drugs in each category are listed.

and has a very low side effect profile. It should not be taken by women who are pregnant or planning to become pregnant.

Calcium Channel Blockers

Calcium channel blockers also represent a commonly used class of antihypertensive medications for people with diabetes. In general, they are well tolerated with few side effects and can be taken once or twice a day. Each calcium channel blocker is slightly different from the others, and it is important for you to ask your caregiver or read about the one you are prescribed. They have a different mechanism of action than the other classes of medications, so they can have beneficial synergistic effects on your blood pressure when combined with the other drugs, especially ACE inhibitors or ARBs. The combination of a calcium channel blocker and an ACE inhibitor is probably one of the more commonly prescribed combinations. Women who are pregnant or trying to become pregnant should not take ACE inhibitors or ARBs as they have been shown to cause problem for the fetus.

Alpha-Blockers

Alpha-blockers represent another class of blood pressure agents that seem especially well-suited for people with diabetes. Once again, the newer drugs listed in **Table 12-3** have few side effects and can be taken once or twice a day at the most. Alpha-blockers can be added safely to other medications such as ACE inhibitors and calcium channel blockers. Alpha-blockers may also favorably affect your cholesterol levels.

It is important to take alpha-blockers exactly as prescribed, especially when you are initiating therapy, because they can cause dizziness upon standing (orthostasis). Most of the time, alpha-blockers are started at bedtime to avoid this problem, which dissipates in a few days.

Centrally Acting Agents

Centrally acting agents, such as clonidine, represent an older class of medications. However, they can be effective to get your blood pressure under control. They are usually not used as first- or second-line therapy because they sometimes cause dry mouth and tiredness. A skin patch for clonidine is available, which may be better tolerated than the pills, and you only have to change the patch every 7 days.

Indoline Diuretic

Indapamide is an excellent additive medication to control the blood pressure. It is a once-a-day drug with no side effects. It is normally not a first-line agent because it is not as potent at lowering the blood pressure and therefore many physicians are not familiar with this drug.

I frequently prescribe indapamide as the third-line agent, after ACE inhibitors and calcium channel blockers.

Thiazide Diuretics and Beta-Blockers

Thiazide diuretics and beta-blockers may slightly worsen your diabetes control and associated conditions such as high cholesterol levels. They were the workhorses of the 70s, 80s, and early 90s; however, they should not be used as first-line therapy, but rather as additional medications to the newer drugs, such as the ACE inhibitors, ARBs, and calcium channel blockers, which do not have these adverse side effects. Don't panic if you are on a thiazide diuretic or beta-blocker since there may be a very good reason why your physician has decided to use this medication. For example, some patients are put on a low-dose thiazide diuretic if there is a kidney problem or if fluid retention is present. I prescribe low-dose thiazide diuretics occasionally if the more standard drugs of choice are ineffective at getting the blood pressure down to goal ranges. Furthermore, some of the newer beta-blockers have been formulated or designed to be more diabetic-friendly (carvedilol or Coreg is one of the newer beta-blockers that is diabetic-friendly). In general, thiazide diuretics and beta-blockers are effective at lowering the blood pressure. Remember that the primary goal is to get the blood pressure down, no matter how you do it!

Controlling Cholesterol Levels

Abnormal cholesterol levels are another major contributor to atherosclerosis, leading to heart attack and stroke. Unfortunately, people with diabetes are prone to cholesterol problems and suffer from clogging of the arteries that deliver blood to the heart, brain, and legs. Once again, like many other complications of diabetes, abnormal cholesterol levels are painless and do not cause symptoms. This can be a dangerous situation.

It is important to clarify what types of lipids or cholesterol exist and the goals of therapy (**Table 12-4**). There are three different types of cholesterol or lipoproteins that are normally measured in your blood in a lipid panel. The LDL (low-density lipoprotein or bad cholesterol), HDL (high-density lipoprotein or good cholesterol), and triglycerides are all forms of cholesterol, but differ in size, shape, density, and have different functions. You should have a lipid panel measuring the different types of cholesterol done once a year or more frequently if you are initiating or adjusting cholesterol medications.

Most diabetes specialists recommend that all people with diabetes get their LDL value below 100 mg/dL if they have had no problems with their heart at all and below 70 mg/dL if they have had a heart attack

Table 12-4

Goals of Therapy for Cholesterol Levels in People With Diabetes

	Total*	HDL	LDL	TG
Heart disease present†	<200	>40 (men) >50 (women)	<70 (well below 100)	<150
No heart disease	<200	>40 (men) >50 (women)	<100	<200

Abbreviations: HDL, high-density lipoprotein (cholesterol); LDL, low-density lipoprotein (cholesterol); TG, triglycerides.

* The total cholesterol may be misleading in determining your risk of heart disease. See text. All values are in milligrams per deciliter (mg/dL).
† Heart attacks, congestive heart failure, strokes, etc.

is the past. One must fast to get an accurate fasting triglyceride value (nothing to eat past midnight with the blood drawn first thing in the morning before eating), which is used to calculate the LDL cholesterol. In reality, you do not have to fast for the total cholesterol and HDL, but they are usually all measured together at the same time anyway.

I use the word "abnormal" when discussing the cholesterol or lipid problems in people with diabetes because it is not simply that the LDL levels are too high or that the HDL levels are too low. There are other characteristics of the different types of cholesterol or lipoprotein that increase the risk of atherosclerosis. For example, the LDL and HDL cholesterols get "oxidized" and "glycosylated" (glucose molecules stick to them), making them more dangerous in terms of causing heart disease. This is why antioxidants and improved glucose control may help lower your risk of a heart attack or stroke in addition to normalizing the absolute levels (**Table 12-5**).

Have a Lipid Panel Done

A lipid panel will consist of four different values (total cholesterol, LDL, triglycerides, and the HDL). The total cholesterol value may be a misleading number in determining your risk of heart disease. The total cholesterol is made up of both the LDL and the HDL cholesterol levels. Since the HDL or good

Table 12-5

Lipid Abnormalities Seen in People With Type 2 Diabetes

- Elevated triglyceride levels
- Low high-density lipoprotein (HDL) levels (good cholesterol)
- "Abnormal" changes in the low-density lipoprotein (LDL) (bad) and HDL (good) cholesterol structures:
  - Oxidized
  - Glycosylated

cholesterol levels are normally low in people with diabetes, the total cholesterol level is lower than it would be in people with high levels of this protective HDL or good cholesterol. Do not be lulled into a false sense of security if your total cholesterol level is less than 200. You may still have low HDL and abnormal LDL levels, thus putting you at extreme risk for heart disease. This is why you should get a lipid panel that includes the LDL, HDL, and triglyceride levels and not solely a total cholesterol level.

What do all of these different and complicated lipid abnormalities mean to people with diabetes? Basically, in the simplest terms, we need to be aware of what our cholesterol levels are and work with our health care providers to reach our target goals of therapy. Unfortunately, there are millions of Americans, with and without diabetes, who have untreated abnormal cholesterol levels in the high-risk range. The reasons for this are many, although patient and physician ignorance and apathy play a big part. In addition, there are no symptoms of high cholesterol levels!

Treatment Options

Meal planning and an exercise program are two of the more potent nonpharmacologic ways to improve your cholesterol levels and are discussed in detail in later chapters. However, it is important to emphasize that people with diabetes sometimes have tough-to-treat cholesterol levels, just as they have tough-to-treat high blood pressure. Diet and exercise will rarely bring abnormal cholesterol levels down into the normal range. Even though oral medications may be needed to reach your cholesterol goals, you must maintain some type of dietary and exercise program. I am not asking you to lose 30 pounds, eat lettuce all day, and jog marathons. I know that lifestyle changes must come gradually, in small incremental steps. In addition, you can improve your cholesterol levels, especially your triglyceride levels, just by lowering your blood glucose values into a more normal range.

I classify abnormal cholesterol levels into three basic categories when I consider pharmacologic therapy:
1. Elevated LDL cholesterol
2. Elevated triglyceride/low HDL levels
3. Elevations in both LDL cholesterol and triglyceride levels and a low HDL level.

This inverse relationship of high triglyceride levels being associated with low HDL levels is a common abnormality in people with type 2 diabetes. Even though low HDL levels are of concern, there is no medication specifically designed to raise HDL levels. However, a secondary benefit of the other medications used to treat high LDL and triglyceride levels is to raise HDL levels modestly. The drugs commonly used to treat high LDL and/or triglyceride levels are listed in **Table 12-6**.

Most diabetes experts agree that the class of drugs called the statins is the most efficient, safe, and effective way to lower LDL levels. The statins work by blocking the key step in cholesterol production in the liver. There are few side effects and they can be taken once a day, usually at bedtime. The statins may also raise HDL levels 5% to 10%. These drugs have been used in millions of people worldwide and are super safe and effective. The statins are responsible for preventing lots of people from getting off the bus due to heart disease and stroke.

An LDL-lowering medication called Zetia (ezetimibe), which works by blocking the absorption of cholesterol that comes from food is now available. It has very few if any side effects and works well with statins to help people get their LDL levels to goal. A combination pill called

Table 12-6
Drugs to Treat Abnormal Cholesterol Levels

Drugs to Treat High LDL Cholesterol Levels
- The "statins:"
  - Rosuvastatin (Crestor)
  - Fluvastatin (Lescol, Lescol XL)
  - Atorvastatin (Lipitor)
  - Pravastatin (Pravachol)
  - Lovastatin (Mevacor, Altocor)
  - Simvastatin (Zocor)
- Niacin or nicotinic acid:
  - Many over-the-counter preparations (nonprescription vitamin)
  - Niacin extended-release (Niaspan) is a newer niacin formulation that is better tolerated
- Bile acid sequestrants:
  - Colestid (colestipol)
  - Questran (cholestyramine)
  - WelChol (colesevelam)

Cholesterol Absorption Inhibitor
- Zetia (ezetimibe)

Combination Drugs
- Lovastatin/niacin ER (Advicor)
- Vytorin (ezetimibe/simvastatin)

Drugs to Treat High Triglyceride Levels
- Lopid (gemfibrozil)
- Tricor, Lofibra, Triglide, Antara (fenofibrate)
- Niacin extended-release (Niaspan) is a newer niacin formulation that is better tolerated
- Omacor (omega-3-acid ethyl esters)

Combination Drug to Treat Hypertension and Abnormal Cholesterol Levels
- Amlodipine/atorvastatin (Caduet)

Abbreviation: LDL, low-density lipoprotein (cholesterol).

Vytorin (exetimibe/simvastatin) is now available. Please see the following section on combination medications.

Niacin can raise blood glucose levels and cause headaches and flushing. Niaspan is a slow-release niacin preparation that is better tolerated than the over-the-counter niacin preparations. Bile acid sequestrants such as Questran and Colestid commonly cause stomach upset and constipation, and can interfere with the absorption and effectiveness of other drugs or medications that you take in the same time period. Niacin and Questran have been prescribed less frequently since the new statins are more effective and easier to take.

High triglyceride levels are best treated with Lopid (gemfibrozil) or Tricor (fenofibrate). These two medications have few side effects and must be taken twice a day. When the triglycerides are initially high (>400 mg/dL), one can see a dramatic drop in the triglyceride levels of up to 40% and a 10% to 25% increase in the HDL levels (when triglyceride levels drop, the HDL levels usually go up and vice versa). I want to emphasize that if your glucose control is poor, it will be difficult to bring the triglyceride levels to normal. Niacin also lowers triglyceride and raises HDL levels.

If one of my patients has both LDL and triglyceride elevations, I decide which abnormality is of the greater magnitude. I normally prescribe a statin when the LDL is the predominant abnormality and Lopid or Tricor if the triglyceride problem looks more out of range (>400 mg/dL). It is not uncommon that I prescribe Lopid or Tricor in addition to a statin, or a statin in addition to Lopid or Tricor, depending on which one I started first. Some statins, such as Lipitor (atorvastatin), Zocor (simvastatin), and Crestor (rosuvastatin), can have a significant impact on triglycerides as well when used in higher doses, and there may not be a need for a second drug. Tricor is a relatively new drug on the market that works in a manner similar to Lopid to bring down the triglycerides, also lowers LDL levels (although not as much as the statins), and may be helpful in people with both LDL and triglyceride elevations. It also can raise HDL levels significantly, which of course is a good thing. It is important to discuss potential side effects of cholesterol-lowering mediations with your caregiver, especially if using different ones in combination.

Combination Blood Pressure and Cholesterol Medications

A combination pill that contains two different blood pressure or cholesterol medications is becoming more and more popular, and there are several benefits. First of all, you do not have to swallow multiple pills and you get the dual action of two different types of blood pressure and cholesterol medications that have been proven to work well together. Last, you will only have one copay and every type of savings can add up, especially if you are on a low fixed income. There is even a combination pill that has an excellent blood pressure medication combined with a statin. **Table 12-3** and **Table 12-6** list the combination blood pressure/cholesterol products currently available.

What About Aspirin Therapy?

There is no question that anyone who is at risk for heart disease should take one aspirin a day with rare exceptions. The evidence in the medical literature is overwhelmingly positive in support of aspirin therapy to prevent heart attack and stroke in people with and without diabetes. Aspirin is an old and inexpensive over-the-counter medication that is often overlooked and underutilized. The exact dose that one needs has not been determined and ranges from 75 to 325 mg/day. I recommend a baby aspirin that contains 81 mg in anyone over the age of 21. I buy my enteric-coated aspirin (easier on the stomach) at big discount stores in large quantities. An aspirin a day helps to keep the heart attack away!

What About Antioxidants?

Antioxidants such as vitamins E and C are not proven therapies to prevent or treat atherosclerosis. However, there are a lot of positive and very little negative data that point to beneficial effects of antioxidants on reducing the risk of atherosclerosis. The exact reasons why antioxidants are beneficial are not known; however, they do help transform the LDL or "bad" cholesterol into a less dangerous form. Antioxidants should never be used instead of proven therapies, such as the statins, to reduce heart disease. Antioxidants should be used as supplements only.

Case Presentation

Steve Edelman (yes, this really is my story) is a 51-year-old white man with a 37-year history of type 1 diabetes, diagnosed at the age of 15. My current degree of control is good, with a glycosylated hemoglobin usually between 6.7% and 7.4% (normal nondiabetic range 4% to 6%). I was found to have protein in my urine in 1987 and was started on an ACE inhibitor. During the next few years, a calcium channel blocker and indapamide were added to control my blood pressure to less than 120/80 mm Hg documented by my wrist-worn home blood pressure monitoring device. I am on three different drugs just to keep my blood pressure normal, but this will reduce my chances of having a heart attack, stroke, or kidney failure.

My high cholesterol levels were first diagnosed in 1992. Grandparents on both sides of my family had heart attacks at an early age (before the age of 60). I do not smoke cigarettes (only an occasional good cigar and I don't inhale) and have not experienced any problems with my heart (knock on wood!). My lipid panel before treatment was as follows: total cholesterol 260, LDL 171, HDL 76, and triglycerides 65. Current risk factors for atherosclerosis include diabetes, family history of heart disease, high blood pressure, and high LDL cholesterol levels. I have four major risk factors for the development of atherosclerosis; however, I have a high level of the protective HDL, which counteracts some of the other risk factors. At least I am not postmenopausal!

My doctor started me on a statin with the goal of getting my LDL at least under 100. The triglycerides are normal and the HDL level is at a beneficial level. I also started taking one enteric-coated aspirin a day (81 mg) and vitamins E (1200 IU/day) and C (2000 mg/day). I am now on a low-dose statin (Lipitor 20 mg), my LDL went down to 99, my triglycerides stayed about the same at 70; however, my HDL rose to the 90s. My total cholesterol also dropped to 238 (remember that when the good HDL cholesterol goes up the total cholesterol tends to go up as well). If my protective HDL had not gone up, then my total cholesterol would have been lower. Thus the total cholesterol can be a misleading number when analyzing changes in cholesterol therapy as discussed earlier.

I was also advised to get a cardiac stress test before starting a strenuous exercise program to make sure that I had no underlying asymptomatic heart disease. It is not uncommon for people with diabetes to not feel the classic chest pain that usually precedes a heart attack as discussed earlier. I also get a cardiac stress test once a year to be on the safe side.

Summary

Heart attack and stroke unfortunately account for a tremendous amount of death and human suffering in people with diabetes. Atherosclerosis is also one of the biggest and most potent reasons why Americans "get off the bus." One of the main problems in diagnosing and treating people with diabetes in a timely manner is the fact that both high blood pressure and abnormal cholesterol levels may not cause any major symptoms unless it is the final event, such as a heart attack or stroke (chest pain and paralysis). This is why both high blood pressure and abnormal cholesterol levels, two of the biggest and most modifiable risk factors for heart disease, have been called the silent killers.

The bottom line is that many of the major risk factors for atherosclerosis discussed in this chapter can be modified to reduce the chances of a stroke or heart attack. You need to be knowledgeable, not only about practical and realistic lifestyle modifications, but also about the most effective and well-tolerated medications to lower your blood pressure and cholesterol levels. In addition, by simply taking one aspirin a day, you may significantly reduce your chances of having a heart attack or stroke. These are the types of important issues that you need to discuss with your physician. Make sure you know your goals of therapy and that you reach and maintain those goals over the long term. It may be a struggle to attain acceptable blood pressure and cholesterol values; however, maintenance of these levels will be relatively simple. Trust me, you do not want to have a heart attack or stroke!

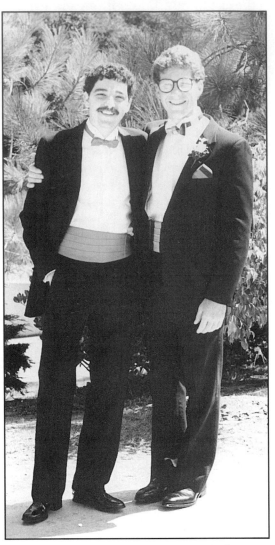

Me and Ken Facter at my wedding in San Diego, August 16, 1987.

13

Be Sweet to Your Feet

by Ingrid Kruse, DPM

Introduction

Foot problems, including foot ulcers, are a major cause of disability in people with diabetes. Even today, diabetes remains the leading cause of foot and leg amputation in the world. Techniques to prevent amputations range from the simple, but often neglected, foot inspection to complicated vascular reconstructive surgery.

In order to take an active role in preventing foot problems, you must first understand why foot problems occur so frequently in people with diabetes. The main reason is nerve damage (neuropathy) but blood flow problems (vascular disease) and poorly controlled diabetes also contribute to the problem. Luckily, all of these are treatable and, more importantly, preventable problems.

Neuropathy

Neuropathy, or nerve damage, will affect approximately 50% of people who have had diabetes for more than 25 years. High blood glucose levels over long periods of time are highly correlated with the development and progression of neuropathy; tight blood glucose control has been shown to reduce the incidence of neuropathy. The Diabetes Control and Complications Trial (DCCT) showed that neuropathy could be prevented in almost 70% of the cases where patients had excellent glycemic control.

Neuropathy typically starts in the toes with some tingling and numbness but can progress up the leg to where people are numb all the way up to their knees. It may also affect the fingers and hands but this is less common. The ability to feel pain is one of our body's main warning systems. It informs the brain that something is wrong somewhere… to ignore pain is never a good thing. Anyone who has forced himself or herself to keep exercising despite being injured or has ignored a toothache knows that things typically get worse when you do that sort of thing.

When you lose the ability to feel pain, an alarm bell will not go off and you will become prone to injury that may go undetected for quite a while. Here is a typical scenario that I have seen many times: Let's say you have developed some numbness in your feet due to diabetes. You are out walking or shopping, and inadvertently you step on a nail. Your nerves won't feel the injury and can't warn you by giving pain signals. By the time you get home, you will have a wound in

your foot and probably some blood on your sock. If you happen to notice the blood when you take off your shoes, you will discover the wound and can take steps to prevent infection by cleansing it and applying a dressing to the wound. However, if you did not notice the blood, or even worse, if you continue wearing the shoe with the nail sticking through it into your foot, you may soon have an infected foot ulcer.

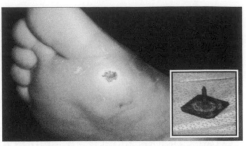

Puncture injury sustained when stepping on a nail or tack.

This is exactly why the daily foot inspection (discussed in detail later in the chapter) is so important and one of your best preventive measures, especially when you already have some nerve damage!

The nerves that are typically affected in diabetic neuropathy are the smallest ones: pain, temperature, fine-touch, and pressure nerves.

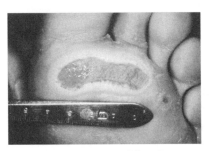

Blistering injury resulting from temperature insensitivity.

It is not uncommon for people to burn themselves and not realize it. Something as simple as sitting too close to an open fire place with your feet propped up and reading a book, or walking barefoot outside on hot pavement, or using hot water bottles on your feet can all have disastrous consequences.

When your feet are numb, you can also fracture (break) a bone without knowing it. Your foot, ankle, and leg will become very swollen and warm; this is called a Charcot's joint. It may take a long time for your doctor to figure out what is going on since there are many reasons for swelling in the feet and legs. The big distinction here is that we're talking about just one foot and leg being swollen, not both. It is important to see your health care provider or podiatrist immediately if this should happen and make sure you get an x-ray to check for fractures. Treatment of Charcot's joint includes taking measures to reduce the tremendous swelling and then keeping the joint protected to let it heal. This means avoiding any kind of weight on it and usually involves the use of a cast or protective brace. Protecting the foot from bearing weight is of utmost importance even if you don't feel any pain when walking; these fractures need to heal! Sometimes a bone stimulator and medication are used to facilitate in healing the fractures. If you continue walking around on an acute Charcot's joint, your foot will become distorted and deformed over time, making it impossible to fit into regular shoes.

Acute Charcot's joints are often missed by doctors since they are not that common, so it is important that you know about them and their presentation.

Diagnosis

How can you tell whether you have neuropathy and how much damage is present? A simple, painless, and quick way to find out is to have your physician check your feet with the Semmes Weinstein monofilament or 10-gram monofilament (**Figure 13-1**). Depending on whether you can feel the pressure from those little nylon filaments on your feet allows you to find out if you have so-called "protective sensation"; that is, enough feeling in your feet to know when some injury occurs. The doctor may also do vibration testing with a tuning fork (which tends to show up earlier than other signs), check reflexes, temperature sense, and pinprick sensation.

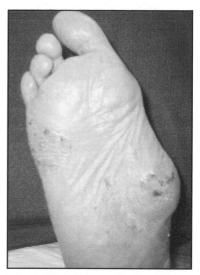

Charcot's joint results in distortion of the foot over time.

Other causes of neuropathy, such as vitamin B_{12} deficiency, should also be excluded before making the diagnosis of diabetic neuropathy.

Painful Diabetic Neuropathy

In some patients with neuropathy, the predominant symptom of their neuropathy is not numbness but pain. This is called painful diabetic neuropathy (PDN). In this situation, the nerves are not damaged to the point where they are unable to feel anything but rather they are irritated and hyperactive, firing all the time and giving your brain pain messages for no good reason. This type of pain is typically worse at night and the most common symptoms include burning pains, sharp shooting pains, stabbing pain, electric shock pain, tingling sensation, cramping pain, hot or cold sensations, feeling tightness in the toe joints or ankles, and hypersensitivity to even light touch, such as bed sheets or socks.

These symptoms can be explained by the predominant nerves that are affected by neuropathy, as mentioned before: pain, temperature, fine-touch, and pressure nerves.

Treatment and Prevention

This neuropathic pain is difficult to treat and patients rarely have complete resolution of their pain. It is usually considered successful if a medication can decrease the pain by 50%. Also, the typical medications used to treat neuropathy take 4 to 6 weeks before they have any effect since the doses need to be increased very slowly in order to prevent side effects. Always consult your doctor before taking any type of medication.

The majority of the medications used to treat PDN fall into two categories: antidepressants and antiseizure medications. Commonly used drugs include amitriptyline, imipramine, and desipramine, which are tricyclic antidepressants (TCAs) and Neurontin (gabapentin), which is an antiseizure medication. There are now two medications on the market that were specifically approved by the FDA for the treatment of PDN. One of them is Lyrica (pregabalin), a second-generation gabapentin that is more potent and causes less sedation (drowsiness) than gabapentin. However, patients on pregabalin must be carefully monitored for possible side effects and adverse events. The typical dosage is 300 mg to 600 mg per day, given in divided doses either 2 or 3 times daily. The other drug

Figure 13-1

Semmes Weinstein Monofilaments

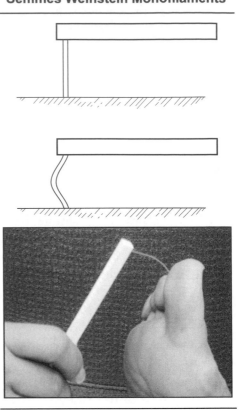

Applying a nylon filament mounted on a holder perpendicularly to the surface of the skin *(top)* with sufficient force (10 grams) to cause the filament to bend *(bottom)* for a duration of approximately 1.5 seconds will determine the existence of neuropathy. Research has shown that a person who can feel the force of the filament will not develop ulcers associated with neuropathy.

232

specifically approved for neuropathic pain is Cymbalta (duloxetine), an antidepressant. Typical dosage is 60 mg to 120 mg per day. Side effects include nausea, dizziness, and somnolence (feeling like a zombie). Patients taking Cymbalta should have their liver enzymes monitored.

In Europe, alpha lipoic acid (an antioxidant) has been used quite successfully by giving it as an intravenous infusion, which showed not only improvement of symptoms but also nerve function. The antioxidant is also available in pill form as a nutritional supplement in the United States.

There are also topical agents (applied directly to the skin) available to treat PDN. One of them is capsaicin cream, a hot chili pepper extract that needs to be rubbed into the entire painful area 4 times a day; one must use gloves while applying it to avoid burning the hands. This may make it logistically difficult for some people to do. The other is the 5% lidocaine patch that was approved by the FDA for treatment of PDN. It has the advantage of having no side effects, therefore, it is safe to use and has shown improvements in pain as well as quality of life in patients with PDN. The patch is simple to apply: peel off the sticky portion and apply to the area where it hurts.

In summary, PDN is a difficult complication to treat. It requires a lot of discussions between doctor and patient to figure out the best medication approach. People diagnosed with PDN need to remember that it typically takes 4 to 6 weeks for any of these agents to start working, and by that, we anticipate on average a 50% improvement in pain. Having falsely high expectations will only lead to frustration.

Our best strategy for combating neuropathy is still strict glycemic control. As mentioned before, not only does this prevent the onset of neuropathy, it has also been shown to slow down the progression of neuropathy by almost 60%! If you only have a little bit of numbness in your toes and really optimize your blood glucose readings, you can stop the neuropathy at this very early stage and prevent any of the problems that accompany nerve damage.

Taking control of your diabetes will indeed prevent complications!

Vascular Disease

Blood flow problems, or vascular disease, is the second most important reason why people with diabetes have foot ulcers that fail to heal and result in amputations. Arteries are the blood vessels that carry blood from the heart to various parts of the body (including the feet) as opposed to veins, which carry the blood back to the heart.

Arteries are usually soft and pliable structures but in diabetics can become rigid and stiff due to excess calcium deposits, which make it difficult for them to push the blood along. Furthermore, blockages can develop in the artery itself (called atherosclerotic plaques), eventually shutting off the circulation through that vessel and thus compromising the circulation to the foot. This is in essence how blood flow problems develop. Once you have a situation where the flow of blood is impaired, this also means that oxygen, nutrients, and even medications (such as antibiotics do not get delivered where they should go). In a foot in which an ulcer and perhaps an infection are present, it will be almost impossible for the wound to heal.

Fortunately, we have made great progress in restoring the circulation to the feet of patients with vascular disease. Bypass surgery can be performed from an area above the blockage all the way down to the foot with great success. More recently, surgeons have started placing stents in the arteries to bypass them, which is a much less invasive surgery and is more easily tolerated by the patient. The above procedures have saved many limbs in people with diabetes.

Having your circulation assessed is an important part of the foot exam. This may simply require checking the pulses, but if they are absent, it may be necessary to do further testing in the vascular laboratory using a Doppler device and other techniques. These are painless tests that give your physician a lot more information about the status of your circulation.

What are the risk factors for developing blood flow problems and is there anything you can do to prevent vascular disease? The incidence of vascular disease goes up with the number of years you have had diabetes, just as it does for neuropathy. It also increases with age in general, and unfortunately, we cannot do anything about those factors. Other risk factors, such as smoking, high cholesterol levels, and high blood pressure, can be addressed and treated. This will then contribute to keeping your blood flowing!

Immunity

I would like to mention a little bit about your immune system. It plays a crucial role in fighting infection and can be adversely affected by poor blood glucose control. If your blood glucose frequently rises above 250 mg/dL, the immune cells (white blood cells) that travel through your bloodstream to the feet in order to fight infection become sluggish and don't move well in a forward direction. Also, their ability to engulf and gobble up the invading bacteria is impaired, and the infection starts raging out of control. Even in a person with well-controlled diabetes, blood glucose commonly goes up when an infection is present. Therefore, you may need to temporarily take extra insulin or a higher dose of oral medications in order to bring it back down. Testing blood glucose frequently is important whenever you are ill. Make sure you discuss with your caregiver how to make adjustments in your medications when you have an infection.

The Daily Foot Inspection

Daily foot inspection is probably the single most important screening tool for preventing serious foot problems in diabetics! It is best done just before you go to bed, since most injuries occur not while sleeping but rather during the day:

1. Wash feet daily with mild soap and dry carefully, especially between the toes, in order to prevent athlete's foot infections.

2. Athlete's foot infection between the toes looks like a crack in the skin or whitish, moist-looking skin. It can also look like little blisters or bumps in the arch area or dry, peeling skin on the bottom of the foot. It may or may not itch. Treat athlete's foot with creams such as Lamisil, Clotrimazole, or Tinactin, and remember to use the cream both in the morning and at bedtime.

3. Inspect for blisters, cuts, scratches, or bruises. Check for cracks in the skin, commonly in the heels. Use moisturizers after bathing.

4. If you have trouble reaching your toes, use a hand mirror or have a family member or friend assist you.

5. Check your shoes for foreign objects, torn linings, or things sticking through the bottom before you put your feet in them.

6. Always wear socks, but avoid socks with holes or mends.

7. Shoes should fit your feet in both length and width, don't go up a half size in length when the shoe is too narrow. Remove the insole of your shoe (good athletic shoes have removable insoles) and place your foot on top of it to see if it is wide enough or make a tracing of your foot on a piece of paper and then place the shoe on top of it. Never try to break in shoes; they should fit perfectly at the time of purchase. Choose a soft leather upper or try athletic shoes and buy them at the end of the day when your feet tend to be more swollen than in the morning. The first time you wear new shoes, wear them only for 1 hour and only around the house. Then inspect your foot for blisters or red areas and slowly increase the wearing time. Medicare will pay for shoes and protective insoles if you are at risk for developing a foot ulcer. See your podiatrist for a prescription.

8. Trim your nails straight across with a slightly rounded edge. If you have neuropathy, vision trouble, or difficulty trimming them yourself (for example, if you have thick fungus nails), see a podiatrist! Please avoid all types of "bathroom surgery," like trying to fix an ingrown nail by yourself—the results can be disastrous!

9. Do not walk barefoot, even in the house, because of danger of stepping on pins, needles, tacks, glass, or other items on the floor.

10. Make the daily foot inspection a regular part of your daily routine, just like brushing your teeth.

Troubleshooting

What should you do when you find a blister or cut on your foot at the time of the daily foot inspection? Cleanse the area with an antiseptic; hydrogen peroxide is a cheap and effective antiseptic that you can buy in any drugstore.

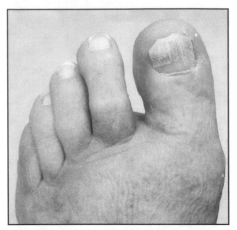

Trim toe nails straight across with slightly rounded corners. Thick, fungus nails should be attended to by a podiatrist!

Inspect the wound for foreign objects, which should be removed. Also be sure to check your shoes, the culprit could be inside.

Apply an antibiotic ointment (such as Neosporin) and cover with gauze and tape, not just a band-aid. If there is any redness around the wound or if there is an odor or pus coming from the wound, you have an infection and need to be seen by your physician for blood cultures, antibiotic pills, and possibly x-rays. Do not ignore a foot infection; it will get worse. If you have fever, chills, nausea, vomiting, or your blood glucose is running unusually high, always check your feet—these may be your only warning signals when an infection is present in your foot.

Summary

Neuropathy and vascular disease are common complications of diabetes but do not have to lead to amputations. Early diagnosis, halting the progression of neuropathy by strict glucose control, and checking your feet daily for injuries will help you minimize problems and treat them effectively. Addressing factors such as high cholesterol, blood pressure, and smoking for your circulation will keep you from developing serious vascular disease. This cannot be stressed enough— controlling your diabetes is of the utmost importance, not only for preventing these complications but also for ensuring that your immune system is functioning at its optimum level and is ready to protect you from infection and aid in healing.

14

How to Preserve the Life of Your Diabetic Kidneys

Prevention, Early Detection, and Aggressive Management—Avoiding Dialysis and Transplantation

Introduction

Diabetic kidney disease is a scary thing. To think about being on dialysis or needing transplantation from a cadaver or living donor is depressing. Unfortunately, diabetic kidney disease causes a tremendous amount of grief and misery for people with diabetes and their loved ones. Diabetes is one of the leading causes of kidney failure in the world.

I remember quite clearly when I studied physiology during medical school in 1978. The professor was citing statistics from old textbooks about the high death rate in people with diabetes. He stated that 50% of people with diabetes die from diabetic kidney disease within 20 years after the initial diagnosis of diabetes. At the time I was 23 years old with 8 years of diabetes behind me. I told myself that I would at least do everything in my power to prevent the development and progression of kidney disease.

In 1982, I discovered that my blood pressure was elevated for the first time and I did not want to take drugs. To me, it was a sign of weakness and vulnerability. The only medication that I regularly took at that time was insulin. This period in my diabetic life was emotionally significant because it marked the first time that I needed medication for a complication of diabetes. Even though I already had retinopathy, I did not need daily drugs after I received laser treatments. I finally slapped myself around and said, "Who are you fooling and what

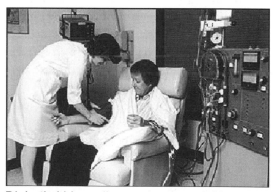

Diabetic kidney disease is preventable and treatable. Avoid end-stage renal disease and dialysis by taking control of your diabetes.

237

are you accomplishing by avoiding an important therapeutic modality to preserve the life of your kidneys?"

The message I have for you in this chapter is: *Diabetic kidney disease is preventable and it is treatable once present.* Through years of clinical research, we now know of several techniques to prevent the onset and delay the progression of diabetic kidney disease. In addition to aggressively treating kidney disease, screening methods for early diagnosis of this problem have been developed. This information is vital to all people with diabetes to avoid end-stage kidney disease (requiring dialysis or transplantation).

Definition

What is diabetic kidney disease, and why do diabetics develop kidney disease? Stating it simply, diabetic kidney disease is the failure of the kidneys to function properly due to poorly controlled blood glucose and elevated blood pressure over an extended period of time. Diabetic kidney disease is also referred to as diabetic nephropathy in the medical literature. The kidneys are important and vital organs responsible for filtering and cleaning our blood. The kidneys are also responsible for maintaining electrolyte balance (sodium, potassium, chlorine, carbon dioxide, etc) and normal fluid levels in our body. Years of chronically elevated blood glucose damages the vital filtering structures of the kidneys. Diabetic nephropathy is called a microvascular complication, because it involves very small blood vessels that feed oxygen and other nutrients to the kidneys as well as the eyes and nerves. This is why the term microvascular complications refers to the kidneys (nephropathy), eyes (retinopathy), and nerves (neuropathy).

Poorly controlled blood pressure, which can be an early manifestation of kidney disease or can be present because it runs in your family, is also very damaging to the kidneys. If left untreated, high blood pressure will greatly accelerate the decline of kidney function. It turns out that high blood pressure also contributes to acceleration of diabetic eye disease or retinopathy.

Inadequate screening for the early signs of diabetic kidney disease, thus delaying proper treatment, is also a serious problem. Remember, high blood pressure and early kidney disease do not occur with any noticeable symptoms, which makes screening of utmost importance. Sensitive tests are now available that can detect kidney disease at an early stage when the damage may be reversible with aggressive treatment. The information and advice in this chapter are simple, straightforward, and relatively easy to follow. It is vitally important that you preserve the life of your diabetic kidneys.

Prevention

Prevention of diabetic kidney disease by maintaining tight glucose control has been convincingly proven by the Diabetes Control and Complications Trial (DCCT) as well as by several other large reputable studies in people with type 1 and type 2 diabetes.

The DCCT conclusively demonstrates the importance of glucose control in preventing the onset and delaying the progression of the classic microvascular complications of diabetes (eye, kidney, and nerve disease) in patients with type 1 diabetes. The importance of glucose control in patients with type 2 diabetes is now widely accepted by physicians as it is in those with type 1 diabetes. The majority of diabetes specialists and other caregivers who are interested in diabetes feel that the duration and severity of hyperglycemia will dictate the rate and extent of microvascular complications, such as eye, kidney, and nerve disease, in all patients with diabetes no matter what type of the disease is present.

If you have high blood pressure from any cause, you may be able to prevent the onset of diabetic kidney disease just by aggressively treating the blood pressure to keep it in the normal ranges or even lower! In addition, it may be possible that two types of blood pressure medication called an angiotensin-converting enzyme (ACE) inhibitor and an angiotensin receptor blocker (ARB) (discussed later in this chapter) can prevent the onset of kidney disease if started early enough. We know that they prevent the progression of kidney disease once you have it, but their role in prevention is not known for sure. The indications to start either of these two types of medication are discussed later in this chapter.

Early Detection

Diabetic kidney disease has a natural history similar to type 2 diabetes in that it takes years to develop and deteriorate to an end-stage situation. The big problem is that in the early stages when aggressive therapy can prevent the progression of diabetic kidney disease, there are no symptoms that can be recognized. If you and/or your doctor are unaware of the screening methods to pick up early problems, by the time you feel poorly from the late stages of kidney disease, you have missed a golden opportunity to catch things early and prevent progression of this potentially devastating complication.

Microalbuminuria

The first measurable laboratory abnormality in the course of diabetic kidney disease is the presence of albumin in the urine in small amounts, which is referred to as microalbuminuria. Albumin is a protein that is normally not found at all or only in very small amounts in the urine. The prefix *micro* refers to the amount (small) of albumin in the urine. People with microalbuminuria have a high likelihood of experiencing decreasing kidney function if left untreated over a period of years.

The important thing to remember is that once microalbuminuria is present, there are therapeutic maneuvers to retard the progression of diabetic kidney disease. Remember that there are no symptoms of kidney disease in the early stages. This is why screening is so important —so that aggressive management can be started in a timely fashion. This is the key to preventing the need for transplantation or dialysis!

You are responsible for getting tested for the presence of microalbuminuria and obtaining aggressive therapy if needed. The test for microalbuminuria is now readily available, but that was not always the case. I will always remember the day when I got a call from a representative of an insurance company from which I was seeking to get life insurance. He said, "Dr. Edelman, I regret to inform you that your application for life insurance was denied because the urine sample we received from you had several thousand milligrams of albumin in it." I was shocked, because I knew this was an indication of fairly advanced kidney disease—way past the microalbuminuria stage. This was another huge wake-up call for me.

If you have type 1 diabetes, you should be screened for microalbuminuria once a year beginning 5 years from the time of your diagnosis of type 1 diabetes. People with type 2 diabetes should be screened every year from the time of diagnosis. There are several different screening tests for microalbuminuria, which usually involve a timed urine collection for albumin (12 or 24 hours). Your physician can also measure a ratio of the albumin in the urine to the creatinine (another substance that goes up with kidney disease) in the blood (**Table 14-1**). The purpose of showing **Table 14-1** is not for you to completely understand or memorize all of the medical jargon but for

Table 14-1

Definitions of Urinary Albumin Excretion Rates

	Urinary AER (mg/day)	Urinary AER (mcg/minute)	Urinary Albumin (mg) to Creatinine Ratio
Normoalbuminuria	<30	<20	<30
Microalbuminuria	30-300	20-200	30-300
Macroalbuminuria	>300	>200	>300

Abbreviation: AER, albumin excretion rate.

you to be aware of the different ways that your kidney function can be evaluated. The albumin-to-creatinine ratio has become the most popular test, because you do not need to do the tedious 24-hour urine collection, and it is fairly accurate. If you do perform a 24-hour urine test, the large urine collection jug must be kept in the refrigerator. (Remember to label it carefully!)

Several new home test kits for microalbuminuria have now been developed. This fantastic advance will really improve the awareness and access to early testing and hopefully appropriate therapy (Google *home microalbuminuria test kits* to get more information). One can also be screened with simple and quick urine dip test strips that measure microalbuminuria in the urine (Micral test strips). These test strips are much different from the older strips. The older strips tested only for gross protein or macroalbuminuria, not microalbuminuria. This older method is too insensitive to pick up small amounts of albumin or protein in a timely manner. If the Micral test is negative, you can be rescreened in 1 year. However, if the screening test is positive or even marginally positive, I recommend getting a albumin-to-creatinine ratio or 24-hour collection for better quantification of protein spillage. Certain situations, such as strenuous exercise, may make your microalbuminuria test positive even though you do not have diabetic kidney disease. Hence confirming the presence of microalbuminuria with at least one additional test is suggested, especially before starting aggressive therapy.

I also feel it is important to repeat yearly microalbuminuria testing, even if you are being treated aggressively. If the microalbumin level continues to increase despite aggressive therapy, that will warrant a closer look by your physician for additional factors that might hasten the decline of your kidneys. Some of these factors include making sure that your blood pressure control over a 24-hour period is adequate, using a special computerized monitoring device and examining any other medications that you are taking that may

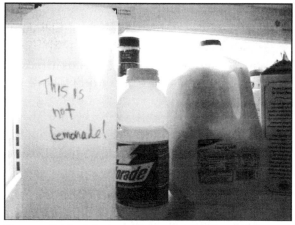

Be careful to label your urine collection jug!

241

damage the kidneys. In addition, if your glucose control is not ideal, this should be an important area of focus.

If your doctor has already informed you of evidence of excessive protein in your urine (another way of saying macroalbuminuria or much more than a little protein in your urine), you are past the microalbuminuria stage. You now need to have regular urine tests to measure how much protein or albumin is in your urine and institute very aggressive therapy to retard the progression.

It is also extremely important to realize that the presence of microalbuminuria or protein in the urine may be a marker for additional abnormalities other than the development of end-stage kidney disease. Microalbuminuria is also associated with the presence of diabetic retinopathy or eye disease, high cholesterol levels, and heart disease.

Blood Pressure Screening

Proper blood pressure screening is also an important tool in picking up signs of early kidney disease. If you have or are at risk for the development of kidney disease, obtain an accurate home blood pressure monitoring device so that you can take your own readings on a regular basis. It is important to measure your blood pressure at home during your normal daily activities and not only in a doctor's office. Home blood pressure monitoring allows for an accurate indication of what your blood pressure values are on the average. Home blood pressure monitoring devices are inexpensive and can be found at most pharmacies, department stores, or medical supply stores. Select one that you feel comfortable using and that has a good warranty. My blood pressure monitor fits quickly and easily on my wrist and appears to be very accurate. It is important to bring your home blood pressure device to your doctor's office once or twice a year so that one of the staff can compare the readings on your machine with the gold-standard method of manually pumping up the sphygmomanometer and listening to the pulse in your arm with a stethoscope. If the values are not within 10% of each other, your machine should be calibrated. If you go to the supermarket or drug store to get your blood pressure checked, be aware that they are not always accurate. Anyone with high blood pressure or hypertension should have their own machine at home, just as every person with diabetes should have their own home glucose monitoring device at home.

Aggressive Management

Diabetic kidney disease is treatable. You can truly make a difference in your risk of developing end-stage renal disease requiring dialysis or transplantation. Four therapeutic strategies have been well proven to prevent the progression of diabetic kidney disease. Two other strategies have not been well proven (cholesterol reduction and the use of antioxidants); however, they may be of therapeutic benefit and will be discussed (**Table 14-2**).

Glucose Control

As previously discussed, the DCCT conclusively demonstrated that intensive glucose control can retard the progression of diabetic kidney disease already present in individuals with diabetes. It does not matter if you have type 1 or type 2 diabetes; glucose control is crucial. Follow the suggestions throughout this book, with the help of your caregivers, to achieve the best control that is possible for you. Get that glycosylated hemoglobin (A1C) value into a near-normal desirable range.

Blood Pressure Control

Aggressive blood pressure control, along with glucose control, is probably one of the more powerful interventions to reduce the progression of diabetic kidney disease. Please do not take this last statement lightly. It is super important!

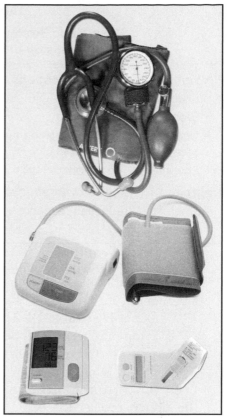

Blood pressure readings can be obtained using various monitoring devices. The "gold standard" is a stethoscope and sphygmomanometer *(top)* as typically used in your doctor's office. Home monitoring devices can be arm cuffs *(center)*, wrist cuffs *(bottom, left)*, or a finger cuff *(bottom, right)*.

The treatment of diabetic hypertension could be the topic of an entire book, but it deserves a few comments here and is discussed further in Chapter 12. First of all, it is important that "normal blood pressure" be correctly defined. Blood pressure goals have been defined differently and have been recently changed by several organizations (World Health Organization, American Heart Association, American Diabetes Association, etc). The American Diabetes Association

243

Table 14-2

Therapeutic Strategies to Prevent or Retard the Progression of Diabetic Kidney Disease

Proven Therapeutic Interventions
- Glucose control
- Blood pressure control
- Use of angiotensin-converting enzyme (ACE) inhibitors or an angiotensin receptor blocker (ARB)
- Low-protein meal plan

Unproven Therapeutic Interventions
- Cholesterol reduction (especially low-density lipoprotein [LDL] cholesterol)
- Antioxidants

---

currently recommends treatment to at least less than 130/80 mm Hg. Many kidney experts say that if you have evidence of protein or albumin in your urine, your average blood pressure should be less than 120/80 mm Hg (**Table 14-3**).

The top number in a blood pressure reading refers to the systolic blood pressure and represents the pressure when the heart is working its hardest to pump out blood to the rest of the vital organs of the body. (Of particular interest is that of the many organs in the body, the kidneys receive 25% of the "cardiac output," which demonstrates how important the kidneys are.) The bottom number refers to the diastolic blood pressure and represents the pressure when the heart is resting, filling up with blood before the next systolic beat. The abbreviation *mm Hg* refers to millimeters of mercury, the universal unit of measuring blood pressure. When your blood pressure is too high, it puts a very large strain not only on your heart and blood vessels but also on your kidneys, brain, and eyes. Elevated blood pressure

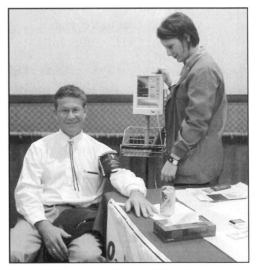

I am taking advantage of the free service of having my blood pressure taken as provided at a TCOYD conference in Amarillo, Texas.

Table 14-3

Goals for Blood Pressure Control

No Evidence of Protein or Albumin in the Urine
- Systolic blood pressure less than or equal to 130 mm Hg
- Diastolic blood pressure less than or equal to 80 mm Hg
  Medical jargon: ≤130/80 mm Hg

Persistent Protein or Albumin in the Urine
- Systolic blood pressure less than or equal to 120 mm Hg
- Diastolic blood pressure less than or equal to 80 mm Hg
  Medical jargon: ≤120/80 mm Hg

---

over the years leads to heart attacks, strokes, and accelerated eye and kidney disease. I have heard many experts say that controlling the blood pressure is as important as controlling the glucose values, and they have lots of clinical research evidence to back them up. Instead of debating which one is more important, how about just spending our efforts on controlling both of them?

Use of Angiotensin-Converting Enzyme Inhibitors

Angiotensin-converting enzyme (ACE) inhibitors represent an entire class of blood pressure–lowering medications. ACE inhibitors have proven effective in preventing and slowing the progression of diabetic kidney disease in terms of reducing albumin (protein) spillage into the urine and lowering blood pressure. ACE inhibitors have also been shown to benefit the kidneys of both type 1 and type 2 diabetics who have microalbuminuria, even when the blood pressure is normal. In this scenario, ACE inhibitors are given in low doses so that the blood pressure does not get too low (this is a rare problem in people with diabetes). In summary, ACE inhibitors protect the kidneys from further decline in function. You need to know if you are a candidate for taking an ACE inhibitor. **Table 14-4** lists some commonly used ACE inhibitors.

An ACE inhibitor is generally considered the first drug of choice for the treatment of hypertension of diabetes but should be used with caution in two types of patients:

- People who have a tendency to have high potassium levels in the blood—This usually occurs in people who have had diabetes for a long time and already have some damage to the kidneys.
- Patients with a condition called renal artery stenosis—Renal artery stenosis basically means clogging (stenosis) of the arteries that deliver blood to the kidneys (renal means pertaining to the kidneys)

- Women who are pregnant or are trying to become pregnant should not take ACE inhbitors or ARBs as they have been shown to cause problems for the fetus.

How do you know if you have one of these two conditions? It is easy to find out if you have a tendency for high potassium levels in your blood. Potassium levels are commonly measured in most laboratory blood screening tests, and you should have several such measurements in your medical chart. If not, then you can get a simple blood test for potassium that does not require fasting. The symbol for potassium (which may be on your laboratory report) is K+. Renal artery stenosis is more difficult to detect, although it is not too common. Usually, if you have stenosis or clogging of your renal or kidney arteries, you most likely will also have problems with other arteries in your body, such as your coronary (heart), cerebral (brain), and lower-extremity arteries. If you have any concerns or questions, simply ask your doctor about these issues. Last, some people may develop a persistent, dry cough while taking ACE inhibitors. This dry cough occurs in approximately 5% of people who take ACE inhibitors. The problem goes away when the ACE inhibitor is stopped, and then an ARB is normally substituted.

Table 14-4

Commonly Used ACE Inhibitors

- Benazepril (Lotensin)
- Captopril (Capoten)
- Enalapril (Vasotec)
- Fosinopril (Monopril)
- Lisinopril (Zestril, Prinivil)
- Moexipril (Univasc)
- Perindopril (Aceon)
- Quinapril (Accupril)
- Ramipril (Altace)
- Trandolapril (Mavik)

Abbreviation: ACE, angiotensin-converting enzyme.

Use of Angiotensin Receptor Blockers

Angiotensin receptor blockers (ARBs) work in a similar manner as ACE inhibitors, and have been shown to protect the diabetic kidney as well. If for any reason you are not able to take an ACE inhibitor, then substituting for an ARB is a great alternative. Many caregivers use ARBs as first-line therapy for people with diabetes and hypertension, which is perfectly appropriate. **Table 14-5** lists the commonly used ARBs.

The bottom line is that all diabetics, with few exceptions, should be taking an ACE inhibitor or an ARB if there is albumin or protein in the urine and/or if the blood pressure is high. Even if your blood pressure is normal and you have microalbuminuria, you should still be taking an ACE inhibitor or an ARB. If your blood pressure is truly normal and you have absolutely no evidence of protein or albumin in your urine, then you do not need an ACE or ARB. Saying this, I know of physicians who put all of their patients with diabetes on an ACE or ARB no matter what. I am not at this stage in my recommendations yet, but since they are safe with few side effects, I do not have any huge objections.

Table 14-5

Commonly Used ARBs

- Candesartan (Atacand)
- Eprosartan (Teveten)
- Irbesartan (Avapro)
- Losartan (Cozaar)
- Olmesartan (Benicar)
- Telmisartan (Micardis)
- Valsartan (Diovan)

Abbreviation: ARB, angiotensin receptor blocker.

Low-Protein Meal Plan

Diets high in protein have been shown to induce and accelerate kidney disease in animal and human studies. Based on the results of several clinical trials, it is recommended that people with diabetic kidney disease should restrict their protein intake to 0.8 grams per kilogram of body weight per day or about 10% of their total daily calories. I tell my patients that this is the equivalent of a small or medium amount of protein only once a day. There is also additional evidence that vegetable protein, such as beans and tofu, may be better than animal protein, and that white meat may be better than red meat. This may relate to the fact that red meat has more fat in it than do other sources of protein.

If you are a "steak and potatoes" type of eater, you should start thinking about reducing the amount of meat in your diet long before any evidence of diabetic kidney disease is present. Big changes in one's lifestyle must come slowly. I grew up eating meat at least 2 times a day. My family always had some type of red meat or chicken for dinner. My lunches usually consisted of a peanut butter and diet jelly or a cold-cut sandwich. In addition, I often had eggs for breakfast. This type of diet is at least 1.2 grams per kilogram of body weight per day or about 20% of my daily calories. I have now slowly adapted to a low-protein diet that I enjoy. I usually now have toast or a bagel for breakfast, a veggie or white meat (chicken or tuna) sandwich for lunch, and a pasta dish for dinner. When I have a veggie lunch, then I have some protein with dinner. When I go out to eat, I satisfy my meat cravings by usually ordering the ribeye or 10-oz filet (medium rare, of course).

Occasionally, I have days when I eat a lot of protein, and other days, none at all. Trust me—I do not turn down a huge slab of roast beef with white, creamy horseradish sauce at a banquet dinner. The key is to practice moderation in the diet, allowing yourself to enjoy what you eat so that sticking to your diet comes naturally, and is not a daily emotional fight or guilt-ridden process. Please refer to Chapter 4 for further discussion on meals.

Cholesterol Reduction

Although not as well proven as the above therapeutic strategies for aggressively treating diabetic kidney disease, there is accumulating evidence that by lowering the cholesterol levels, especially the LDL (or bad cholesterol) level, the progression of kidney disease is reduced. The "statins" are the most effective class of medications for reducing your LDL cholesterol level. They are easy to take (once a day, usually at bedtime) and have little or no side effects (**Table 14-6**).

Reduction of LDL cholesterol has been strongly proven to reduce heart disease in people with diabetes and can only be beneficial. If it turns out that one can also reduce the decline of kidney function by lowering cholesterol levels, then by doing so I will have done both my patients and myself an extra service. I do not recommend taking any cholesterol-lowering medication if your LDL cholesterol level is at the desired goal. Normal cholesterol levels and statin therapy are discussed in Chapter 12.

Table 14-6

"Statin" Medications Available for Lowering Cholesterol*

- Atorvastatin (Lipitor)
- Fluvastatin (Lescol)
- Lovastatin (Mevacor, Altocor)
- Pravastatin (Pravachol)
- Rosuvastatin (Crestor)
- Simvastatin (Zocor)

* Discussed in detail in Chapter 12.

Antioxidants

The role of antioxidants in the treatment of diabetic kidney disease and other microvascular complications is not yet defined. Many of the studies that have shown benefits of antioxidants are from test tube and animal studies and only recently from studies in people with diabetes. There is also a body of literature hinting that antioxidants may have benefits against heart disease by improving the character of cholesterol particles so they do not cause heart disease as aggressively. At the same time, recent studies have also shown they do not help, and some suggest there may be negative associations with other conditions in people who take antioxidants. It is tough literature to decipher and understand.

I do not push vitamins on my patients, although if they ask me for permission to take antioxidants or for my advice regarding vitamins, I usually suggest vitamins C and E. I know of no adverse effects from taking 400 to 800 international units (IU) of vitamin E and/or 1000 mg of vitamin C per day. When purchased at discount stores in larger quantities, vitamins C and E can be fairly inexpensive.

Antioxidants are not proven to retard kidney disease!

Case Presentation

Mary is a 24-year-old woman who was diagnosed with type 1 diabetes at age 12. She is currently on a long-acting insulin analogue (Lantus [glargine]) once a day given at bedtime and a fast-acting insulin analogue (Apidra [glulisine]) before meals. She checks her blood glucose sporadically when she "feels" it is high, with most of the morning blood glucose levels greater than 180 mg/dL, and she had a recent A1C of 8.6%. Her last dilated eye examination was 2 months ago and showed early diabetic retinopathy or eye disease. She reports that both feet are a little numb and tingle at night. She continues to exercise regularly, running 5 to 10 miles per week, and is at her ideal body weight. She is following a high-protein diet that she read about in a sports magazine several years ago. She does not smoke.

Over the course of the past year, her blood pressure has risen from a baseline of 110/70 mm Hg to 135/80 mm Hg. A urinary albumin-to-creatinine ratio measured 4 months ago was 50 mg/g (normal range <30, see **Table 14-1**). She takes no medication other than insulin.

Case Discussion

This woman is a poorly controlled type 1 diabetic who is at signficant risk for the development of end stage diabetic complications. She has microalbuminuria, which is the first clinical sign of diabetic kidney disease, and her blood pressure is elevated compared with her usual baseline. Many physicians would consider 135/80 mm Hg as normal, but compared with her usual blood pressure of 110/70 mm Hg, it is definitely high. In addition, her glucose control is not adequate, and she also has evidence of eye and nerve disease from poorly controlled blood glucose levels. Mary has evidence of all three major microvascular complications, and this should be a huge wake-up call for her and her physician.

249

Treatment of this patient's early diabetic kidney disease required a multifaceted approach, including improved glucose control, dietary changes (such as reduced daily protein intake), and aggressive treatment of her high blood pressure with an ACE inhibitor or an ARB. She agreed to:

- Test her blood glucose more regularly
- Consider getting a continuous glucose monitoring device
- Follow a low-protein diet
- Start taking an ACE inhibitor.

I encouraged her to keep a close eye on her blood pressure levels at home with a blood pressure cuff. If her blood pressure is not close to 120/80 mm Hg, adding a second blood pressure medication will be warranted for sure.

Summary

Diabetic kidney disease is preventable and treatable. The two most powerful and proven methods of preventing diabetic kidney disease is to maintain strict glycemic control and blood pressure control from the time of diagnosis. Early detection is of vital importance in order to initiate aggressive treatment early. Yearly microalbuminuria testing is currently the most sensitive technique for detecting early kidney damage, and it is also a marker for other conditions, including heart disease. Once the presence of microalbuminuria and/or high blood pressure has been detected, aggressive therapy with a number of proven strategies should be instituted as soon as possible. These strategies include:

- Glucose control
- Blood pressure control
- Use of ACE inhibitors or ARBs
- A low-protein meal plan.

Two additional therapies, but not as well proven, include lowering cholesterol levels and the use of antioxidants. You can make a difference in your life and the life of your diabetic kidneys. You can prevent the need for dialysis or transplantation.

15

For Your Eyes Only

Don't Lose Sight of the Problem

by Steven V. Edelman, MD
and Paul E. Tornambe, MD

The Main Message

Diabetic retinopathy is the result of microangiopathy, abnormal sorbitol pathways, glycosylation of the retinol basement membranes, and possibly the oxidation of cellular and molecular structures of the orbital layers—we scared you, didn't we? We are not going to make you read a chapter on the pathophysiology of diabetic retinopathy. You can get this type of information from any medical textbook on diabetes. We would rather tell you the most important sight-saving information that you should know as a person living with diabetes.

Get a dilated eye examination at least once a year by an eye specialist who is very familiar with diabetic eye problems! This is the main message of this chapter. Just by getting your eyes carefully examined annually, you can lessen or prevent your chances of going blind or becoming visually impaired. If everyone with diabetes took this simple advice, the incidence of blindness would be a fraction of what it is today. Today, diabetic retinopathy is unfortunately the leading cause of blindness in the United States.

The American Diabetes Association recommends a dilated eye examination once a year but does not specify who should administer the examination. The person who may be making sight-saving decisions about your eyes could be an ophthalmologist, a primary care physician, a nurse practitioner, or an optometrist.

Traditionally, an ophthalmologist with a special interest in diabetic eye disease or retinopathy should be the person looking after your eyes, especially if you already have documented problems. Although it is true that there are some optometrists and other caregivers who are capable of picking up the early signs of retinopathy, many do not have this type of expertise. We send all of my patients to an ophthalmologist who has the most experience with diabetic retinopathy. Early detection and aggressive treatment are the keys to avoiding serious problems.

It is important to pick up the early changes in the eye that are a result of diabetes because there are many measures that one can take to prevent the progression to blindness (**Table 15-1**). Remember—there are no symptoms of diabetic retinopathy until it is at an advanced stage when aggressive therapy may not be effective in saving your vision. This is why regular screening is so important.

Table 15-1

Measures That You Can Take to Prevent Blindness Once You Have Diabetic Retinopathy

- Get your blood glucose level under the best control possible
- Make sure that your blood pressure is in the normal range
- Visit an ophthalmologist with a special interest in diabetic retinopathy as often as prescribed (at least once a year)

An Eye Doctor's "Bird's-Eye" View

Diabetes is a disease of small blood vessels. The eye contains many small blood vessels, so the eye is frequently involved in diabetes. The eye is an organ of vision. Like the photographer's camera, light enters the eye from the front through the cornea (like the camera lens) and the picture is taken on a fine membrane (like the film) called the retina. The information is then transferred to the brain by way of the optic nerve. The retina contains millions of nerve fibers which are nourished by very small blood vessels. These blood vessels become involved in diabetes.

Sadly, most diabetics go blind for one reason: they are brought to the attention of the eye specialist too late. The National Eye Institute (NEI) sponsored an extensive study of diabetic retinopathy, results of which were published in 1976. The study proved that with appropriate and timely laser treatment, the risk of severe visual loss from diabetes can be reduced by 70%.

There are two forms of diabetic retinopathy: a background form and a proliferative form. In type 1 diabetes, retinopathy can begin as early as 5 years after the diagnosis of diabetes is made. Therefore, a teenager who has had diabetes for 5 years must be evaluated at least yearly by an eye-care specialist to check for diabetic retinopathy. For people with type 2 diabetes, screening should start at the time of diagnosis since it is possible that the diabetes has been around for years before the diagnosis.

In background diabetic retinopathy, the retinal blood vessels leak fluid and sometimes bleed. If the leakage develops close to the area of central vision, reading vision will be compromised (**Figure 15-1**). The NEI trial has proven that laser treatment can stop the progression of dia-

Figure 15-1
Compromised Reading Vision With Proliferative Diabetic Retinopathy

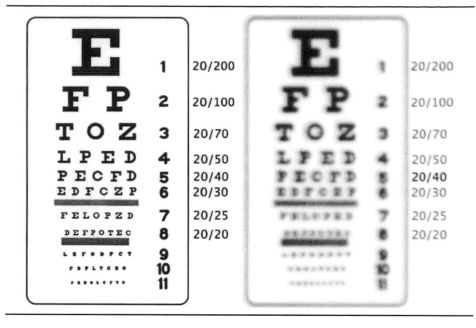

betic retinopathy. However, as the person with diabetes gets older, other blood vessels start to leak, and several laser treatments may be required over a lifetime. This is why we advise that people with type 2 diabetes have an eye examination as soon as diabetes is diagnosed as they may have had borderline disease for years and the eyes might already be affected.

Proliferative diabetic retinopathy is a more rapidly progressive form of diabetic retinopathy. As the small blood vessels in the eye fail to carry oxygen to the retinal tissue, the tissue releases VEGF. This substance tells the body to make blood vessels so more oxygen can be brought to the retina. Unfortunately, the blood vessels that the body makes inside the eye are weak and fragile, and they tend to break and bleed easily. Again, laser treatment is effective in directly cauterizing these vessels, and it also improves oxygenation to the retina, which prevents VEGF production. If laser treatment is not applied, the blood vessels continue to bleed, scar tissue forms, and the retina is torn as the scar tissue contracts. The retina will then separate from the back of the eye (retinal detachment) and die, resulting in blindness.

Vitrectomy is an operation developed in the 1970s, which, using space-age technology, can remove the blood and scar tissue and restore the retina to its proper position. Again, if instituted early enough, blindness can be prevented. During vitrectomy surgery, instruments less than

1 mm in diameter are inserted into the eye. The blood is vacuumed out of the eye and the scar tissue is removed with microscopic forceps and scissors. Laser can then be applied internally to stop the bleeding. The operation takes several hours but is usually done on an outpatient basis. It is effective in more than 90% of cases.

Currently, medications are being developed to inject into the eye in order to prevent scar tissue formation. We will see more pharmacologic manipulation of disease within this next century. VEGF inhibitors are just the beginning. We will also likely define the gene(s) that causes this disease and will either manipulate the gene or produce the substance that the gene doesn't make to prevent the complications of diabetes.

For the time being, there are three things you can do to minimize the damage to your eyes caused by diabetes: First, if you think you do not have diabetes but have a family history of diabetes or are experiencing symptoms of thirst, frequent urination, and weight loss, you may have diabetes. Early detection and appropriate treatment will significantly reduce the incidence of diabetic complications. If you have diabetes, make sure your first- and second-degree relatives get regular screening. Second, if you have diabetes, make every effort to control it tightly. The National Institutes of Health completed a very important study that proved, beyond a doubt, that tight blood glucose control reduces the incidence of blindness, heart disease, and peripheral neuropathy. Third, get a dilated eye exam by someone who knows what he/she is looking for at least once a year! Tight blood glucose control, close medical supervision, and regular dilated exams will decrease the complications of diabetic eye disease. Just do it!

Diabetic Retinopathy and Laser Therapy

Diabetic retinopathy is caused by years of excessively high blood glucose or sugar levels. Glucose sticks to and damages many of the structures of the body; however, certain organs are more susceptible to the adverse effects of prolonged hyperglycemia, including the eyes, kidneys, heart, and nerves. The specific structure of the eye that is damaged is called the retina, which is one of many important layers that make up the eye. Diabetic retinopathy results in the development of new blood vessels in an attempt to supply more oxygen-rich blood to the damaged retina; however, these new blood vessels are fragile and break easily. When these abnormal blood vessels break, they bleed into the center of the eye (vitreous hemorrhage). The vitreous is normally full of clear fluid and when blood inappropriately enters this liquid cavity, it becomes cloudy red and vision is severely impaired. If the bleeding stops either on its own or by laser therapy, the blood will slowly sink to the bottom of the eye like the oil in salad dressing, and vision will slowly improve over weeks to months.

One of the biggest advances in diabetes therapy has been the development and availability of laser therapy for the treatment of retinopathy. This type of laser therapy is very different from the corrective laser surgery that allows people to be glasses-free. Laser therapy alone is responsible for preventing severe visual impairment and blindness in millions of Americans. Laser therapy must be done in the early stages of retinopathy, before the abnormal blood vessels break and long before there are any noticeable eye symptoms. The basic concept behind laser therapy is that when the ophthalmologist aims and shoots a laser beam into your eye, the energy generated works to coagulate (or seal up) the leaky blood vessels. Laser therapy is also used to purposefully destroy the outer areas of the retina in order to reduce the body's adaptive drive to deliver blood to those areas. In this manner, the number of abnormal vessels will decline, reducing the chance for a bleed or vitreous hemorrhage. The outer areas of the retina are mostly responsible for peripheral vision and are not vital to maintain adequate sight. In addition, night vision may be diminished after extensive laser therapy. Reduced peripheral and night vision is a small price to pay to prevent total blindness.

Exciting New Developments for the Eye

It is also exciting that new medications are being tested and developed that may help prevent the progression of microvascular complications, including retinopathy. The most exciting drugs are called protein kinase C (PKC) inhibitors. The clinical trials are currently ongoing and the PKC inhibitors may not only prevent and/or reduce retinopathy, but they may also be protective to the nerves, kidneys, heart, and blood vessels. Unfortunately, these new drugs have not passed the strict FDA review process yet.

A new set of drugs may change the way we manage diabetic retinopathy. At the time of this writing, doctors are learning how to use these drugs called VEGF inhibitors (Avastin [bevacizumab], Lucentis [ranibizumab], Macugen [pegaptanib sodium]). VEGF (which stands for vascular endothelial growth factor) stimulates abnormal blood vessels to grow into the eye (proliferative diabetic retinopathy) and VEGF also stimulates normal blood vessels in the eye to leak (diabetic macular edema). At the moment, these drugs must be injected into the center of the eye, sometimes more than once. In the case of proliferative retinopathy, a single injection has been shown to dramatically stimulate complete regression of the new proliferative vessels in 5 days (**Figure 15-2A** and **15-2B**). After a month or two, the drug wears off and the blood vessels return. This treatment "buys time" for the patient and doctor to apply laser treatment or perform a vitrectomy operation more safely with less chance of bleeding. Interestingly, sometimes an injection of this drug in one eye improves the disease in the fellow eye. We do not know exactly what the reason is for this crossover effect. Laser is still necessary, but in severe cases, this treatment will give retina surgeons a better chance to save more advanced cases.

Drugs to Treat/Prevent Diabetic Retinopathy

Diabetic retinopathy may be defined as normal blood vessels, which have been damaged and now leak fluid, lipid, and blood (background diabetic retinopathy) or the development of new abnormal fragile blood vessels, which "break" and can bleed significantly (proliferative diabetic retinopathy). What causes diabetic retinopathy? Well, elevated blood glucose in diabetes leads to the overaction of a protein called PKC beta. PKC beta plays an important role in damage to small blood vessels that can lead to increased vascular permeability (leakage). This prevents enough oxygen and nutrients from getting to retinal tissue. Lack of oxygen releases another protein called VEGF, which makes blood vessels leak even more and stimulates the proliferation of abnormal fragile blood vessels,

Figure 15-2

Use of VEGF Inhibitors With Proliferative Diabetic Retinopathy

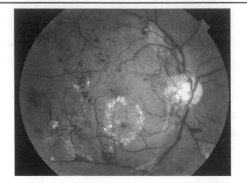

A. Note blood vessels on the optic nerve of this eye prior to treatment with Avastin

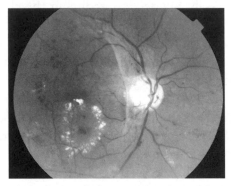

B. Five days after injection of Avastin into the eye, the blood vessels on the optic nerve have regressed completely

Abbreviation: VEGF, vascular endothelial growth factor.

which then bleed. A new class of drugs taken orally inhibits the action of PKC B, thus damage to the blood vessels is minimized and retinopathy is less likely to develop and advance. In recent clinical trials, these drugs have decreased the incidence and severity of swelling in the retina (macular edema) but did not prevent eyes from developing proliferative diabetic retinopathy. However, as mentioned earlier, another class of drugs called VEGF inhibitors, which are injected into the eye, cause a dramatic regression in proliferative diabetic vessels. Thus we have drugs that alter the course of diabetic retinopathy. This is just the beginning of new drugs, which will allow us to pharmacologically treat and possibly prevent diabetic retinopathy!

People with diabetes should also be aware that Avandia could cause macular edema and decreased vision. If patients taking Avandia have ankle edema and decreased vision, they should consider stopping Avandia. The same swelling noted in their legs can develop in their macula.

The Story of My Eye Problems

I (Steve Edelman) distinctly remember when I first developed eye problems. It was in the fall of 1983, after 12 years of living with diabetes. A classmate of mine, John, was a big burly guy who gave me the biggest bear hug of my life after one of our successful intramural softball games. Several hours later, I noticed my vision was blurry and the straight lines of one of my textbooks looked wavy. Another close classmate, Patty, drove me to an ophthalmologist; after a brief examination, he told me I had diabetic retinopathy. Patty cried and I started worrying about going blind. This was the first dilated eye examination of my life. My primary care doctor had never sent me for a dilated eye examination. Remember that in 1983, the Diabetes Control and Complications Trial (DCCT) was just getting started and many physicians were uninformed about any preventive strategies.

Unfortunately, the retinopathy progressed. One morning in March of 1986, I awoke unable to see out of my left eye. All I could see was a dense red haze. After several months of waiting for the blood to sink, I received laser therapy. It was difficult to work long hours as an endocrinology fellow and be handicapped and distracted during every waking minute of every day. I was able to read and study only with the aid of a big magnifying glass. A big red blob that moves around in your visual field is hard to ignore.

Over the next several years, I had three more eye hemorrhages, but I thank my lucky stars that they did not occur at the same time. One of the bleeding episodes was during a family vacation in Germany. I was really a lot of fun during that trip! After what seems like a zillion dilated eye examinations and over 2000 laser zaps to each eye, my eyes have stabilized and I have not had a hemorrhage since 1993 (knock on wood).

I consider myself lucky to have good vision as I write this book. I am able to drive (not according to my wife) and carry on a normal visual life. In exchange, I am happy to live with reduced peripheral vision and poor night vision. When I go into a dark movie theater, it is pitch black to me for a long time as my eyes are slow to adapt. Many of my eye problems could have been avoided if I had been more actively involved in my own care as a young adult.

Summary

The bottom line is that it is your responsibility to get a dilated eye examination at least once a year, preferably by someone familiar with the complications of diabetes in the eyes. This person must be an ophthalmologist if you already have eye problems. You can prevent blindness. Don't lose sight of the problem!

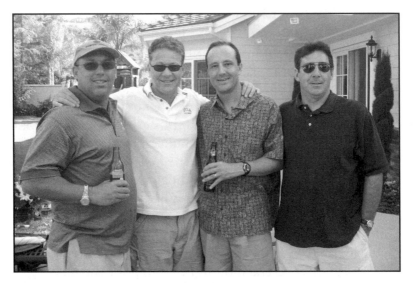

Me and my buddies *(from left to right)* Mike Spinazzola, me (Steve Edelman), Rob Merkin, and Bob Weinberger.

16

Diabetes Can Affect Your Musculoskeletal System

Stiff Hands, Trigger Fingers, and Aching Joints

by Rachel Peterson Kim, MD
and Steven V. Edelman, MD

Introduction

The musculoskeletal system is quite commonly affected by diabetes. The term "musculoskeletal system" refers to your joints, muscles, tendons, ligaments, and bones. Diabetes can cause a number of changes in the musculoskeletal system, which is usually a surprise to people with diabetes as well as to their caregivers. These changes can result in a variety of symptoms and conditions of which you should be aware. Some musculoskeletal conditions are unique to people with diabetes, whereas others are the same as those seen in people without the disease; however, they may occur at a higher frequency among people with diabetes. Importantly, many of these conditions are treatable, but you must first recognize and identify them, which has traditionally been the main problem. This chapter will review some of the more common musculoskeletal problems seen in people with diabetes.

Hands

The hands are commonly affected in diabetes. This can be quite problematic, as our hands clearly play an integral role in our daily personal and professional life. Diabetes can affect the hands in a number of ways.

Diabetic Cheiroarthropathy (Limited Joint Mobility)

The syndrome of limited joint mobility (also known as diabetic stiff-hand syndrome or diabetic cheiroarthropathy) is very much what it sounds like. There is limitation of joint movement, especially of the small joints of the hands, with a decreased ability to bend and/or straighten the fingers. The skin often becomes thickened, waxy, and tight. It is generally a painless condition and tends to affect all four fingers. The "prayer sign" observed in this condition is an inability to flatten the palms together completely, with a visible gap remaining between the opposed palms and fingers (**Figure 16-1**). Limited joint mobility occurs in both type 1 and type 2 diabetes, and the risk increases with increasing hemoglobin A1C values as well as with increased duration of diabetes. Limited joint mobility is difficult to treat and generally irreversible. Optimizing control of blood glucose is advised. Physical and occupational therapy with passive stretching of the palm may be of benefit when limited joint mobility affects the feet. It may also be associated with an increased risk of foot ulcers.

Flexor Tenosynovitis

Flexor tenosynovitis (or trigger finger) is a frequent musculo-skeletal complication of diabetes. Affected people complain of a catching sensation, or locking, of the finger(s). It is often painful, and there may be a nodule that can be felt on the palm at the base of the affected finger. The finger may actually become stuck in a flexed or bent position, requiring the use of the other hand to straighten it out (**Figure 16-2**). Trigger finger is more common in long-standing diabetes (**Figure 16-3**). A local steroid injection may be adequate treatment, at least temporarily, but sometimes minor outpatient surgery is required for trigger finger.

Figure 16-1

The "Prayer Sign" of Diabetic Cheiroarthropathy

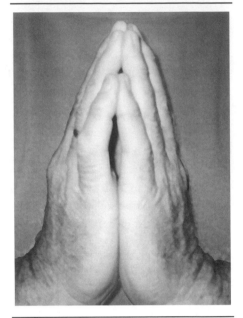

Diabetic cheiroarthropathy limits the ability to bend or straighten the fingers. Predictive of other diabetic complications, this syndrome tends to correlate with the duration of diabetes.

Dupuytren's Contracture

Dupuytren's contracture results from a thickening, shortening, and fibrosis of the connective tissue (fascia) just under the skin of the palm. The result is a pulling downward of the fingers (particularly the fourth and fifth fingers). Bands, bumps, or nodules are often felt along the palm. The frequency of Dupuytren's contracture increases with the duration of diabetes. It has a variable course. For mild cases, passive stretching of the digits and palms a few times a day is recommended (you can use a tabletop). For more advanced cases in which function is

Figure 16-2

The Trigger Finger of Flexor Tenosynovitis

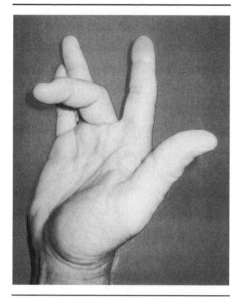

Flexor tenosynovitis is a catching sensation or locking of the finger(s) associated with pain and sometimes requiring use of the other hand to straighten the affected digit.

the duration of diabetes. Affected people often notice a burning pain, pins-and-needles sensation, or loss of sensation in the thumb, index, and middle fingers as well as half of the ring finger. The pain may radiate up the forearm and may be worse at night. It is usually made worse by activities such as driving, holding a newspaper or book, typing, or using a knife and fork. There may be associated loss of dexterity or weakness of the hand. If CTS is not severe, initial treatment consists of using

affected and/or there is significant pain, steroid injections may be tried, but are not very effective in long-standing cases. Surgery may be done for extreme cases, but the recurrence rate is high.

Carpal Tunnel Syndrome

Carpal tunnel syndrome (CTS) is seen in up to 20% of people with diabetes. It is due to compression of the median nerve as it passes through the wrist into the hand. In people with diabetes, this compression may be due to structural changes in the connective tissue of the wrist caused by high blood glucose. The finding of CTS is related to

Figure 16-3

Trigger Finger Coupled With Arthritis

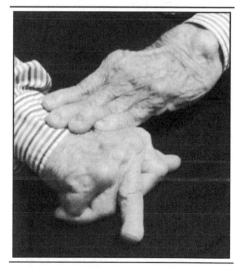

A patient with a long history of type 1 diabetes and arthritis, displaying trigger finger in all of her fingers except the middle one in her right hand.

wrist splints. Anti-inflammatory medications may also be tried (such as ibuprofen). Local steroid injection of the carpal tunnel is another option. For severe or refractory cases, carpal tunnel release surgery may be performed.

Shoulders

Adhesive Capsulitis

Adhesive capsulitis (frozen shoulder) has been reported in roughly 20% to 25% of people with diabetes. In this condition, the capsule that surrounds the shoulder joint becomes stiffened and tightened, resulting in restricted range of motion of the joint. Affected people notice stiffness, decreased movement, and sometimes pain in the shoulder. Treatment involves gentle stretching and range-of-motion exercises, often through physical therapy. Pain-relieving medications and/or steroid injections into the joint may also be used. The cause of this stiffening and contraction of the shoulder joint capsule is not well understood. It is generally reversible and responds well to appropriate treatment.

Reflex Sympathetic Dystrophy

Reflex sympathetic dystrophy (RSD) or "shoulder-hand syndrome" is another shoulder condition seen in people with diabetes. However, it may affect other parts of the arms or legs as well. Typical symptoms include severe pain or a burning sensation in the affected arm from the shoulder down to the hand. There may be associated swelling; skin changes such as shiny skin, changes in hair growth, and color or temperature changes of the affected area: Increased sensitivity to temperature and touch may also be seen. Trauma may precipitate RSD, but the cause is not always known. Anti-inflammatory medications, other pain relievers, and oral steroids have been used in conjunction with physical therapy for this condition. Sympathetic nerve blocks (blockade of some of the nerves of the sympathetic nervous system that supply the affected area) with numbing medication given by injection, usually performed by an anesthesiologist, may also be helpful.

Feet

People with diabetes must be meticulous about foot care. Injuries to the feet often go unnoticed in people with diabetes due to underlying peripheral neuropathy and the associated decreased sensation in the feet. For this reason, inspecting your feet on a regular basis is critical to prevent infections that may develop silently without any symptoms.

Diabetic Osteoarthropathy

Diabetic osteoarthropathy (also known as Charcot's joint or neuropathic arthropathy) is a chronic, severe, destructive form of arthritis associated with loss of sensation in a joint from underlying diabetic peripheral neuropathy. The foot is most commonly affected. This condition is quite rare, affecting approximately one in 700 people with type 1 or type 2 diabetes. Although the exact cause is uncertain, it is postulated that repeated inadvertent microtrauma to the joint, which goes unnoticed due to the underlying neuropathy and decreased sensation, results in laxity, instability, and degenerative changes with resulting deformity. Usually there is no history of overt trauma or injury, such as falling off a curb. There may be skin changes overlying the affected area, including redness, swelling, bruising, and ulcers. The diagnosis is confirmed with x-rays. Treatment includes avoidance of weight-bearing on the affected area, appropriate shoes, and possibly bisphosphonate therapy. Surgery is usually avoided in most cases.

Muscles

Diabetic muscle infarction (loss of adequate blood supply to an area of muscle, with resultant death of tissue) is a rare condition. It occurs spontaneously, without a history of trauma, and tends to affect people with a long history of poorly controlled diabetes. This condition is seen more commonly in people using insulin who also have other microvascular complications, such as neuropathy, nephropathy (kidney disease), or retinopathy (eye disease). Typical symptoms include the abrupt onset of pain and swelling of the affected muscle groups, such as the thigh or calf. Investigations are done to exclude other conditions, such as tumors, muscle infection or abscess, blood clots, localized muscle inflammation, or infection of the underlying bone. Muscle biopsy may be needed to confirm the diagnosis. There is no known cause of diabetic muscle infarction. Treatment consists of rest and pain relief. Routine daily activities may be painful but are not thought to be harmful. Physical therapy may cause worsening of spontaneous diabetic muscle infarction. The condition tends to slowly resolve over weeks to months in most cases.

Case Presentation

Steve is a 51-year-old physician who has been living with type 1 diabetes for over 30 years (yes, it is me again). In 1997, I started to develop a catching sensation in my right middle finger as I opened and closed my fist. This catching sensation developed into a painful locking of my finger when I bent it, and I had to use my left hand to unlock it. I developed a nodule on the upper part of my palm just below where the middle finger leaves the palm. I am also unable to align my palms and fingers together so that there is no gap between them (you can basically drive a truck through my gap). Those are my hands in the trigger finger and positive prayer sign photos (**Figures 16-1** and **16-2**).

I have both the syndrome of limited joint mobility and a trigger finger. For my trigger finger, I saw an orthopedic surgeon who injected the joint with steroids that helped for a few weeks but really screwed up my blood glucose for a few days. Eventually the problem got so painful and debilitating that I had hand surgery; it was an outpatient procedure lasting about 30 minutes (I required only local anesthesia with numbing medication).

The surgery involves simply cutting a cylindrical sheath in which the finger tendon travels back and forth when you flex your finger. With a trigger finger, the sheath gets too narrow or is swollen; the tendon slides through fine when you flex your finger but gets stuck when you try to straighten it. By cutting the sheath, the blockage is fixed (**Figure 16-4**).

I eventually went through the same situation with two more surgeries. My left thumb started to lock up last year, but when I had to take anti-inflammatory drugs for several months for a knee problem, the triggering went away... at least for now.

Summary

Diabetes does commonly affect the musculoskeletal system. These conditions can have a significant impact on the quality of daily life of people with diabetes. However, many of these complications are treatable, with resultant improvements in quality of life and more independence in activities of daily living. Become aware of the possible ways in which diabetes may affect your musculoskeletal system, and discuss these symptoms with your primary care physician or rheumatologist.

Figure 16-4

Surgical Procedure to Relieve Trigger Finger

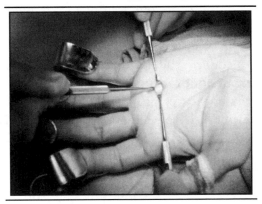

Steve Edelman's hand is shown here with the sheath being isolated so that the surgeon could cut it, relieving the trigger finger.

17

Diabetes Can Affect Your Stomach

by James D. Wolosin, MD

Introduction

Gastrointestinal (GI) disorders are common and those individuals affected by diabetes are certainly not immune to these problems. The medical term "GI" or "GI tract" refers those areas of the body from your mouth and throat, past your stomach and small intestine, and ending with the colon (large intestine) and rectum (**Figure 17-1**). The liver, gallbladder, and pancreas are also considered to be part of the GI tract as they are closely linked with digestive function.

Any discussion of GI manifestations of diabetes should first deal with the reality that most of us will experience, at some time in our life, common nondiabetic-related problems with our GI tract, whether it be ulcer disease, gallstones, irritable bowel syndrome, food poisoning, or some other malady. Up to 75% of people visiting diabetes clinics will report significant GI symptoms. Common complaints may include constipation, abdominal pain, nausea, vomiting, and diarrhea. Treatments provided in these situations are often no different between diabetics and nondiabetics. Nonetheless, it is apparent that in both the short and long term, poorly controlled diabetes can lead to specific GI problems.

As with other complications, the longer you have diabetes and the poorer the glucose control, the more severe the GI problems may be. Many GI complications of diabetes seem to be related to abnormal function of the nerves supplying the gut. Just as the nerves in the feet may be affected in the condition known as peripheral neuropathy, involvement of the intestinal nerves may lead to enteric neuropathy. This neuropathy may lead to abnormalities in intestinal motility (movement), sensation (pain), and secretion/absorption (digestion of foods). The purpose of this chapter is to familiarize you with the GI problems that you may experience living with diabetes (**Table 17-1**).

Throat and Stomach

Esophagus

The esophagus is the muscular tube that connects the mouth with the stomach and serves as an active conduit through which food is propelled. As we age, abnormalities of esophageal movement or motility

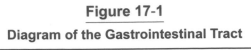

Figure 17-1

Diagram of the Gastrointestinal Tract

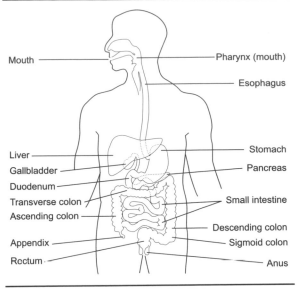

Mouth — Pharynx (mouth)
— Esophagus
Liver —
Gallbladder —
Duodenum —
Transverse colon —
Ascending colon —
Appendix —
Rectum —
— Stomach
— Pancreas
— Small intestine
— Descending colon
— Sigmoid colon
— Anus

become more common; the medical term for this is presbyesophagus or esophagus of the elders. This may be more common in diabetes, but it tends to cause only minor symptoms in most people. The most common esophageal problem seen in people with diabetes is yeast infection or candidiasis. Yeast loves sugar. When blood glucose levels are consistently high, yeast can grow in numerous areas, including the mouth, esophagus, intestine, vagina, and skin. Treatment is usually easy as there are numerous medications available to treat this including nystatin (various manufacturers and brand names) and Diflucan (fluconazole). When acid backs up into the esophagus from the stomach, heartburn occurs. This is no more common in diabetics than nondiabetics unless there is a component of delayed emptying of the stomach. Up to 30% of the general population experiences some degree of heartburn or gastroesophageal reflux disease (GERD). Treatment of GERD may include changes in diet/lifestyle, medications, elevation of the head of the bed, and occasionally surgery. Numerous effective medications are available including Zantac (ranitidine), Pepcid (famotidine), Prilosec (omeprazole), Aciphex (rabeprazole), and others.

Table 17-1

Gastrointestinal Problems in Diabetes

- *Mouth*: thrush
- *Throat*: thrush and reflux or heartburn
- *Stomach*: ulcers, gastroparesis (delayed stomach emptying)
- *Small intestine*: bacterial overgrowth, delayed emptying, and celiac sprue
- *Large intestine or colon*: neuropathy
- *Pancreas*: exocrine insufficiency
- *Liver:* fatty liver
- *Diabetic medications that may affect the stomach*: sulfonylureas, Glucophage, Glyset, and Precose

Delayed Stomach Emptying (Gastroparesis)

After eating, the stomach distends with food and digestive acid, then slowly contracts to mix, grind, and digest the meal. This involves a delicately coordinated process called peristalsis during which waves of muscular contractions force the food toward the outlet of the stomach. The contractions are coordinated with opening of the pylorus or "exit valve" of the stomach. The end result is gradual emptying of the stomach. In individuals with a long-standing history of diabetes, damage to the nerves supplying the stomach (eg, the vagus nerve) and damage to the stomach muscles can lead to gastroparesis or impairment in stomach emptying. This can be very difficult to deal with because erratic stomach emptying leads to unpredictable food absorption and blood glucose levels that are difficult to control. This is particularly true in people with diabetes treated with insulin where low blood glucose may occur following a mealtime injection of insulin followed by slow emptying of food from the stomach. Gastroparesis may cause bloating, distention, abdominal pain, nausea, or vomiting. Food and acid may back up into the esophagus (bottom part of the throat), leading to symptoms of heartburn and regurgitation. Fatty foods and very fibrous foods normally exit the stomach slowly and may be poorly tolerated in people with diabetic gastroparesis. Consumption of frequent small meals may provide some symptomatic relief. It is important not to stuff yourself at any meal.

Medications such as Reglan (metoclopramide) stimulate the stomach (gastric) nerve endings damaged by long-standing diabetes and may improve delayed stomach emptying. Erythromycin is an antibiotic that has unique properties that stimulate stomach motility and may be beneficial in select individuals. Propulsid (cisapride) may also help accelerate stomach emptying but is now only used in special circumstances because of cardiac side effects. Motilium (domperidone) is another agent that accelerates emptying of the stomach and is better tolerated than Reglan; however, it is not available in the United States (it is available in Canada and Mexico). Botox injections into the pylorus have been used successfully in some cases to enhance stomach emptying. Finally, a gastric pacemaker has recently been introduced that may help some individuals with diabetic gastroparesis. Newer agents that enhance stomach emptying will hopefully be available in the near future. Most important, careful attention to blood glucose control is essential.

Ulcer Disease

Ulcer disease is a common problem in people with or without diabetes and affects up to 10% of the population at some time during their life.

Acid irritation of the stomach or esophagus leads to heartburn, indigestion, and a burning sensation in the upper abdomen (dyspepsia). Ulcers can occur either in the stomach or duodenum (the first part of the small intestine). *Helicobacter pylori*, the bacteria responsible for many ulcers, is no more common in people with diabetes than in the general population. In fact, diabetes itself does not increase one's risk of developing ulcers. Individuals with ulcers and ulcerlike symptoms are treated in the same fashion whether or not they have diabetes. Treatment is geared toward suppression of gastric (stomach) acid secretion with H_2 blockers (Tagamet [cimetidine], Pepcid, Zantac, and Axid [nizatidine]) or the more potent proton pump inhibitors (Prilosec, Aciphex, Protonix [pantoprazole], Nexium [esomeprazole], and Zegerid [omeprazole/sodium bicarbonate]). This allows the acid-irritated lining of the intestine to heal. If *H pylori* is present, you will need to be treated with antibiotics as well.

Yeast Infections of the Gastrointestinal Tract

People with diabetes may develop yeast infections in the GI tract, especially when blood glucose is running high. When yeast infections occur in the mouth, it is called oral thrush and is characterized by a thick white coating of the tongue and throat, along with pain and burning in the mouth and throat. The infection may extend further down the throat and cause intestinal bleeding, heartburn, and difficulty swallowing. This type of extensive yeast infection is usually diagnosed with an endoscopic examination of the upper GI tract. Treatment is highly effective and is focused on the eradication of the yeast infection with medicines such as nystatin, Nizoral (ketoconazole), and Diflucan. Controlling the blood glucose is of utmost importance since the yeast loves a sweet environment. That is why women with poorly controlled diabetes experience vaginal yeast infections so frequently.

Small Intestine

Bacterial Overgrowth Syndrome

In some cases of long-standing diabetes, the enteric nerves supplying the small intestine may be affected, leading to abnormal motility of the small intestine. This leads to slowing of food transit through the intestine and some stagnation. This may result in an overgrowth of naturally occurring bacteria, leading to symptoms such as abdominal discomfort, bloating, diarrhea, and weight loss. Individuals who have had prior intestinal surgery may be at increased risk for this. The diagnosis of this condition may be difficult as it is hard to culture the contents of the small bowel accurately. Various breath tests may be helpful in diagnosing this condition, but more frequently, physicians may try a course of treatment with antibiotics to see if this helps. While just about any antibiotic can be helpful in lowering the bacterial count in the intestine, a newer antibiotic called Xifaxan (rifaximin) has certain unique advantages in treating this condition. It is a nonabsorbable antibiotic (active only in the intestine) and has a very broad spectrum of activity against the bacteria in the intestine. In addition, medications that promote more rapid motility in the small intestine may be of benefit in clearing out the overgrowth of bacteria.

Diabetic Neuropathy of the Small Intestine

At times, damage to enteric nerves may lead to a chronic abdominal pain syndrome similar to the pain that may occur in the feet of people with peripheral neuropathy. This condition may be difficult to treat but will sometimes respond to pain medications and tricyclic antidepressant medications, such as Elavil. Tricyclic antidepressants act on the sensory nerves to decrease pain sensation and increase pain tolerance. Other medicines with possible benefit include Tegretol (carbamazepine), Dilantin (phenytoin), and Neurontin (gabapentin), but these medications have a higher incidence of side effects. Unfortunately, narcotic addiction may be common in patients with this type of painful neuropathy as it may be difficult to treat.

Celiac Disease

Celiac disease (also known as celiac sprue) is a rather uncommon disorder of digestion that is caused by a reaction to gluten, a protein commonly found in wheat, barley, rye, and sometimes oats. Although it may occur in up to 0.5% of the general population, the disorder is more common in type 1 diabetics, and approximately 6% may be affected. Why this occurs is uncertain. There is clearly a genetic or inherited component to the condition and up to 10% of first-degree relatives of a patient with celiac disease may also be affected.

Celiac disease is not considered a true food allergy, but when people with this condition consume gluten, their immune system is activated, leading to damage to the lining of the small intestine. Because the body's own immune system is triggering this damage, celiac disease is considered to be an autoimmune condition. The type of damage that occurs to the small intestine is unique and leads to changes that can be easily identified by a biopsy of the small intestine. There is flattening and inflammation of the characteristic fingerlike projections coating the lining of the small bowel (villi). When this damage occurs, food and nutrients cannot be absorbed properly and inadequate absorption occurs (malabsorption). This leads to multiple symptoms, including diarrhea, bloating, abdominal pain, weight loss, and fatigue. Stools may become grey and oily in appearance due to inadequate absorption of fats. Lack of proper nutrition may lead to anemia, vitamin and protein deficiency, and thinning of the bones (osteoporosis). In children, growth retardation is a frequent problem. A rare skin condition called dermatitis herpetiformis may occur in conjunction with celiac disease.

Unfortunately, the symptoms of celiac disease are nonspecific and are similar to those seen in more common conditions such as irritable bowel syndrome. This frequently leads to a delay in the diagnosis of celiac disease. When this condition is suspected, the first tests should include blood tests for antiendomysial, antitissue transglutaminase, and possibly antigliadin antibodies. These blood tests are relatively accurate in diagnosing this condition. In addition, a biopsy of the small intestine may be advised. All of these tests may become negative or normal if a gluten-free diet is eaten.

The only treatment for celiac disease is to avoid consumption of all gluten. Unfortunately, gluten is present in a large amount of the food that we consume. Wheat, rye, barley, and oats are very common and are present in foods such as grain, pasta, cereal, cakes, and bread. Gluten is commonly used as a thickener and is present in many gravies and sauces. The good news is that many foods are gluten free, including fresh meat, fish, and chicken, as well as fruits and vegetables. Over the past 10 years, awareness about gluten sensitivity has increased and there are now specialty stores that supply gluten-free breads and pastas. Many foods are labeled as gluten free in stores. There is a large amount of information available on the Internet as well *(www.celiac.org, www. csaceliacs.org)*.

Celiac disease is a relatively uncommon cause of intestinal problems that occurs more frequently in individuals with type 1 diabetes. Patients with diabetes who are experiencing intestinal problems should be screened for celiac disease. A simple blood test can determine whether there is a concern for this very treatable condition.

Colon or Large Intestine

There is limited information available regarding the effects of diabetes on the colon (or large intestine). Neuropathy may affect the nerves of the colon, leading to some decrease in motility. Constipation is one of the more common GI complaints seen with neuropathy of the colon. Proper evaluation must first ascertain that there are no structural abnormalities of the colon, such as mechanical blockage. Fiber supplementation with bran or psyllium products (Metamucil, Citrucel, Konsyl), as well as a high-fiber diet, increases the water content of the bowel movement and may relieve constipation. Mild laxatives, such as milk of magnesia or Dulcolax (bisacodyl), will often help as well. Zelnorm (tegaserod) accelerates colonic movement and may increase the frequency of bowel movements.

Diabetic Diarrhea

As many as 20% of people with a long-standing history of diabetes may experience frequent, unexplained diarrhea. Diabetic diarrhea is a syndrome of unexplained persistent diarrhea in people with a long duration of diabetes. This may be related to problems in the small bowel or colon. Abnormally rapid transit of fluids may occur in the colon, leading to increased bowel movement frequency and urgency. In addition, abnormalities in the absorption and secretion of colonic fluids may develop, leading to increased bowel movement volume, frequency, and water content. Diabetic diarrhea may also be due to neuropathy, leading to abnormal motility and secretion of fluid in the colon. In addition, there are a multitude of intestinal problems that are not unique to diabetes that can cause diarrhea, the most common of which is the irritable bowel syndrome.

Evaluation and treatment of diarrhea is similar in people with or without diabetes. If the basic medical evaluation of diarrhea is unable to target a specific cause for the diarrhea, then treatment is tailored toward providing symptomatic relief with antidiarrheal agents such as Lomotil (diphenoxylate/atropine) and Imodium (loperamide). Fiber supplementation with bran, Citrucel, Metamucil, or high-fiber food items may also thicken the consistency of the bowel movement and decrease watery diarrhea. In addition, antispasmodic medicines such as Levsin (hyoscyamine), Bentyl (dicyclomine), and Donnatal (belladonna/phenobarbital) may decrease stool frequency. Finally, in severe cases, injections of a GI hormone (Sandostatin [octreotide]) have been shown to significantly decrease the frequency of diabetic diarrhea. The bottom line is that you need to work with your caregiver to find the most effective treatment strategy that works best for you. Tighter control of blood glucose may be beneficial in this situation.

Pancreas

The pancreas is the organ that secretes insulin, the hormone that helps to control the blood glucose levels in the body. This is called the endocrine function of the pancreas. However, the pancreas also has an exocrine function (ie, secretion of digestive enzymes directly into the intestinal tract to aid in the breakdown and absorption of carbohydrates, proteins, and fats). Up to 80% of individuals with type 1 diabetes will have some degree of impairment in pancreatic exocrine function, but this is rarely significant enough to lead to any clinical problems with digestion. The pancreas has a tremendous reserve, and a modest reduction in pancreatic enzyme secretion rarely leads to difficulty in food breakdown or absorption. The exocrine function of the pancreas may also be affected in some patients with type 2 diabetes but to a lesser extent. The symptoms of pancreatic exocrine insufficiency include watery diarrhea, floating bowel movements in the toilet bowl, and cramping after eating. The treatment is simply to take pancreatic enzyme pills with each meal. The results of therapy are usually quite good. In individuals who have had chronic problems with inflammation of the pancreas or have had surgical removal of the pancreas, diabetes may ensue due to a lack of insulin secretion from the gland. Insulin therapy is generally required in these situations.

Liver

We have entered a new era in which obesity has become much more prevalent and with it has come an epidemic of diabetes. One of the very first abnormalities that arise in the metabolic syndrome that is associated with obesity and adult-onset diabetes is the development of nonalcoholic fatty-liver disease. This syndrome is associated with obesity, elevated cholesterol/triglycerides, and insulin resistance. Fat is deposited within the liver and leads to abnormalities similar to alcohol-related liver disease. While up to 25% of the American public have this condition, only a small percentage (less than 5%) go on to the more advanced stage of nonalcoholic steatohepatitis or NASH. These numbers are much higher in obese individuals and those who have type 2 diabetes. NASH is associated with progressive liver disease and may even advance to cirrhosis or liver cancer.

Fatty liver has become one of the more common causes of abnormal liver tests. Common symptoms include right-upper abdominal pain and fatigue. Treatment usually is centered on weight loss and good control of blood glucose levels. Medicines such as Actos (pioglitazone) and Avandia (rosiglitazone) may help lower elevated insulin levels in type 2 diabetes and may lead to improvement in the fatty-liver syndrome. Glucophage (metformin) may also be of benefit in treating fatty liver but further research is needed before this can be recommended as a routing treatment.

Fatty liver is often one of the first signs that an individual is developing diabetes and can be a wake-up call to change one's lifestyle to help prevent the development of diabetes.

Gallstones

Diabetic patients seem to have an increased incidence of gallstones and other gallbladder problems, but these problems, much like fatty infiltration of the liver, are primarily related to the obesity associated with type 2 diabetes and not the diabetes itself. Obesity leads to secretion of bile (the fluid that goes into the gallbladder) by the liver that is oversaturated with cholesterol. This bile tends to form tiny cholesterol crystals in the gallbladder that eventually grow into gallstones. Gallstones are also common in the general population, with a 15% lifetime risk.

People without diabetes with gallstones have traditionally been advised to avoid surgery for gallstones (cholecystectomy) unless symptoms of gallbladder disease develop. Typical symptoms include intermittent right-upper abdominal pain, nausea, and jaundice (skin and eyes turn yellow). In the past, people with diabetes have been instructed to have surgery for gallstones whether or not they had symptoms because of a concern for an increased risk of complications, such as infection or rupture of the gallbladder. However, more recent experience with modern medical and surgical care would indicate that this is not the case. Thus people with diabetes and gallstones should be managed in a fashion similar to nondiabetics. Surgery is generally recommended only for those individuals whose gallstones are causing symptoms.

Gastrointestinal Side Effects of Medications Used to Treat Diabetes

Patients with diabetes are treated with a wide range of medications designed to control blood glucose and, although most are well tolerated, some may have significant GI side effects. Any discussion of the GI complications of diabetes would be incomplete without mention of the potential side effects of some of these medications. Insulin itself is generally well tolerated and free of any significant GI side effects. This topic is also discussed earlier in the chapter on oral agents.

Sulfonylureas

Orinase (tolbutamide) and Diabinase (chlorpropamide), which are older sulfonylurea drugs, may be associated with nausea, vomiting, diarrhea, and loss of appetite, although this occurs in less than 5% of patients. Newer, second-generation sulfonylurea drugs, such as DiaBeta (glyburide), Micronase (glyburide), and Amaryl (glimepiride), are rarely associated with intestinal problems; nausea, diarrhea, and abdominal pain occur in less than 2% of patients.

Glucophage

Glucophage (metformin) may be associated with significant intestinal symptoms, such as diarrhea, loose stools, nausea, gas, and appetite suppression, in up to 20% of patients. These symptoms tend to occur shortly after the medication has been started and improve with time. Starting with a low dose of medication and slowly increasing it may minimize symptoms. Intestinal symptoms are rare in patients taking the medication long-term. Occasionally, a metallic taste in the mouth may occur.

Precose and Glyset

Precose (acarbose) and Glyset (miglitol) act to lower blood glucose levels by preventing the breakdown and absorption of dietary carbohydrates. GI side effects are common due to the malabsorption of carbohydrates and the presence of undigested sugars in the small intestine. These include gaseousness, diarrhea, and abdominal discomfort. Slow titration is important to reduce these side effects (see Chapter 6).

Summary

So what can you do to help prevent the GI problems that may sometimes develop with diabetes? First and foremost, take care of yourself and use common sense. Tight control of your blood glucose will help prevent the complications of enteric neuropathy and worsening of your bowel function. Eat sensibly and follow a low-fat, high-fiber diet. Avoid overeating, weight gain, and obesity since these are independent risk factors for the development of some GI problems, especially gallstones and fatty liver. Obesity is a major contributing factor associated with type 2 diabetes and a low-fat, low-calorie diet may lead to better blood glucose control and subsequently to a decreased incidence of long-term complications. Pay careful attention to your diet and try to avoid any food items that tend to precipitate symptoms. Fatty foods in particular may delay emptying of food from your stomach and will contribute to bloating, nausea, and vomiting in some individuals. Stress management is important as emotional factors will often affect GI motility and exacerbate intestinal problems. Remember, GI problems are extremely common both in the general population and in individuals with diabetes. Many of these problems are readily treated by primary care physicians, diabetologists, and gastroenterologists. Do not hesitate to discuss these problems with your physician, especially if the problems are persistent or are associated with other significant health-related conditions.

18

Caring for Your Teeth and Gums

An Imperative Task for People With Diabetes

by Mayssoun S. Khoury, DDS,
Cyndee R. Fena, RDH, MT,
and Steven V. Edelman, MD

Introduction

Diabetes is strongly associated with many inflammatory conditions. Among these is periodontal disease, which is considered the sixth major complication of diabetes.

This chapter will clarify the bidirectional relationship between diabetes and periodontal disease, discuss the additional oral problems associated with diabetes, and explain various effective measures that help prevent and treat such problems.

What Is Periodontal Disease?

Periodontal disease is a painless process that damages the supporting structures of the tooth (gum, bone, and ligament tissue that fasten the tooth to the jaw bone). It is estimated that 80% of the adult population in the United States has periodontal disease.

Periodontal disease causes more loss of teeth than tooth decay and is considered more serious because it is almost symptom-free until its destruction becomes severe. Once you have this condition, it is almost impossible to eradicate it with preventive procedures only. However, early detection and continued treatment can slow down the destructive process.

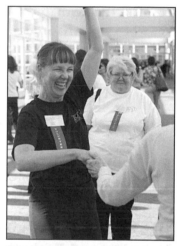

Cyndee Fena had an infectious enthusiasm for life and was our head volunteer at TCOYD. Unfortunately, she passed away from a severe hypoglycemic reaction in 2006.

Periodontal disease is called plaque disease because plaque is the main reason for this condition to appear. What is plaque? Plaque is a thin coat or layer which comes from saliva and forms on the tooth surfaces and traps many bacteria. Fortunately, it can be removed by proper brushing and flossing.

When a person with poorly controlled diabetes does not brush or floss thoroughly, a sticky layer full of bacteria (plaque) starts to build up on the surface of teeth. With the help of nutrients from the high content of sugar in saliva and the host food, the bacteria begin to grow. In a few days, the plaque can turn into calculus (a hard substance that gathers under the gum line). As plaque continues to form over the calculus, the gums become red, sore, swollen, and bleed easily from brushing and flossing. This first stage of periodontal disease is called gingivitis. With gingivitis, there are often no pain signals to alert the person with diabetes. Gingivitis can be treated completely by effective oral hygiene procedures, but if left unchecked, it can become quite serious.

As periodontal disease progresses, inflamed gums pull away from the surface of the crown and root of the tooth, forming a pocket where bacteria accumulate and destroy the ligament tissue and the bone; this is when periodontitis occurs. At the final stage, the supporting structures are eroded; the tooth becomes loose and is eventually lost.

Table 18-1 lists periodontal disease signs and symptoms that you should be aware of.

Table 18-1

Periodontal Disease's Signs and Symptoms

- Gums bleed from brushing and flossing
- Teeth look longer due to receding gum lines, and they become sensitive
- Bad breath or bad taste forms in the mouth
- Teeth become loose and separate
- The person's bite changes when teeth close against one another
- The fit of dental appliances may change (partial dentures)

Bidirectional Relationship Between Diabetes and Periodontal Disease

Diabetes reduces the body's resistance to infection. This explains why periodontitis is a common problem in individuals with diabetes, especially among people with poorly controlled diabetes. Moreover, recent research implies that chronic periodontal disease may be a risk factor for developing diabetes by allowing bacteria to enter the bloodstream and activate the immune system. These active cells produce inflammatory signals that have destructive effects throughout the body, including the pancreas. Periodontitis can also complicate the management of blood glucose levels.

This bidirectional relationship requires treatment of two chronic diseases (diabetes and periodontitis). This critical task can be accomplished by increasing awareness on the part of people with diabetes, physicians, dentists, dental hygienists, and diabetes educators.

Additional Oral Problems That Can Occur in People With Diabetes

In addition to periodontal diseases, there are other oral problems that can affect diabetic patients, including the following:

- Dry mouth (xerostomia): Many individuals with poorly controlled diabetes experience dry mouth as a result of salivary gland dysfunction or the dehydration effect of the diabetes process itself. It can also be a side effect of medications that are often prescribed for individuals with diabetes (drugs used to treat high blood pressure, swelling of legs, neuropathy, and depression). Dry mouth predisposes patients to an increase of plaque accumulation (which enhances the development of dental cavities and periodontal diseases), decrease of taste sensation, difficulty in swallowing, and inflamed painful oral mucosa.

  The appropriate management for dry mouth caused by diabetes is to control the diabetes. However, to alleviate the dryness, people with diabetes are advised to wash their mouth with fluoride mouth rinse (alcohol-free), drink a lot of liquid and refrain from using drinks containing caffeine, use artificial saliva or saliva stimulants, and chew sugar-free gum. **Table 18-2** shows the suggestions for dry mouth management.

Table 18-2

Dry Mouth Management

- Wash the mouth with fluoride mouth rinse (alcohol free)
- Drink a lot of liquid (avoid drinks containing caffeine)
- Use artificial saliva or saliva stimulants
- Use sugar-free chewing gum

- Oral fungal infection (candidiasis) and delay of wound healing: As a result of high blood glucose levels, the reduced saliva flow rate and the high content of sugar in saliva create an attractive environment for fungal infections, especially among those who wear dentures (due to improper cleaning of the dentures), those who smoke, and those who are often required to take antibiotics.

  Oral fungal infection produces white patches in the mouth that may be sore or may turn into ulcers. Any oral ulcer that does not heal within 2 weeks should be seen and examined by one's dentist.

The management of oral candidiasis requires good oral hygiene. This includes gently cleaning the involved tissue, applying topical antifungal agent, properly cleaning the dentures, avoiding smoking, and improving glucose control.

- Decrease of taste sensation is a symptom often affecting individuals with diabetes, and may result from a change in salivary chemistry, dry mouth, or the presence of oral fungal infection.
- Oral neuropathy, although a rare complication of diabetes, is often manifested by numbness or burning sensation in the mouth or on the tongue and lips (similar to neuropathy in the feet). This condition is usually worse in individuals with poor diabetes control.
- Halitosis (bad breath) is another common condition in the general public as well as in people with diabetes. Diabetes leads to several abnormalities that can cause the development of oral malodor, such as ketoacidosis (which produces a very distinct acetone fruity sweet odor) and dry mouth. Also, gingivitis and periodontitis are considered common causes of halitosis.

Identifying the cause of halitosis helps to develop the appropriate treatment plan. If the bad breath originates from poor diabetes control, then we should look first into improving the glucose control. If the bad breath originates from periodontal disease, then we should start treating this inflammatory condition by promoting improvement of oral hygiene and tongue brushing. **Table 18-3** lists the additional oral problems associated with diabetes.

Table 18-3

Additional Oral Problems Associated With Diabetes

- Dry mouth
- Oral fungal infection and delay of wound healing
- Decrease of taste sensation
- Oral neuropathy
- Halitosis

How Can You Keep Your Teeth and Gums Healthy?

To keep their teeth and gums healthy, individuals with diabetes should follow the general guidelines listed in **Table 18-4** and discussed below:

- *Control blood glucose level.* Because of the bidirectional relationship between diabetes and periodontal disease, the person with diabetes should be aware of the signs and symptoms of these two conditions and understand that neglecting oral health will eventually develop oral infection that might interfere with management of diabetes.
- *If you are a smoker, avoid smoking.* Tobacco is one cause of periodontal disease. Smoking can be associated with gum recession,

pocket formation, and the loss of bone and teeth. This explains why smoking cessation programs are essential for the successful treatment of periodontal disease.

- *Eat a well-balanced diet.* Nutrition is important for the maintenance of oral tissues, and the nutritional factor is related to preventing infection and enhancing wound healing.

- *Apply good oral hygiene.* Oral hygiene is considered the cornerstone of prevention. Since every mouth is different, your dentist needs to personalize an oral hygiene regimen for you. The general guidelines in basic oral hygiene are the following:

- *Brush your teeth twice daily.* Brushing removes plaque and food particles from the sides of the teeth and stimulates the gums. It is advisable to use a soft or extra-soft toothbrush positioned at a 45-degree angle so it can scrape under the gums as you brush away from the gum line while applying gentle force. Once you finish brushing, you should brush your tongue gently to freshen your breath. Change your brush when the old one loses its original shape or stiffness. Soak your brush once a week in hydrogen peroxide or an antiseptic mouthwash to clean it of bacteria. Unless your dentist recommends a certain type of toothpaste, use whatever kind you enjoy, but it should contain fluoride. Many individuals prefer electric toothbrushes. Ask your hygienist about the proper way of brushing using a powered toothbrush.

- *Floss at least once daily* (**Figure 18-1**). It has been shown that after teeth are brushed, 40% of the tooth is still unclean. Flossing finishes the job that brushing starts.

Table 18-4

General Guidelines to Keep the Teeth and Gums Healthy

- Control diabetes
- Avoid smoking
- Eat a well-balanced diet
- Apply good oral hygiene (effective brushing, flossing, and mouth rinsing; if you wear dentures, clean them properly)
- Visit your dentist 3 or 4 times a year for professional teeth cleaning, cavity control, monitoring, and possible periodontal treatment

Figure 18-1

Proper Flossing Technique

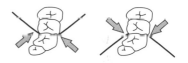

Wrap floss around half of the tooth, maneuvering the floss through the space while scraping the plaque off from the gums to the top of the tooth. Repeat for each tooth sharing a space.

It removes plaque and food particles from between the teeth and around the gums. The proper flossing method is as follows: Take an 18-inch piece of dental floss and be sure to move along the floss (or to a new place on the floss) for every new area you are cleaning so you are not transferring plaque and bacteria into other areas. Keep your fingers close to the teeth and gently maneuver the floss through the space between them. Wrap the floss around half of the tooth and scrape the plaque off from the gums toward the biting surfaces of the teeth. It does not matter what kind of floss you use. When choosing dental floss, you should always consider your specific oral condition, for example, ribbon floss can be used to clean around dental implants. For individuals who have periodontitis with deep pockets, dental floss may not be able to reach; it is advisable to use a WaterPik irrigation device in conjunction with tooth brushing.

– *Be careful with mouthwashes.* Some contain fluoride to protect the teeth from decay and some have an antibacterial effect to control gingivitis. Be careful with mouthwashes that have a high content of alcohol, since these can be hard on your gums (alcohol can sometimes make the gums blister and peel). Unless your dentist suggests a specific mouthwash or toothpaste, you should choose oral care products that display the American Dental Association's Seal of Acceptance. Hydrogen peroxide mixed half and half with water is an inexpensive and effective mouthwash. Because the bacteria that cause periodontal disease are anaerobic (live best where there is no oxygen), they cannot survive when exposed to the oxygen in hydrogen peroxide. It is advisable to wash your mouth twice daily for 30 seconds each time.

– *If you wear dentures, clean them properly.* Dirty dentures are sources of bacteria and fungi which may cause unpleasant odor and localized or systemic fungal infection. Patients are advised to take good care of their dentures and the soft underlying tissues and to perform regular oral self-check to detect and treat any irritation.

• *Have your teeth cleaned regularly.* You should visit your dentist at least two times a year. The frequency of cleaning may increase three to four times a year if you are diagnosed with periodontal disease and your diabetes becomes out of control. If after periodontal probing your dentist finds that you have periodontal disease and gum treatment is necessary, consultation with your physician is desirable. You may need antibiotics before any future dental treatment because you are more susceptible to infection after cleaning, especially if your blood glucose level is not under control. Since your ability to fight off infections is compromised by high blood glucose levels, it is important to get your glucose level under control prior to any dental appointment. If your gum infection is severe, you may need to make a change in your insulin or medication dosage to better control your diabetes.

To decrease the risk of an episode of low blood glucose (hypoglycemia) in the dental office, appointments should be scheduled after meals, preferably in the morning. Depending on your type of diabetes, be cautious when scheduling an appointment during your lunch break or late in the day (before dinner) when your blood glucose level may become low, especially if your dental procedure interferes with eating. You should bring your own glucose meter to your appointment so that you can check yourself if needed. Avoid long appointments. If several procedures must be done to complete your dental work, spread them out over several visits. This is especially helpful in individuals with type 1 diabetes on a multiple-injection insulin regimen and who have had hypoglycemic episodes in the past. **Table 18-5** lists some important precautions to take when visiting the periodontist, dentist, or hygienist.

Table 18-5

Precautions to Take When Visiting the Dentist

- Make your appointment at an appropriate time, especially if you are on insulin therapy
- Bring your glucose meter to your appointment
- Get your blood glucose under adequate control prior to your dental appointment if possible
- Avoid long appointments, especially if you are on insulin therapy

Questions Your Dentist May Want to Ask You

Your dentist needs to be provided with important information about your diabetes at each appointment to avoid any potential problems:

- Do you take any oral medications and/or insulin to control your diabetes?
- How much, what kind, and how many times a day do you take oral diabetic drugs and/or insulin?
- When have you last eaten today? What was your last glycosylated hemoglobin (A1C) value, and when was it taken?
- What other medical conditions do you have?

Having this information available before your appointment will make it go faster and easier. Print it out on a sheet of paper to leave with your dentist to review and put in your chart.

Case Presentation

Steve Edelman is a 51-year-old man who has lived with type 1 diabetes for the past 36 years. He is a busy physician and was told by his dentist that he had periodontal disease. The dentist pushed a thin metal probe along his teeth next to his gums and measured how far the probe penetrated (the probe, when it penetrates deeply, indicates periodontal disease). Steve's blood glucose control was adequate (A1C 7.2%), although he did not floss regularly (usually only during the week preceding and just after his dental appointment!). Steve always seemed to become motivated after his appointment to floss regularly but that lasted no more than 4 or 5 days. His usual time to floss was at bedtime and although he had good intentions, Steve was usually too tired and told himself he would do it the next night, which never happened. After extensive periodontal work, lots of time at the dental office, and a huge bill that was not covered by his dental plan, Steve decided to change his ways.

Steve finally learned how to brush his teeth correctly. He also flosses regularly after dinner instead of at bedtime. Steve keeps an extra toothbrush, mouthwash, and dental floss at work and in his car for those days that he feels really motivated. His breath has improved and his dentist noticed a marked improvement in his periodontal disease. He also has his teeth cleaned 3 times a year instead of twice a year.

Summary

As the Surgeon General's *Report on Oral Health* states, good oral health is integral to general health. The mouth reflects general health and well-being. Therefore, taking control of your teeth and gums is important. Like so many complications of diabetes, periodontal disease can creep up on you slowly until the condition is fairly severe. Preventive measures include regular proper brushing, rinsing, and especially flossing your teeth. It seems that the major challenge is to develop good dental habits that you can perform regularly on an ongoing basis and not just a few days before your scheduled dental appointment.

Q: What does the dentist of the year get?
A: A little plaque.

19

Taking Care of the Skin You're In

Dry Skin, Rashes, and Other Skin Disorders That Affect People With Diabetes

by Janet M. Trowbridge, MD, PhD

My life has not been directly touched by diabetes. However, I have learned a great deal from my patients who have presented with many manifestations of diabetes. I have also had the pleasure of training under Dr. Edelman at UCSD. So here goes.

There are a number of skin conditions that affect people with diabetes. They have impressive polysyllabic names like necrobiosis lipoidica diabeticorum, diabetic dermopathy, and acanthosis nigricans, and are best diagnosed and treated by a dermatologist. **Table 19-1** lists some dermatologic conditions that affect people with diabetes.

This list is by no means comprehensive. Ironically, dermatologists sometimes find the first clue that diabetes might be affecting a person. That's because, ultimately, the skin is a canvas on which the body's inner workings are projected. The skin is an amazing organ. In fact, your skin is your body's largest organ. It is a critical part of your body's immune system. Since uncontrolled diabetes can lead to poor immune function, the skin's myriad functions can be impaired. So while you care for your heart, kidneys, and lungs, you should also remember to take care of your packaging. Your skin is your first line of defense against a very harsh world.

Table 19-1

Some Skin Conditions Associated With Diabetes

- Xerosis (dry skin)
- Yeast and fungal infections
- Acanthosis nigricans
- Necrobiosis lipoidica
- Eruptive xanthomas
- Scleredema diabeticorum
- Neuropathic ulcers
- Diabetic dermopathy
- Granuloma annulare

Think about it! Your skin has to protect you from extreme changes in temperature and humidity. Your skin is also front and center for mechanical trauma like abrasions and burns. Finally, skin breaks are the portal by which a plethora of wee beasties enter and cause a great deal of damage. The environment is full of bacteria, fungi, and viruses just waiting for the chance to break though the skin's barrier and set up shop. We call these "opportunistic infections." Many organisms, especially yeast and fungi, are plentiful in our environment and usually don't get the chance to cause much trouble. That's why wound prevention and especially foot wound prevention is so critical. As a dermatologist, I see a lot of feet, and a common complaint from patients with diabetes (as well as the general public) is toenail and foot fungus.

Toenail Fungus and Athlete's Foot

The name says it all, almost, because in addition to fungal growth, we also see yeast and bacteria in this setting (**Figure 19-1** and **Figure 19-2**). The concept is that microtrauma creates a warm, moist, inviting environment (think Miami!) for potential pathogens. Once fungi set in, the nail becomes yellow, thickened, brittle, and difficult to cut. The skin on the foot and between the toes can become scaly and inflamed, resulting in tissue breakdown.

This is a setup for a wound. The best treatment is—you guessed it—prevention. Regular podiatric care is a must. Never, ever try to cut, file, or otherwise do battle with nail fungus. An easy means of prevention is keeping feet dry, wearing cotton socks, and keeping toenails trimmed short.

Figure 19-1
Athlete's Foot (Tinea pedis)

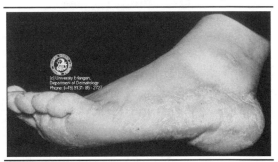

Treatment

An agent like urea, which is available with a prescription (one brand is Carmol-40), is great for keeping the nail thin and pliable. It is also good to use in combination with topical antifungals if fungus gains a foothold. I have people alternate the Carmol with an antifungal

Figure 19-2
Toenail Fungus

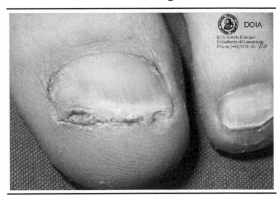

solution or cream. There is even a clear antifungal nail lacquer on the market. This regimen is also great for scaly, itchy feet, which we call a "moccasin" distribution; it is incredibly common. You can alternate an antifungal cream like clotrimazole, which is available over the counter, with urea. Despite what you see in television and magazines ads, oral antifungals are not a panacea for fungal infections. The cure rate is far from 100%! Because many of these agents have side effects like liver damage and because they can interact with other more critical medications, I try to avoid them.

Fungus and Yeast Elsewhere (Think Other Moist, Warm Regions)

The body has other warm, moist real estate too. And under the right circumstances, yeast and fungus will move in. What does fungus look like? Affected areas are usually round, red, and scaly. The outer borders look raised and are redder than the center that may even start to look like normal skin. It is often very itchy and tends to spread slowly over time.

Yeast, or Candida, is pinkish and moist appearing. It favors what are called intertriginous areas, basically areas where skin touches skin, such as the genitals, groin, armpits, and the skin under the breast (**Figure 19-3**) or belly. A telltale sign that an itchy area is caused by yeast is the presence of little red pustules studding the edge of the affected area. Thrush refers to yeast infection in the mouth.

Figure 19-3

Inframammary candidiasis

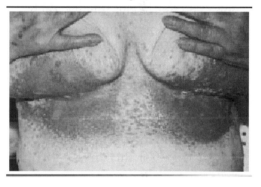

Treatment

Prevention is the cornerstone. Keeping moist areas as dry as possible is the key. Patting dry and air-drying after bathing and using drying powders, such as Zeosorb or Zeosorb-AF (AF stands for antifungal), can help. Wearing cotton clothing is also helpful. As with all skin issues in a person with diabetes, you must be certain to seek out help if an infection is suspected because this might signal that your diabetes is poorly controlled. If so, you are poorly equipped to fight off the wee beasties. An over-the-counter topical antifungal/antiyeast, such as Lotrisone (clotrimazole) or Nizoral (ketoconazole), is often sufficient. However, in some cases, a physician may prescribe an oral medication such as Diflucan (fluconazole) or Sporanox (itraconazole) if the fungal or yeast infection is extensive.

Acanthosis Nigricans

I mentioned earlier that sometimes dermatologists are the first to diagnose diabetes and this is one of the tip-offs. Brown color and a velvety textural change of skin around the face, neck, underarms (**Figure 19-4**, *top*), and groin is most commonly found in association with diabetes and obesity. The elbows, knees, toes, and fingers (**Figure 19-4**, *bottom*) may also be affected. The change can be subtle or extreme and is not uncommon. It often precedes the other telltale signs of the disease. Why this happens is not entirely clear. The most common explanation holds that high levels of insulin lead to these skin changes.

Treatment

Weight loss is often a good way to stop and even reverse these skin changes. Controlling diabetes might also help. However, there are no guaranteed fixes for this one. The use of keratolytics, such as urea and ammonium lactate, might decrease the thickness of the skin. Retinoids might also help. In general, this is mostly a cosmetic concern. So here I am saying it again: Prevention is the key. If diabetes runs in your family, be on the look-out for this one.

Figure 19-4

Acanthosis Nigricans

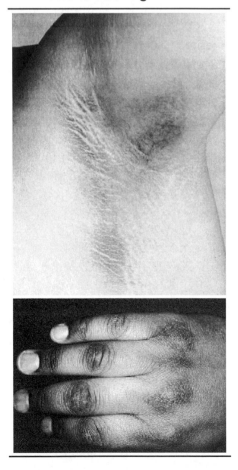

Diabetic Dermopathy for "Shin Spots"

Diabetic dermopathy refers to the brown to dull red, round, often indented spots on the shin that occur after minor trauma (**Figure 19-5**). Shin spots probably represent impaired skin barrier and repair functions that I previously mentioned. Other than being unsightly, they are not dangerous. There is no treatment other than (you guessed it) not getting them in the first place. Long pants and compression stockings if you suffer from poor circulation can help, as can glucose control and being careful!

Necrobiosis Lipoidica Diabeticorum

How's that for a name? Most dermatologists call this NLD because pronouncing it all at once can be difficult and it sounds rather serious. NLD refers to yellowish to orange areas on the shins or legs (**Figure 19-6**). They are firm to the touch and may be shiny and slightly depressed with raised borders. NLD is not usually painful or otherwise symptomatic. The skin appears thin and sometimes tiny blood vessels are visible. These areas are very fragile and may bleed and ulcerate under minimal trauma. In general, the lower leg heals poorly and these are particularly difficult to treat. A small proportion of chronic ulcers may progress to a type of skin cancer called squamous cell carcinoma. NLD is three times more common in women than men.

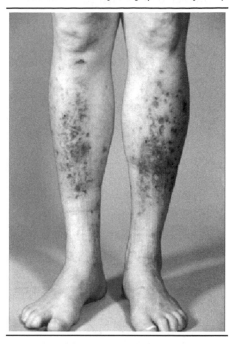

Figure 19-5

Diabetic Dermopathy (Shin Spots)

Treatment

High-potency topical steroids such as clobetasol have been used successfully to treat early NLD. Injecting steroid directly into the area is also sometimes helpful. Topical retinoids have also been used. Oral medications such as aspirin, dipyramidole, and pentoxifylline are also worth a try. These treatments are based on the concept that NLD is caused by microvascular damage (like many of the other manifestations of diabetes), so making the blood thinner and blood elements such as platelets more slippery, better flow can be accomplished and perhaps healing can proceed. Once NLD has taken hold, it is imperative that the utmost care be taken to avoid injuring these highly fragile areas.

By this time, you may be wondering just what dermatologists are good for other than giving long names to things since the last three disorders I told you about have unclear causes and no great treatments. Do not despair, as there are a couple of diabetes-related skin problems with bona fide cures!

Eruptive Xanthomas

Xanthomas are cholesterol deposits in the skin. They often occur suddenly in crops and without warning. Red to yellowish papules can occur anywhere on the body (**Figure 19-7**). They may be itchy but commonly cause no symptoms other than shock at their sudden appearance. This is another skin condition that leads dermatologists to diagnose diabetes. A common scenario is for an apparently healthy person to walk into the office, present an elbow, hand, or buttock and say, "This just popped up." Eruptive xanthomas are caused by uncontrolled glucose and lipids. They occur in people without diabetes as well. Blood tests after fasting will reveal the culprit!

Treatment

Treatment includes bringing the glucose and most often triglycerides under control with diet and medication. Xanthomas will regress once this is accomplished, usually leaving no scars unless the areas have been scratched or picked.

Figure 19-6

Necrobiosis Lipoidica Diabeticorum

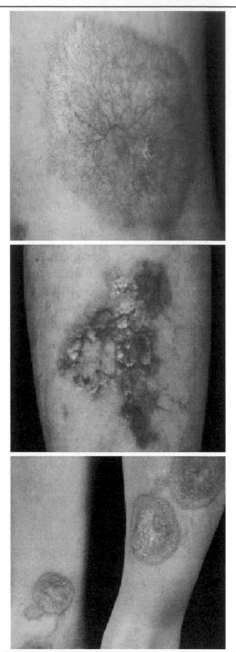

288

The Big Itch and How to Prevent and Tame It

The most common dermatologic complaint of people with and without diabetes is itchy skin. A sudden increase in pruritus or itch may signal

worsening liver or kidney function and should be brought to the immediate attention of your health care provider. Once an internal

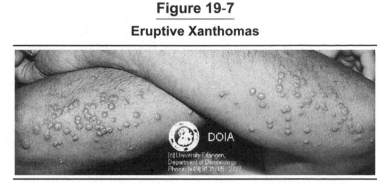

Figure 19-7

Eruptive Xanthomas

cause has been ruled out, managing the itch most commonly precipitated by dry skin is a stepwise approach.

The bad news is that itchy skin can be an annoying and chronic condition that left untreated can lead to damaged skin from constant itching and rubbing. And damaged skin leads to infection! Also, the more you scratch, the more you will itch! There is something peculiarly satisfying about scratching an itch. That's because we have nerve endings in our skin that once stimulated by the scratch send our brain a positive message. Resisting the urge to scratch can be very difficult.

The good news is there are a variety of simple strategies you can follow to beat the itch. First, remember that your skin is the body's largest immune organ and serves as a first-line barrier against a harsh environment. Helping your skin serve its barrier role and preventing that pesky itch is as easy as this:

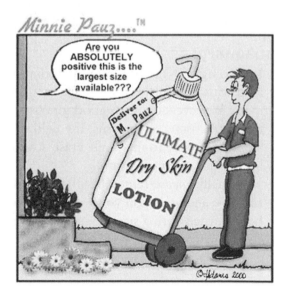

1. Moisturize, Moisturize, Moisturize! Moisturize from within and without. Drink water. Use a humidifier. Apply a moisturizer daily. There are many, many

moisturizers on the market. Pick one you will use. It need not be fragrant or fancy. Frost yourself! Some of my favorites are by Neutrogena, Cetaphil, and Eucerin, but I am always trying new brands. For tough spots like feet and elbows, your doctor might prescribe compounds containing urea or lactic acid. Amlactin contains the latter agent and is available without a prescription. A great, but sticky, moisturizer is called Aquaphor. It is basically high-test Vaseline. Putting it on at night under your jammies is an easy way to grease up worry free at night. Crisco and olive oil work well too, but are not recommended if you have pets.

2. Avoid hot showers, excessive sun, synthetic clothing, and powerfully chlorinated hot tubs and pools. Resist the urge to become pruney. It also helps to skip the postbathing towel rub. Drip dry and grease up while there is still a little moisture on your skin. Soak, then grease!

3. Do not scratch. Scratching leads to skin damage and guess what? More itching. Put down the back scratcher and pick up the moisturizer. Products like Sarna and Eucerin Calming Cream can help soothe and relieve the itch. If prevention fails, your doctor can prescribe an antihistamine or other medications designed to treat the itch, especially if it is preventing you from getting rest.

Remember, it is important to keep in mind that intractable itching can be a sign of serious disease such as liver or kidney problems or even malignancies. So if you have frosted, hydrated, and generally babied your skin barrier and the itching persists, seek the advice of a medical professional.

Summary

In closing, I'd like to remind you that many skin disorders are associated with diabetes, but most are harmless. Most are preventable and many are reversible with good glucose control and careful skin care. In terms of cosmetic concerns, the field of dermatology is advancing fast so we may be able to magically erase acanthosis nigricans and necrobiosis lipoidica in the near future.

Finally, please remember that your skin is your largest organ. Give it the care and attention you reserve for your finest garment and you will be rewarded with a strong, supple, gorgeous wrapper.

20

Obstructive Sleep Apnea

It Can Take Your Breath Away

by Aaron B. Morse, MD, FCCP
and Julia Sarmiento

What's a Chapter on Sleep Apnea Doing in a Book About Diabetes?

Obstructive sleep apnea is a very common disorder affecting a large percentage of the population. Most people with sleep apnea snore and complain of daytime sleepiness and fatigue, but sleep apnea can do a lot more than make you feel lousy during the day. It can kill you.

Like diabetes, it is often seen in people who are overweight. It is common in diabetics, with several studies suggesting an incidence of 20% in type 2 diabetes. Also, like diabetes, it can contribute to a number of cardiovascular problems, so the combination of sleep apnea and diabetes is particularly dangerous. There is evidence that sleep apnea can make diabetes worse, and treating sleep apnea may, in some cases, improve diabetic control. When you finish reading this chapter, you will know everything you ever wanted to know about sleep apnea but didn't know what to ask, and you will be better able to take control of your health.

How Does Sleep Apnea Occur?

Basically, the soft tissues in the throat relax and block the throat when we breathe. This sets off a panic response in the brain resulting in un-conscious arousals from sleep as well as repetitive drops in blood oxygen level. All of the problems that occur with sleep apnea come from these events, which can occur hundreds of times per night without any aware-ness on the part of the individual.

The process begins during inspiration when we actually suck the tongue and soft tissues into the throat. Snoring represents partial closure of the throat, where the soft tissues vibrate and make noise. Snoring, however, is not a disease, but a social problem. While it can produce sleep disorders in bed partners, it does not affect the person who snores. Many people who snore are completely unaware of it and may even deny it, though they chase others out of the room. The human throat, however, is a soft, floppy tube, which allows this obstruction to occur (**Figure 20-1**).

Figure 20-1
What Happens During Upper Airway Obstruction

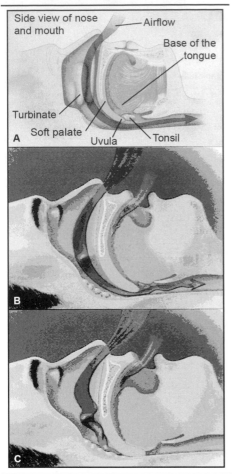

A) Side view of the normal human nasal, oral, and pharyngeal anatomy; B) Snoring results when air flow is partially blocked due to the tongue and soft tissues being sucked down into the throat; C) During sleep apnea, air flow is completely blocked by this soft tissue obstruction.

It turns out that humans are unique in the animal kingdom in being susceptible to sleep apnea, because we need this floppy tube to speak. Without it, we would be barking at each other. The downside is the risk for sleep apnea. (How about a bit of trivia: The only exception is the English Bulldog who, unfortunately, can get sleep apnea and still can't speak).

You will see that this simple event precipitates multiple physiologic, metabolic, and cardiovascular consequences. Sleep is supposed to be a time of quiet for the brain and the body. While the exact purpose of sleep is unknown, we do know that brain waves slow and become more regular. Pulse, blood pressure, respiratory rate, and metabolic rate also drop.

A sleep study on a person with sleep apnea demonstrates multiple changes happening at the same time: Airflow stops, oxygen level drops, heart rate speeds up, brain waves quicken, and the brain briefly awakens. Blood pressure can shoot up to high levels during apneas. This is like being strangled all night long... 30, 40, or 50 times per hour or more! For people with severe sleep apnea, breathing and sleeping become mutually exclusive: You can't do both at the same time. Brief episodes of sleep are like swimming underwater, and arousals are like coming up for a few breaths before diving down to sleep without breathing again. Instead of resting, the brain is involved in an unconscious struggle to keep the throat open. In addition to drops in oxygen, these events are characterized by surges in panic hormones such as adrenalin. Trying to breathe against a closed throat can also produce large pressure swings in the chest that can affect the heart.

If you think this is pretty bad for the heart and blood vessels, you're right. We know that sleep apnea can contribute to the development of high blood pressure, stroke, heart arrhythmias, congestive heart failure, and heart attacks. Stress hormones can raise blood glucose, and sleep apnea is known to cause insulin resistance. There is evidence of increased blood coagulation, and it is possible that sleep apnea may also contribute to obesity.

Signs and Symptoms of Sleep Apnea

There are a number of signs and symptoms that can be present with sleep apnea. Some of the more common appear in **Table 20-1**.

Obesity

Obesity is one of the more important risk factors for sleep apnea. It turns out that fat is deposited in the throat as well as everywhere else, narrowing the throat and making collapse more likely. This being said, there are plenty of thin people with sleep apnea. This is most commonly seen in small-boned people (especially women) with fine facial features, overbites, or recessive chins, as shown in the photos (**Figure 20-2**).

In addition, sleep apnea may contribute to obesity, though this is less well established. People with sleep apnea are less active, resulting in decreased energy expenditure. There is also evidence that sensitivity to an appetite-suppressing hormone (leptin) is reduced, causing increased appetite and weight gain. This sensitivity returns with treatment.

Table 20-1

Symptoms of Obstructive Sleep Apnea

- Obesity (17-inch neck in males, 16-inch in females)
- Snoring—often heavy and/or witnessed apneas
- Gasping and choking during sleep
- Excessive daytime sleepiness
- Restless sleep
- Irritability
- Depression
- Memory loss
- Lack of concentration
- Morning headache
- Nocturia (nighttime urinating)
- Sexual dysfunction
- Esophageal reflux (heartburn)

Snoring

Snoring is very common and is often described as loud or constant. Occasionally the bed partner notices the patient actually stop breath-

Figure 20-2

Upper Airway Anatomy in a Thin Woman With Sleep Apnea

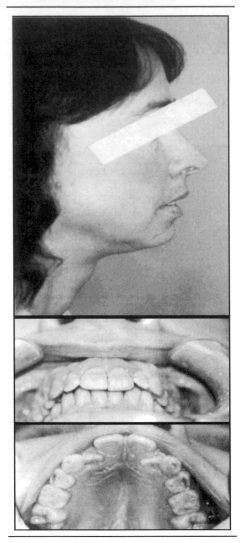

Anatomic abnormalities in a woman with symptoms of sleep-disordered breathing. This woman had a respiratory disturbance index of less than 5 and daytime tiredness. Note her slim neck *(top)*, overbite *(center)*, and high ogival hard palate *(bottom)*.

Annals of Internal Medicine; April, 1995.

ing or gasping in his/her sleep. While snoring is considered one of the major features, it is often not reported because the spouse sleeps through it. We frequently see patients who deny snoring and when studied in the sleep laboratory, shake the walls!

Excessive Daytime Sleepiness

Excessive daytime sleepiness and/or fatigue is often what causes you to seek medical attention. Interestingly, men more commonly describe sleepiness and women complain of fatigue. This may be why the diagnosis is missed more often in women. A common complaint is waking up unrefreshed even after a seemingly good night's sleep. These symptoms are often attributed by the person (or even the doctor) to other medical problems (such as diabetes), stress, depression, etc. I commonly hear "It's just because I'm getting older." We occasionally see patients who have had extensive evaluations for uncommon conditions, including brain scans, extensive blood testing, and multiple other evaluations before the common problem of sleep apnea is even considered. While there are a number of causes of sleepiness and fatigue, sleep apnea is often last on the list of possible diagnoses.

To make things even more complicated, people often underestimate their level of sleepiness, because the symptom develops so slowly that they get used to a certain level of daytime dysfunction. We assume that everybody is as sleepy in the morning as we are. I recently saw a university professor with high blood pressure and snoring who was dragged in by his wife. When he denied sleepiness, his wife pointed out that he falls asleep in a chair whenever he sits down. He had 47 apneas per hour, which is very abnormal.

Restless Sleep

Patients often complain of restless sleep. (What would you do if you were being strangled all night long?) This may be noted only by the bed partner or the bed being torn up in the morning. With treatment, sleep is calmer and quieter. I have occasionally heard of a patient's bed partner panicking because they were afraid the person had died—the snoring and thrashing in bed were gone.

Nocturia

Nocturia (getting up frequently to urinate) is common in sleep apnea and is also often attributed to other things such as prostate problems or diabetes. It turns out that the large pressure swings that occur in the chest can fool the heart into thinking that the body has too much fluid. It then produces a substance that increases urine production (for those who care, it's called atrial natriuretic peptide). Esophageal reflux (heartburn) can occur due to these pressure changes, which can cause stomach acid to be sucked up into the chest.

Other Symptoms of Obstructive Sleep Apnea

Other symptoms that are common are due to the sleep fragmentation induced by the frequent nocturnal arousals. These include irritability, depression, memory loss, lack of concentration, and sexual dysfunction.

How Do I Know if I Have Sleep Apnea?

The most important part of making the diagnosis is thinking of it. Because sleep apnea is so common and is responsible for many health problems, a brief sleep history during a doctor's visit is as important as taking blood pressure. Even though awareness of this condition is increasing among doctors, a routine sleep history is still not very common and 75% to 85% of people with this disorder go undiagnosed and untreated. This is particularly discouraging because treatment is so effective. The variability of awareness of sleep apnea among doctors is striking. In a study done in a 55,000-member HMO, only six of 55 primary care doctors ordered 50% of the sleep studies.

Sleep apnea should be suspected in anyone with unexplained sleepiness and fatigue, especially if there is a history of snoring. Because 80% of people with high blood pressure that is difficult to control have sleep apnea, this is an important clue. Most high blood pressure is "essential," which means no underlying treatable cause is identified. Among underlying treatable causes, sleep apnea is the most common. It is also present in a high percentage of individuals with congestive heart failure, and treatment of sleep apnea can dramatically improve heart function. While obesity is a significant risk factor, a number of nonobese people have sleep apnea because of their facial structure (ie, recessive chin). I have known of people who have been told by their doctor "You can't have sleep apnea because you're not fat."

All this means is that you may have to advocate for yourself (or your bed partner) if you suspect sleep apnea. You need to tell your doctor what your symptoms are and why you think you may have this condition. Don't let anybody dismiss chronic sleepiness and fatigue as getting older or working too hard, especially if there are other signs present.

If the diagnosis is suspected, a sleep study should be performed. The gold standard for the diagnosis is a sleep study performed overnight in a sleep laboratory (known as polysomnography). Many sleep labs have become more like hotel rooms than hospital rooms. A number of physiologic parameters are monitored during sleep, including airflow, oxygen level, and respiratory effort, to determine if apneas are really occurring. Brain waves are measured to assess the quality of sleep and detect arousals induced by apneas. Heart rate and body position, among other things, are also measured.

Because this condition is so common, however, there is a great need for simpler approaches so that more people can be evaluated and effectively treated. Home monitors are becoming more accurate and sophisticated and are being used more commonly. They generally measure almost the same things as the in-lab studies, usually without brain waves. They are most appropriate when the likelihood of moderate to severe sleep apnea is high.

Like any test in medicine, however, the level of expertise and involvement of physicians interpreting the study is most important and may be more relevant than the type of test being performed. Consideration of the clinical context and knowing something about the individual's history is important. A physician knowledgeable in sleep disorders should be involved with your care and the interpretation of your sleep study at some level.

How Is Sleep Apnea Treated?

Making the diagnosis is just the beginning. Losing weight, avoiding alcohol and sedatives, stopping smoking, and avoiding sleeping on your back are general recommendations for alleviating sleep apnea. Improving nasal congestion may help with people who have mild sleep apnea.

The most widely used treatment is continuous positive airway pressure or CPAP. With CPAP, a mask is worn usually on the nose and is attached to a small air compressor which blows air through the nose and uses pressure to keep the airway from being sucked closed during inspiration (**Figure 20-3**). CPAP is almost 100% effective, has no significant side effects, and is relatively inexpensive (a CPAP machine costs about as much as 3 months of medication for a moderate asthmatic). There are very few treatments in medicine that have all those attributes! In addition, people with symptoms of sleepiness and fatigue often experience dramatic and immediate improvement after CPAP is started. There is evidence that CPAP also is effective at reducing or eliminating most of the cardiovascular risks, may improve control of diabetes, and reduces or eliminates the increased risk of premature death associated with sleep apnea.

Figure 20-3

How CPAP Works

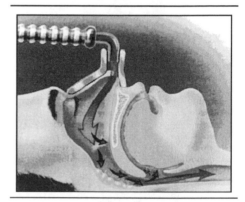

Abbreviation: CPAP, continuous positive airway pressure.

Air pressure applied through the nose by the CPAP prevents the throat from being sucked closed during inspiration.

The greatest challenge in the treatment of sleep apnea with CPAP is compliance—that is, actually using the device, and there has been a great deal of progress in this area. Improvements in technology have dramatically improved the comfort and convenience of CPAP machines and masks.

The first CPAP machines were vacuum cleaners turned backwards, and earlier commercial models were big, bulky, and noisy. Today, the most commonly used CPAP machines are virtually noiseless, can weigh as little as 3 pounds, and almost fit in the palm of your hand.

There are a large variety of CPAP masks available. Some fit around the nose, some fit in the nostrils, and some can include the nose and mouth for people who are mouth breathers. Selection of the most appropriate mask is purely personal, must be individualized, and greatly increases the likelihood of success (**Figure 20-4**).

Figure 20-4
Examples of CPAP Masks

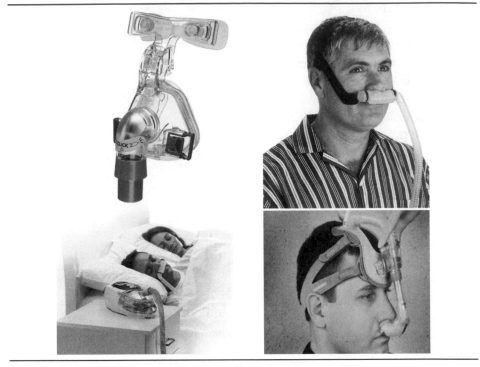

Abbreviation: CPAP, continuous positive airway pressure.

The most important factor in making CPAP comfortable and effective, however, is close follow-up by doctors and sleep technologists who are experienced and knowledgeable in treating patients with this condition. Until recently, almost all of the emphasis has been on diagnosis, with little attention paid to what happens after the CPAP prescription is written. The most common scenario, even today, is performing the sleep study, making the diagnosis, and referral to an equipment company for management, often with little or no additional follow-up.

The sleep-medicine community is beginning to "wake up" (sorry about the pun) to the realization that sleep apnea should be treated like a chronic disease, similar to high blood pressure, diabetes, or asthma. A number of studies have demonstrated long-term compliance rates are better with close follow-up and individual attention. In our center, we try to review the physiology, clinical implications, cardiovascular risks, epidemiology, and treatment options with every patient. In addition to follow-up visits with the doctor, we involve a nurse practitioner, respiratory therapist, and sleep technologist in an extensive compliance follow-up program. Hopefully, more sleep laboratories that currently focus mostly on testing will evolve into sleep centers that provide comprehensive care for patients with sleep apnea and other sleep disorders.

Because CPAP is so effective, and because close follow-up and some trial and error may be necessary to make CPAP comfortable, no one with sleep apnea should give up on CPAP until this has occurred. That being said, there are a significant number of sleep apnea patients who, even after intensive effort and high motivation, cannot adjust to CPAP. For these individuals a number of alternative approaches exist.

The only accepted nonsurgical approach to treating sleep apnea is a dental mandibular advancement device. This looks somewhat like the mouth guard worn by football players and works by pulling the jaw and tongue forward, providing more room in the back of the throat and decreasing the likelihood of obstruction by the tongue (**Figure 20-5**). It is custom-fitted by a dentist. The device is generally well tolerated with only occasionally minor side effects. The success rate is 30% to 60% and it is most effective for simple snoring or mild sleep apnea.

Figure 20-5
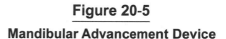
Mandibular Advancement Device

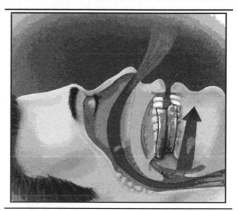

The mandibular advancement device advances the jaw forward, pulling the tongue out of the path of airflow.

A number of surgical approaches exist with varying success rates. One of the more commonly done surgeries, uvulopalatopharyngoplasty (that's a long one!) or UPPP, involves trimming of the uvula, part of the soft palate, tonsils, and other loose tissues in the throat (**Figure 20-6**). The success rate is 40% to 60% and is limited when there is obstruction at the base of the tongue, which is not improved by this procedure. More extensive procedures that involve jaw surgery are sometimes used. Before CPAP was available, the only definitive "cure" for sleep apnea was tracheotomy which is still appropriate for some people. Tracheotomy is a permanent

Figure 20-6
Uvulopalatopharyngoplasty (Removal of Uvula)

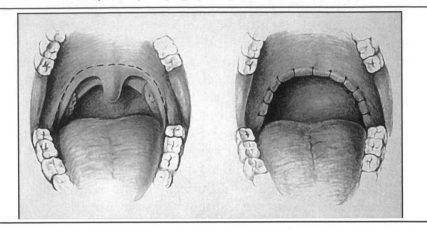

hole in the throat that allows air to completely bypass the obstruction. Now, doesn't CPAP sound easier?

Summary

There are a number of lessons for you to remember from this chapter:

1. Sleep apnea is a common disorder and is a common cause of sleepiness, fatigue, and cognitive decline.
2. Sleep apnea is a contributing factor in a number of medical and cardiac problems, including high blood pressure, heart attacks, stroke, congestive heart failure, diabetes, and premature death.
3. People with sleep apnea have a high incidence of motor vehicle crashes.
4. Treatment of sleep apnea reduces or eliminates virtually all clinical consequences.
5. Sleep apnea needs to be treated as a chronic disease with close follow-up after diagnosis.
6. A brief sleep history should be as much a part of a doctor's visit as a blood pressure check.

21

Using Your Computer to Take Control of Your Diabetes

by Timothy S. Bailey, MD, FACP, FACE, CPI

Introduction

We know that blood glucose control predicts risks for eye, nerve, and kidney damage, and now even heart attack. To better manage your blood glucose levels and find more appropriate insulin or medication doses, your doctor and nurse educator have probably suggested many times that you keep a record of your readings. They have probably even handed you countless varieties of logbooks that over the years have kept local paper recyclers in business.

Logbooks are a time-honored way for people with diabetes to communicate what is going on in their life with their diabetes caregiver. The recording/logbook theory goes as follows:

- You keep a record of everything that affects your blood glucose since the last visit
- You understand your diabetes better after recording these events
- Your doctor, after finding the time to look at your record book, understands exactly what is going on and prescribes a change in therapy that will improve your diabetes control
- The blood glucose levels are better controlled due to more appropriate treatment

Have you considered using a computer to track and manage your blood glucose levels? A computer can help you:

- Collect data from blood glucose meters, certain insulin pumps, and other new devices such as continuous glucose monitors (CGMs)
- Create charts and graphs that reveal trends and patterns in your blood glucose values for better treatment
- Provide an accurate record that both you and your caregiver can use to improve your readings.

A variety of computer programs have been available since the 1980s to assist with diabetes management. Similar to the way a computer organizes your financial data, it can also organize your blood glucose data. Don't miss out on this great tool that can help you to help yourself understand your diabetes. Today's meters, pumps, and continuous monitors can automatically upload blood glucose values and other data right into your computer.

Get Ahead With Today's Meters

Whether you realize it or not, most of the newer blood glucose meters store information about the tests you perform and also let you recall the date and time that you checked it. Some meters keep track of the control and check-strip quality-control tests to ensure the accuracy of your meter. More advanced meters even store data such as low blood glucose reactions, insulin doses, activity levels, the amount of carbohydrates consumed, and even your A1C levels. CGMs, such as the Dexcom STS, Freestyle Navigator, and the Medtronic Guardian RT, can generate 288 readings a day.

Tapping into the information in your meter requires a cable to connect it to a PC and software that can analyze your data. Each meter has a proprietary cable, meaning you will need a different cable for each brand of meter you wish to upload. Cables may be obtained from each meter manufacturer and usually come with software. The cable connects the meter's data port to your computer's serial port (a plug that is distinct from the printer port and is usually located on the back panel of your computer), USB port, or a small box that communicates over the phone or Internet independent of a computer. For those of you with Macintosh computers, there are fewer options, as most software is designed to work under Windows. You need to check your meter's downloading capability.

If you are in the market for a new meter, consider the following features in making your selection:
- How easily does this meter store the data I need?
- How well does it display the data I collect and can I use this to improve my control?
- What information can I store (blood glucose values, medication dose, food intake, activity, etc)?
- How much information will the meter hold?
- What do I need to connect the meter to my computer (and what will it cost)?
- What software is available that will "talk" with it?

A comparison of available blood glucose meters can be found at *www. diabetes.org/diabetes-forecast/resource-guide.jsp.*

Uploading Other Devices

Continuous glucose monitors that measure blood glucose as frequently as every 5 minutes are now available. For short-term control decisions, the trend line, trend arrows, and alerts from one of these devices work well. For a bigger picture to see patterns in your readings, however, a computer download really helps you to organize all the data.

Today's smart insulin pumps are loaded with the data you need to manage your diabetes, such as basal and bolus insulin doses, grams of carbohydrate eaten, and often the blood glucose data from a meter or continuous monitor. They have a data port and, therefore, uploading capabilities. They can provide printouts of the doses of insulin you take and general pump settings.

Other "smart" diabetes devices, such as insulin pens that record time, insulin doses, and carbohydrate intake, and smart phones that also test and transmit your blood glucose values and contain a large food database are now possible. Smart devices will turn your treatments and carbohydrate intake into a complete record. This will let you record more easily, as well as let you analyze your information will less effort. Combined with a health care provider, a fully automated device will assist you in achieving much better control of your diabetes.

Remember that uploading your data is not the end but the beginning of your quest for control. Keep your thinking cap on, along with an open mind and your best analytic tools handy when you review your data. (You DO want to do this!)

Put the Internet and Your Computer to Work

Once your meter is connected to your computer, you need software to make the magic of uploading occur. Until recently, you had to purchase software. Each device company (eg, Roche, Bayer, LifeScan, and Abbott) developed software systems that only work with their meters. These were designed primarily with the physician in mind and so far have still not gained a dominant following with either physicians or patients. The proprietary nature of these programs precludes their effective use in situations where different brands of meters are being used, such as occurs in many diabetes clinics or homes. In response to this need, several independent companies have developed programs that upload multiple meter types. A good list of available software can be located at *www.mendosa.com/software*.

The newest development in uploading is brought to you courtesy of the Internet. Web-based tools for diabetes record keeping are now available. Most of these are free and only require a web browser and Internet connection. These systems allow you to access your information from anywhere—with some, you can even use your cellular phone. An additional benefit is the ability to share information and communicate with your caregivers. However, as with online banking and shopping, you need to ensure the security of your data.

To evaluate the trustworthiness of a website, start with the privacy policy. It must be clear that your data will only be shared with your caregiver and only with your explicit permission. Then read more about the company to see if its purpose is something you agree with. Next, register anonymously—the best sites will allow this, further increasing your confidentiality. Finally, enter your data and take advantage of the tools available with the suggestions below.

How Software Helps Reveal Glucose Patterns and Variability

There are many graphs that you can use to better understand your blood glucose readings. Here are a few that are becoming standard in the diabetes information field:

Standard ("Modal") Day

This graph arranges blood glucose readings from the meter so it looks like a whole week or even months of values happen in 1 day. This chart is important because it shows at what time of the day blood glucose levels are in or out of control. This helps you and your health care professionals pinpoint what may be causing the problem. This chart also has a goal area (the shaded area) so it is easy to tell at a glance if a blood glucose value is too high, too low, or within the goal range.

Before-Meal Glucose and After-Meal Glucose

These are pie charts that show the percentages of time that blood glucose levels are high, low, or within the blood glucose goal range. These charts are great motivational tools because they immediately show how well you're doing and help keep you on track. They also help health care professionals see how meals are affecting your blood glucose.

Combination Line Graph

This type of chart shows the different factors that affect your blood glucose, including medication dosage (including basal rates for pumps), food (carbohydrates consumed), events, and exercise.

Glucose Line Chart

All of your blood glucose levels are graphed in chronological order in a glucose line chart. It lets you see long-term trends in your blood glucose and whether you're in or out of your goal range.

Glucose Statistics

The latest concern in diabetes monitoring is glucose variability. Until recently, the focus of all efforts was to improve A1C (which reflects the average glucose). It might appear obvious to you that the ups and downs of blood glucose matter. However, the notion that this is important to developing long-term complications is relatively new.

So how can we get a handle on this? One approach is to look at the glucose line chart. You can get an overall impression that the more jagged the lines appear, the more variability there is. A better approach is to use something from statistics called a standard deviation.

Standard deviation (SD) reflects the spread around the average with a single number. You can calculate this based on values from entire days or just specific times of day (eg, before-breakfast readings). Dr. Irl Hirsch of the University of Washington created a useful and easy benchmark—the SD multiplied by 2 should not exceed the mean. For super control, the SD multiplied by 3 should be less than the mean. If your standard deviation is high, this means that better coordination of meals, activity, and treatment might be needed.

We will now examine some of these graphs in action in a person with diabetes.

Case Presentation

Dan is a 39-year-old man who developed type 1 diabetes at age 11. He has been followed annually by his family physician since he was a child and was told of the development of background retinopathy 6 years ago by his eye doctor. He recently read an article in a magazine about the chronic complications of diabetes and is concerned that the blurring of his vision over the past few weeks could be due to his diabetes. Both feet have been burning and tingling at night for several months. Additionally, he has occasional nightmares and has been given juice at night several times by his wife because he appeared confused. He has been faithfully taking two daily mixed injections of NPH and Regular insulin (25 N and 20 R every morning and 20 N and 15 R every evening). A1C values have been between 9% and 10% (normal range <6%) on most occasions, and he has made every attempt to follow a healthy diet. He monitors his blood glucose level every morning and states that it is usually 100 to 200 mg/dL. He exercised daily in the past, but attributes his current sedentary lifestyle to the demands of his present employment.

Dan's wife bought him a new blood glucose meter last month that stores his blood glucose information, insulin doses, and carbohydrate intake. He hooked up his meter to his personal computer, using a data cable and a new software package that he had heard about from his diabetes educator. He then entered his blood glucose goals that he had decided on in consultation with his physician and diabetes educator. The information contained in his meter is uploaded to the computer.

With the click of a button, you can display a choice of pie graphs. This one (**Figure 21-1**) shows how Dan is doing overall—in this case, 28.4% of his readings were within his goal range, 61% were higher, and 10.6% were lower. He wants to increase the slice of the pie representing his goals.

Using his computer, Dan decides to analyze his blood glucose patterns by creating a chart showing a standard (modal) day. Here it appears as if the whole weeks or months of values all happened in 1 day. This chart shows that he is checking his blood glucose levels at breakfast and dinner and makes it clear that they are running high. You can also see that he has never checked his blood glucose during the night or at lunch (**Figure 21-2**).

Figure 21-1
Pie Graphs

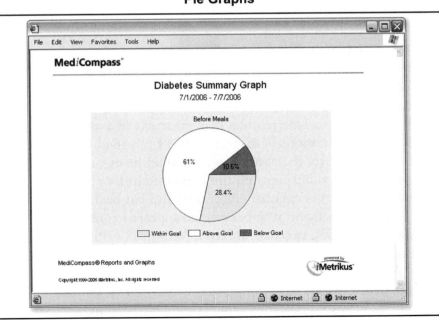

Figure 21-2

Blood Glucose Patterns Analysis

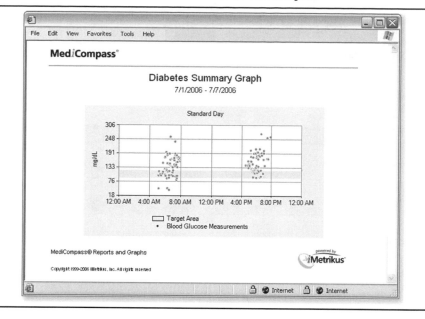

Dan now decides how he will fix those high morning blood glucose levels. His diabetes educator says that he will need to have a good sampling of blood glucose levels before his medication doses can be adjusted with confidence. He decides to test his blood glucose at least four times a day to learn more about his diabetes patterns. He checks his blood glucose several times halfway between bedtime and breakfast (often about 3 AM) as well as several times 1 to 2 hours after meals. He fires up his computer, plugs in the meter, and uploads it to display this new information.

Figure 21-3 shows the logbook automatically generated by the computer program from information in Dan's meter. Such a logbook can be printed out easily and quickly to bring to your next appointment.

Another way to examine the patterns is to click on the button for the computer to do a blood glucose frequency analysis (**Figure 21-4**). This shows Dan where the blood glucose readings cluster according to time of day. You can see that 50% of the blood glucose levels during the night were below 70 mg/dL. Also 5% of the before breakfast and 30% of the before lunch glucoses were also below 70 mg/dL. After breakfast, 85% of the values were between 160 and 200 mg/dL. Compared with simple averages, this better illustrates the distribution of blood glucose levels over multiple ranges.

Figure 21-3

Logbook Generated by Computer From Meter

Medi*Compass

Patient Name: _____   Patient ID: _____

Glucose Logbook
7/6/2006 - 7/12/2006

Date	Before breakfast	After breakfast	Before lunch	After lunch	Before dinner	After dinner	Bedtime	Night
7/12/2006	150 6:18AM		52 10:56AM		142 6:00PM			
7/11/2006	105 5:22AM	167 9:07AM	85 10:31AM		123 6:04PM		179 8:43PM	52 2:59AM
7/10/2006	126 5:58AM	176 7:27AM	46 11:26AM		134 5:55PM			
7/9/2006	152 5:43AM		208 11:30AM		192 5:39PM	272 6:36PM	196 10:23PM	70 3:41AM
7/8/2006	146 6:33AM		74 11:59AM	196 12:13PM	180 6:27PM			
7/7/2006	172 7:10AM	163 7:10AM			198 6:06PM			
7/6/2006	169 6:52AM				204 5:13PM			

MediCompass® Reports and Graphs

Copyright 1999-2006 iMetrikus, Inc. All rights reserved

powered by **iMetrikus**

Figure 21-4

Glucose Frequency Analysis

Patient Goals

*Night	*Before breakfast	*After breakfast	*Before Lunch	*After Lunch	*Before Dinner	*After Dinner	Bed Time
12:00 AM	6:00 AM	8:00 AM	9:30 AM	1:00 PM	2:30 PM	7:00 PM	8:30 PM
80-150	80-120	100-150	80-120	100-150	80-120	100-150	100-140

Glucose Frequency

Blood Glucose	*Night Ct.	%	*Before breakfast Ct.	%	*After breakfast Ct.	%	*Before Lunch Ct.	%	*After Lunch Ct.	%	*Before Dinner Ct.	%	*After Dinner Ct.	%	Bed Time Ct.	%
>350	0	0%	0	0%	0	0%	0	0%	0	0%	0	0%	0	0%	0	0%
>250-350	0	0%	0	0%	0	0%	0	0%	0	0%	0	0%	1	33%	0	0%
>200-250	0	0%	0	0%	1	5%	0	0%	1	7%	0	0%	2	10%	0	0%
>160-200	0	0%	6	30%	6	85%	0	0%	2	66%	6	30%	2	66%	4	66%
>140-160	0	0%	4	20%	1	14%	2	15%	0	0%	3	15%	0	0%	0	0%
>105-140	2	33%	5	25%	0	0%	2	15%	1	33%	8	40%	0	0%	1	16%
>70-105	1	16%	3	15%	0	0%	4	30%	0	0%	1	5%	0	0%	1	16%
0-70	3	50%	1	5%	0	0%	4	30%	0	0%	0	0%	0	0%	0	0%
All	6		20		7		13		3		20		3		6	

MediCompass® Reports and Graphs

Copyright 1999-2006 iMetrikus, Inc. All rights reserved

powered by **iMetrikus**

Dan brought these with him to his next appointment with his physician and diabetes educator. They recommended that he move his dinner NPH insulin from dinner to bedtime so that the NPH would peak later to avoid low blood glucose levels in the middle of the night. They also suggested changing Regular insulin to a new rapid-acting insulin and decreasing his morning and dinner shorter-acting insulin doses by 2 units and that he try to decrease his food intake at lunch. The diabetes team suggested that he track his food intake by counting carbohydrates. Dan let them know that he had also decided to try exercising daily in the afternoon.

Dan uploaded his meter a week later and viewed the glucose line graph shown in **Figure 21-5** on his computer. The difference that these changes made over time is clearly seen. Dan is so pleased with his improvements that he sends these graphs every 2 to 3 weeks to his physician directly from his computer. His physician is also pleased with this information and sends Dan encouragement and suggestions for further refinement of his blood glucose control.

The MediCompass software used in this example is produced by iMetrikus *(www.imetrikus.com)*. Similar graphs are available in other software.

Figure 21-5
Glucose Trend Over Time

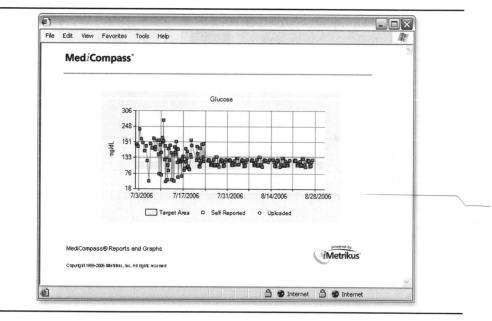

Online Resources for Patients and Health Care Providers

In the past, it was traditional to list resources for patients separately from those aimed toward health care professionals. With the explosion in information available to all (with an Internet hookup), this distinction is less clear. The best sites will have links or jumps to other interesting locations. Be sure to discuss what you find with your health care professional before changing your treatment.

Summary

With a little initial effort from you, your computer can provide a far more complete and accurate record than a conventional logbook or diary. You will learn to recognize important trends in your diabetes. It will also empower you to better communicate with your health care professional and receive better advice. You will have taken the next step in successfully taking control of your diabetes.

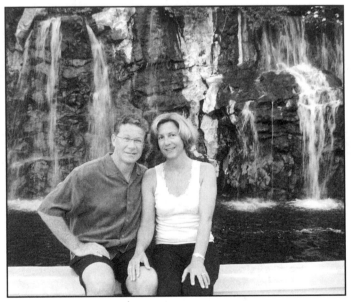

Steve and Ingrid Edelman in Hawaii, 2006.

22

Diabetes in the Workplace

by Urban Miyares

Introduction: Diabetes Saved My Life

In 1968, the word "diabetes" was foreign to me. I didn't know anyone who had the disease. It was never mentioned at family gatherings, in school, or among my friends. I don't even remember ever being questioned by a doctor if there was a family member with diabetes, even when I was drafted into the US Army. But in 1968, as a 20-year-old sergeant with the 9th Infantry Division in Vietnam, I was suddenly introduced to diabetes.

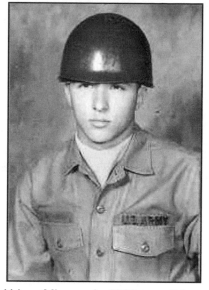

Urban Miyares in 1968 as a 21-year-old sergeant with the 9th Infantry Division in Vietnam.

Over a 2-week period in August of 1968, I was experiencing extreme thirst, dizziness, blurred vision, and severe stomach cramps, with constant bouts of nausea and vomiting. I had little appetite but a tremendous thirst. The sensation to urinate was constant. I could go to sleep anytime and anywhere, including during a night ambush. In the field with my platoon, I was worried, feeling that something was definitely wrong, and maybe I wasn't going to make it back home—a feeling many get in a combat situation. I went to sick call whenever we returned to base camp, and the diagnosis was always heat prostration, battle fatigue, or peptic ulcers. Medicine and rest were prescribed, but I was back out in the field quickly with my platoon for our next mission. The company commander and first sergeant warned me about malingering, with a threat of "The doctor better find something wrong with you, or else...!" Weak, constantly wanting to sleep and drink, losing weight rapidly... it was a life-and-death situation for me and the others in my platoon. If I couldn't do my job, others would die. I was sick, really sick, and no one knew why. The next morning after yet another sick-call visit, with no rationale by the doctor other than heat prostration, we choppered into the Delta with a number of other platoons to check on a reported enemy infiltration in a village we had been to before. Walking toward the village in the heat, the pungent odor from the rice paddy, and flies bathing in our perspiration, I had to stop often to vomit from the nausea. Dizzy, exhausted, and sick, I suddenly heard the hollow sound, the thump of mortars being launched in the distance, and then yelling, gunfire, and the whistling sound of a mortar shell passing overhead. The last thing I remembered was falling face first into the water of the rice paddy.

Two days later, I woke up in a Saigon military hospital. I vaguely remember opening my eyes to bright lights—thought I was in heaven at that moment—hearing a gorgeous young lady with blonde hair dressed all in white—saying in a soft and concerned voice "You're OK, Sergeant Miyares." I fell back to sleep instantly. When I awoke later, I could see drawn white drapes on either side of me, tubes attached to my arms and connected to plastic bags filled with liquid, hanging from poles by my bed. I instantly lifted the sheets to see if I still had my legs. No amputation, thank God. I was feeling pretty good, at least better than I had in the previous weeks, and I didn't have a constant urge to urinate. Soon a different nurse came by and told me I had been in a diabetic coma... and the doctors would be by to talk to me.

This was my first introduction to the word, and I believed it was an illness I must have caught in Vietnam, and soon, with medications, I would be back in the field with my platoon. Little did I know that this was my "silver bullet," my ticket back to stateside, and a reuniting with my new bride. JoAnn and I had wed just prior to my shipping off to Vietnam. Doctors later came to my bedside and tried to explain what my type 1 diabetes was all about, making assumptions about the cause and effects of the disease. I would learn so much more later and how my life would take a sudden turn. The next day I had a visitor come to my bedside, a soldier from the 9th Infantry who wanted to check on me. He then told me I was lucky, damn lucky, as they thought I was dead in the field, hurriedly throwing me in a body bag for an airlift, only to later discover at base camp that I was alive. From the time I passed out in the field to when I awoke in the hospital, two unaccounted for days had passed. I never did find out who that soldier was, but 35 years later I discovered who the medic was that found me in the body bag. We've been communicating and recently had a fantastic face-to-face reunion in San Diego.

Looking back on what happened, and what might have been in 1968, diabetes definitely saved my life.

The World's Greatest Gift

When you're sick and you've gone through a shocking life experience, such as the tragedy of war, becoming philosophical would appear to be the norm. For me, I tried to justify all that had happened in my life, and discovered that we all get "gifts" throughout our life, from the gift of birth to the gift of death. Yes, death.

Returning back to the States from Vietnam, after a 2-week stop in a military hospital in Japan, I was treated for my diabetes at Valley Forge Hospital in Pennsylvania. It was a long 5 months and the treatment for diabetes was archaic, especially when you compare it with today's health care practices, medications, and devices for the disease. Then, it was low-calorie diets (I was prescribed a 700-calorie-per-day diet), taking multiple injections, containing hundreds of units of insulin daily (the injection syringe of glass and a thick needle requiring pre-boiling for sterilization, and a daily sharpening of the needle with an emery board). It was a painful ritual, leaving black-and-blue marks on my arms, legs, and stomach from repeated injections. Glucose blood tests were then only done in the hospital, with the laboratory providing the results. At home, we had to test our sugar and ketone levels with a sample of collected urine, tested in a chemistry-like experiment (test tubes, sugar test strips, and tablets) with the findings often being inaccurate. Little was known about the disease in those years, as the quick diagnosis of the cause was hereditary, and the treatment was extreme—starvation, no sugar, moderate activity, desk-type jobs, etc. It wasn't until years later that I discovered the possible real cause of my getting diabetes, and why all the complications I experienced exploded so quickly. Sometimes it's just not your fault... and then, sometimes it is.

I had lost 67 pounds since the onset of the disease, still weak (yet craving calories), my daily insulin regimen at hundreds of units, taken in multiple injections daily. In a counseling session, the military doctor told JoAnn and me that due to my "uncontrollable" diabetes condition and extreme insulin resistance, I could expect to live or be productive for, at most, 20 years. (Welcome to the 1968 world of diabetes care and management.) It was then JoAnn and I decided that if I had only 20 years left, let's make them the best 20 years of our life, one day at a time.

Diabetes, a disease that was then considered devastating, was to me a gift. It brought me back home from a war, alive. I had a partner who was willing to share the next 20 years with me, in spite of my medical challenges. If I lived longer than 20 years, we both won. I still had a future, even if it was a short one. I was ready to take on whatever life threw me because of this gift. I quickly developed a healthy attitude to enjoy and experience life and not be scared of any of its challenges or outcomes. And there were surely challenges to come, which I didn't realize at the time. Now to get a job.

Note: Within 6 months of the diabetes diagnosis, I began experiencing some of the complications of the disease. I began with peripheral neuropathy and, by the fifth year, the beginnings of vision loss, impotence, and other complications were already showing their signs. And the doctors continued to say I was doing fantastic.

Entering the Workplace

With a medical military discharge (coldly) mailed to me and still having difficulty managing my diabetes, finding employment, especially a prescribed desk job, was difficult. Having only a high school diploma (being drafted soon after graduation), work experience being in food service and sales, and being outdoors and playing sports as passions, working in the office environment was truly a challenge. It was a time, 1968-1969, when the emotions of our country over the Vietnam War had many veterans hide their patriotism and Vietnam experience in the closet. But I hit the New York City job market and quickly found employment through a friend. Working for a stock brokerage firm on Wall Street in New York City, I began a career as a margin clerk—a profession that soon became obsolete with the introduction of the portable calculator and later the computer. I worked in secrecy, not mentioning anything about having been in the military and Vietnam, and kept my stash of needles, insulin, and emergency sugar in my desk drawer. The company had a mandatory health insurance program and all employees were required to take an exam and be enrolled in the program.

I worked intensely, often arriving early and staying later than I was paid, regardless of how I felt, to validate how important and valuable an employee I was. I managed to sidestep the required medical insurance exams for almost a year, as I was sure with the diagnosis of diabetes, I would not qualify for the mandatory coverage and be fired. Couldn't afford to lose a job as I had a family to support. JoAnn was pregnant with our son, Urban Paul. Then, one day I was called into the manager's office with a supervisor in attendance, and I was fired! When I asked for the reasoning, as I was confident my work was exemplary, they told me someone discovered the needles in my desk drawer. I then went on to mention I had diabetes and revealed my military background. "That's it, you're gone. We're not going to have any drug-toting, baby-killing Vietnam vet in this company," he said. I was suddenly unemployed. In 1 year, I was fired from two jobs because I had diabetes. The first job being the US Army and the second being that stock brokerage firm. Welcome home, vet.

Note: Soon after my medical discharge, I quickly changed the doctor-prescribed diet guidelines for my diabetes management and performed work activities that were not recommended. With this self-management course, I gradually added weight and felt better. My diabetes control improved and the number of units of insulin I required each day decreased dramatically, even though I was consuming more calories.

That first employment experience was the start of my workplace journey with diabetes. It forced me to switch into the self-employment arena, although I've had a number of jobs on the side over the years to help pay the bills (many of these jobs not being exactly what the doctor ordered). Entrepreneurship has been with me ever since... and I'm thankful for it. It's allowed me to control my life each day, providing the needed flexibility to better manage my health, and giving me the motivation to continue seeking new challenges in life.

Opportunities and Obstacles in the Workplace

Over the years, diabetes and the many complications I have had from the disease, as well as other nondiabetes-related medical challenges, have definitely changed my approach to work. In the beginning, neuropathy, causing pain and discomfort in my legs, forced me to modify some of my workplace activities. Later, sight loss and eventual total blindness created some unique challenges in the sighted and healthy world of business. Then add to this a stroke, hearing impairment, gastroparesis, kidney transplant, thyroidectomy, and other medical issues not to mention post-traumatic stress disorder, created a distinct way I had to learn how to competitively participate and perform in the workplace... especially with the effects of the new medications prescribed. Yet, for me, by being the owner of the company, the biggest opportunity was "control." Control of the workplace, time, and direction that I and my business would take. It's been a blend that has worked wonderfully for me, although I would have loved to have had a job that would challenge and satisfy me, pay me a fair salary, provide little or no stress, and give my family the long-term security needed. But such an employment offer never presented itself, and I was on a time clock: 20 years. No time to look for that "perfect employer."

A couple of years after returning from Vietnam, I requested vocational rehabilitation counseling for assistance in helping me with my entrepreneurial endeavors. After testing, the vocational rehabilitation counselor told me that because of the severity of my disability and its prognosis, he recommended that I stay home and collect my disability payments, as it was not worth their expense to educate and train me for a job I probably could not keep. And I should "get my head out of the sand, as self-employment was not a realistic option." Years later, when I achieved business success (Inc. magazine's "Entrepreneur of the Year" and recognition by US Presidents, Congress, SBA, etc), I mailed copies of these stories to this vocational rehabilitation counselor. He, too, much like the doomsday military doctor from Valley Forge Hospital, gave me a gift that forced me onto another track of life. Thank goodness I didn't listen to either one of them.

The single biggest obstacle with diabetes in the workplace is that it's a hidden disability. And because you (may) look good, healthy, and perform well, you really don't have it "that bad." It's when you are not in control of your diabetes, that you are "sick." Being sick and having a disability are two entirely different things. It is when you are sick that the obstacles are created in the workplace, in most instances.

*"The key to a healthy business is
a healthy business owner and healthy employees."*

For many, diabetes is often an embarrassment, something to hide. In the workplace, hiding the disease may be hazardous to yourself and to those around you. From my background as an employer, knowing that an employee has diabetes (or any other hidden medical condition) is critical. Depending on how well the employee controls his/her disease or other medical condition, combined with their personality, communication, and social skills with others, is more important than their ability to perform a job. I have, in the past, redefined someone's job description based on their diabetes and their other talents and traits, looking for the best productivity. Over the years, I've seen a number of employees and two partners diagnosed with diabetes while on the job. In each case, the diagnosis was devastating to them, with each suddenly making rash decisions (unjustifiably in my opinion) about work and their future. And the employees I've had in the past who were not in control of their health didn't last long in the company. They just did not have the attitude needed to take care of themselves or the job responsibility: Performance was down, absenteeism was higher, excuses were ever constant, and fellow employees felt uncomfortable around them.

There is no reason why anyone with diabetes needs to experience the negative, discriminating employment situation I had in the late 1960s. Current laws for the workplace and advancements in controlling and managing diabetes should not hamper or mitigate one's performance or acceptance in the workplace. Having diabetes does not necessarily mean that you should display the scarlet letter "D" on your forehead, announcing: "Hey everyone, I have diabetes." Instead, diabetes should be viewed as but one of many challenges you and others face in the workplace. No big thing—at least you know what is wrong with you, and have the tools and the ability to manage its maintenance.

Many obstacles are created, however, and not justified for people with diabetes, especially newly diagnosed cases. Some of these obstacles lead to inappropriate career changes, overmodification of the workplace environment, dramatic changes in workplace needs and requirements, sale of a business (if self-employed), and other dramatic and drastic actions. Such obstacles are artificially created and fostered by emotion and fear, not education and a true understanding of the disease. To live with diabetes successfully, you need to create a sincere, not phony, attitude that having the disease is a fact of life that you can readily control, regardless of complications or other medical challenges, especially in today's advancing medical environment. At least you now know what is "broken," and you can fix it to keep on running just as well as before if you're willing to take the time to manage the disease. You, too, just might discover diabetes, and the requirements for a healthy life, are a gift.

Frequently Asked Questions About the Workplace

1. I have just been diagnosed with diabetes. What type of jobs can I now do?

   Answer: The type of job, career, or business you can do is entirely dependent upon you, your diabetes control, and other factors that may have nothing to do with diabetes. Having diabetes seldom affects your employment options. And if it does, and you truly have a passion for a specific workplace activity, become the business owner, and then hire others to perform the job function you are unable to do yourself.

2. Now that I have diabetes, my current employer is unwilling to accommodate my unique needs and challenges. What can I do to not lose my job?

Answer: A first question is "What accommodations do you need because of your diabetes, and can you modify your needs to meet the requirements of your employment?" Too often people with diabetes suddenly put unwarranted pressure on an employer because of their diabetes, such as having (frequent) doctor visits during the workday, taking more frequent breaks (for blood testing, snacking, bathroom, etc), or having other demands. As an employer, I have found that employees making such demands are often those not in control of their diabetes... and, in some instances, employees who are too much in control of the disease —keeping an extreme, compulsive-like control of their diabetes to the point of constantly having low blood glucose, a frequent (almost hourly) blood-testing regimen, and other behaviors. In the workplace, you need to identify a balance that works best for you and your doctor and does not compromise your workplace duties or put undue pressure on your employer.

3. What type of business can I own having diabetes?
   Answer: Any type of business you would like to own, even if it's a business in which you would not qualify, due to your diabetes, to be an employee. In business, you can either create a job for yourself or create employment for others, with you overseeing or managing their activities and the affairs of the business. Businesses such as trucking companies, ambulance services, airplane charters, and demolition all are owned by people with diabetes. There is not an industry that does not have a business owner with diabetes. It's all up to you.

4. I'm now in school and have had type 1 diabetes since I was 12 years old. What type of career should I focus on?
   Answer: It's a wonderful time to have diabetes, with all of the medical breakthroughs and practices in treating the disease, along with your ability to manage and control your health. The career outlook is wide open for you, and you will discover that whatever area you focus on, you will probably discover others with diabetes already in the field—whether they entered the field with diabetes or acquired the disease after already being in the field. Just keep good control of your diabetes and you'll do fine.

5. I'm approaching 60 years of age and was just diagnosed with type 2 diabetes, high blood pressure, cholesterol, and a heart condition. I'm too young to retire but not disabled enough to collect disability. Should I stay at my current job?
   Answer: Your first job is to take care of your diabetes. This begins

with education and then taking the proper actions to improve your health. You're now starting a dramatic lifestyle change, and it's going to be difficult. But it is needed and the end results are most rewarding. Once you've taken control of this, you may discover work to be both enjoyable and therapeutic. Many, in their retirement years have been diagnosed with diabetes and have gone on to continue work and even start businesses. Being active is key to good health with diabetes, so stay active, keep working, and stay involved in some enjoyable activity. Never retire is my motto… and if you volunteer, you may discover you're working harder and longer hours than when you were employed.

Note: There are many federal and state laws regarding employment of those having disabilities in the workplace, with diabetes generally recognized as a disability, even though you may not have any associated complications of the disease. These laws are to protect you, especially if you believe you have been unfairly treated or dealt with in an employment (job interview or workplace) situation. But if your management of the disease is not under good or medically acceptable control, you may be compromising the benefits you have under current laws. For additional information, read the Americans With Disabilities Act (ADA) and your state's laws and regulations regarding the employment of people with disabilities.

Get Even: Outlive Your Doctors

OK, so you have diabetes. You're confused, maybe angry, questioning your future…your life. Worried that you may become impotent, acquire kidney disease, go blind, have an amputation, or experience some other malady. Concerned that you won't be able to do the same work as before. Your social life is now devastated, and you're going to have to settle and compromise your goals, dreams, and plans. Get over it. It's not going to happen unless you let it. There is no reason you cannot live a rewarding, successful, and healthy, if not healthier, and longer life, than without the disease.

For me, and because of diabetes (some say it's my attitude), I've lived a much more rewarding and exciting life than I would have without the disease. I've been able to serve my country, proudly. I have been fortunate to meet many wonderful people and have met many of our nation's leaders in government and noteworthy Americans spotlighted in stories, on television, or in the movies. As a business owner, hundreds have relied on my performance in the workplace to support their families, dreams, and goals. I've had the opportunity to test myself in athletics—as a former US National Alpine Ski Champion and offshore racing sailor, having raced across the Pacific Ocean twice. I'm a husband, a father, and grandfather. To me, I've lived a few lifetimes in my short existence already, and there is so much more to do. Now planning the next encore, continues to add challenges and rewards of life for me, and I'm far from ready to retire on my past laurels. All of this is because I have diabetes.

If I had listened to the doctors in 1968, I can't imagine what my life would have been like. But what did they really know back then? Diabetes stinks. There is no question about it. But it's not the end of everything. Getting angry is good sometimes, provided you're able to channel the anger into something productive. For me, the outlet is… Outlive Your Doctors!

Agent Orange and Diabetes

Agent Orange was a defoliant used in the Vietnam War and also at times during the Korean War. The medical findings are still out on whether or not Agent Orange is a direct trigger or cause of diabetes (type 2 diabetes is identified at this time) or any other medical conditions. But data collected on those exposed to Agent Orange and other evidence indicate that the chemical dioxin (used in Agent Orange) possibly could be a factor in the onset and diagnosis of (type 2) diabetes. (Note: Approximately 7% to 9% of the general population in America has diabetes, but 20% of the veteran population is diagnosed with diabetes.)

If you are an honorably discharged veteran who now has type 2 diabetes, and served in either Vietnam or Korea, whether or not you have another disability or saw combat, it is recommended that you seek the assistance of a qualified military service organization or contact the Department of Veterans Affairs (VA) to investigate if you qualify to make a claim for service-connected benefits for your type 2 diabetes.

Summary

People with diabetes can have exciting, successful, and productive lives in sports, the workplace, and life. It's up to you alone to make the decision to make changes and take control of your diabetes. You have diabetes, and along with it is change. Change in your health care routine, change in diet, and a new addition of medications to your lifestyle, along with a change in your daily activities, attitude, personality, social activities, relationships, and other traits are in order. Change is difficult, but look at it as a gift, with rewards yet to come.

If you already have complications from the disease or possibly another disability along with diabetes, aggressively controlling your diabetes could possibly slow down the progression of diabetes-related complications or even reverse them (as it has my neuropathy) and improve the management of other medical conditions you may have. It's hard work, but worth it... if you have developed the right attitude.

Getting an attitude is one thing, living it is another. Develop and live the attitude of good health, control, and making a serious effort to be an active part of the future, not a spectator. Accept and welcome challenges. Test your limits and enjoy life. And above all else, try to see a gift in everything and everyone, whether good or bad... including diabetes.

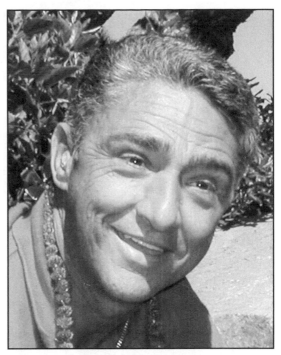

URBAN MIYARES is a nationally recognized blinded Vietnam veteran with type 1 diabetes, an entrepreneur, motivational speaker, writer, media personality, and world-class athlete. Miyares is founder of the charitable Disabled Businesspersons Association, co-founder of Challenged America, and mentor with YEP! (Young Entrepreneur Program).

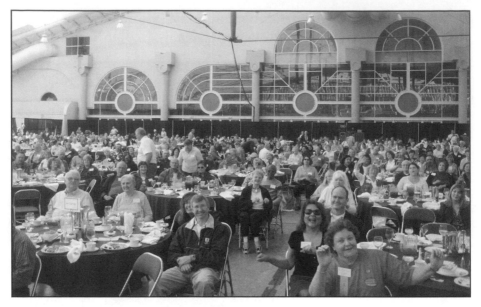

Lunch time at a TCOYD conference.

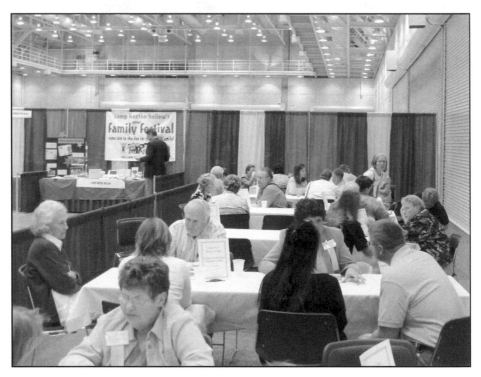

Personalized dietary counseling at a TCOYD conference.

23

Managing Managed Care

Legal Issues for People With Diabetes

by Kriss S. Halpern, JD

Legal Lessons: Getting Chemstrips Used to be Tough

Chemstrips (blood glucose test strips) were what got me started. Chemstrips and a lazy insurance company that took a while to notice I'm a lawyer and was going to keep pushing them until I got some decent medical care in return for the premiums I paid each month.

For 10 years, I had been a volunteer with the Diabetes Control and Complications Trial (the DCCT took place from 1983-1993), the largest study ever conducted in the treatment of diabetes (discussed in Chapter 1). The study was paid for by the National Institutes of Health. We were given an unbiased array of great health care providers, the best drugs and tools available without regard to cost, and as much help as we needed to manage our blood glucose levels as well as we could.

Most of us in the experimental group—the half of the study volunteers working on achieving tight blood glucose control and getting this awesome care—were able to keep our A1Cs below 7% for nearly 10 years. When the study ended, it was announced that there was overwhelming proof that tightly controlled blood glucose levels dramatically decreased the likelihood of long-term complications (*New England Journal of Medicine*, September 1993). Then those of us in the study were sent back to the real world. That's where my trouble with Chemstrips began. But before I tell that story, there is some critical health care evidence I want to share.

Although there is still research taking place in a follow-up study to the DCCT called Epidemiology of Diabetes Interventions and Complications (EDIC began in 1994 and is ongoing), that study is designed only to measure our health and record results, not to help us manage our diabetes or provide much in the way of ongoing care. In EDIC, we visit a test center once a year and they perform a daylong series of health tests and have us fill out an array of questionnaires. In the DCCT, we visited a test center once a month and had as much health care assistance as we needed or wanted at any time. The EDIC follow-up to the DCCT study has provided a great deal of important information about diabetes.

Two aspects of that information are particularly fascinating to me and relevant to my work as an attorney helping people with diabetes.

First, in the years since the DCCT ended in 1993 and all participants were advised and taught to practice tight blood glucose control as a critical way to avoid serious long-term complications, both the former tight-control group (which kept blood glucose levels as measured by glycosylated hemoglobin [or A1C] an average of approximately 7% during the 10-year DCCT study) (**Table 23-1**) and the former standard-control group (which had an average A1C of 9% during the 10-year DCCT) have maintained their A1Cs at the same level on average—around 8%—for the 10 years following the DCCT. Thus the former tight-control group experienced approximately a 1% increase in blood glucose levels on average, while the former standard-control group decreased their A1C about 1% on average.

Second, although the standard- and the tight-control groups have now been maintaining similar blood glucose levels

Table 23-1

Explanation of Glycosylated Hemoglobin (A1C)

A1C Value	Blood Glucose Value
6%	135 mg/dL
7%	170 mg/dL
8%	205 mg/dL
9%	240 mg/dL
10%	275 mg/dL

A glycosylated hemoglobin (or A1C) test measures blood glucose, determining the average amount of glucose present in blood over the previous 2 to 3 months.

on average since 1993, the complications measured have continued to show dramatic benefits for the former tight-control group in comparison with the former standard-control group. Although both groups have had similar A1Cs on average for more than 10 years, the significant difference in A1Cs over the initial 10-year period studied has continued to have dramatically different results, showing superior health in the tight-control group members. (For example, *New England Journal of Medicine*, December 22, 2005: "Intensive treatment reduced the risk of any cardiovascular disease event by 42%… and the risk of nonfatal myocardial infarction, stroke, or death from cardiovascular disease by 57%.")

This evidence supports two conclusions critical to my work and to your knowledge about taking control of your diabetes:

- Obtaining a safe level of tight blood glucose control provides ongoing benefits that continue throughout a lifetime
- Achieving a safe level of tight blood glucose control is extremely difficult to accomplish without the assistance of a highly motivated health care team and easy access to proper drugs and medical tools.

My own experience is a prime example of the difficulty in achieving high quality care in the real world. When the DCCT ended and I turned to an HMO to provide my diabetes care, they sent me a lovely welcoming package with sweet pictures of all kinds of good-looking happy people of all races and ages who looked overjoyed to be receiving such great medical care. Clearly, I was a lucky guy. I looked through their hospital plan options and chose one. I checked out their primary care doctors and picked one. I made an appointment, was sent an approval letter, and made my way to his office. That's where the happy HMO world ended for me.

The hour-long wait was no fun. When I was finally permitted to meet my new doctor, I told him about my experiences with the DCCT. More accurately, I should say, I tried to tell him. He really didn't give a damn. Instead, he told me, I was now under his care and I was now going to be on the protocol approved by the HMO. Wait a second, I responded, this study just proved that all persons with diabetes need to be maintaining tight control; that doing so means a likelihood of far fewer long-term complications. Uh huh, he said, but we have a system here. That's nice, I said, but mine works better and mine's the one I'm using. As you might imagine, HMO doc and I didn't get along too well. I paid my $25 and got the heck out of there. As an aside, it was a good thing I'd gotten some extra insulin and Chemstrips and other medications from the DCCT when it ended or I'd have had to pretend that this doctor was competent long enough to at least get some prescriptions out of him.

So I switched primary care doctors. The next one was thoughtful and willing to listen and work with me. He gave me the benefit of his knowledge and education without assuming dictatorial authority over my diabetes care. He allowed me to have input and control over my own medical treatment and he discussed his thoughts and opinions with me and allowed me to discuss mine with him. And he did so without taking an exorbitant amount of time that would impede his ability to earn a living and treat a full schedule of patients. Among the things he provided were prescriptions for all of the diabetes care medications and tools I'd learned I needed from my experiences in the DCCT. And even though not all of those medical tools required prescriptions to be purchased, I knew my HMO required a prescription if they were going to pay for them.

Armed with my half-dozen prescriptions I went off to the pharmacy. I got most of what I requested that day. Except for the Chemstrips. This was in 1987… before the DCCT results became well known. I called my HMO. They told me Chemstrips weren't covered. I wrote my HMO and explained why they should be. I quoted and sent them copies of their own promises about the great health care coverage they provided. I asserted that these representations were contractual obligations. I sent them a copy of the *New England Journal of Medicine* article where the DCCT results were printed so they could see the obvious benefits to providing quality care. I threatened to take whatever legal action was necessary to obtain coverage. I explained that providing proper medical care as proven by the DCCT could save them money. This last one apparently caught their attention.

It took a while. I had to keep making calls and taking notes of who I spoke with and what they said and who I could write to next. I got my primary care physician to send a letter explaining why Chemstrips were necessary for proper care. To make that a little easier for him, I wrote it myself and faxed it to him (today, it could be e-mailed). But, hey, he reviewed it, and most importantly, he printed it on his letterhead and signed it. Over the next 6 months, my HMO not only agreed to pay for my Chemstrips, they added Chemstrips to their formulary so all persons with diabetes on their plan would receive them with a prescription.

That was my first critical lesson in how to take control: Know what you need; see if your doctor agrees that this is what you need; if your doctor agrees, get him or her to say so in writing; find out where and how to demand what you need; keep appealing until you get it. I have used this same basic strategy time and again. If your requests are proper, this generally works. Depending on the cost of the request and the health care plan, it can take a greater or lesser amount of effort. But fair requests properly made generally get covered. It is, of course, a lot easier if you are not the first to try. Because so many diabetes-related drugs and management tools are introduced and many of them are expensive when they first come out, these techniques are not going to become unnecessary anytime soon. It used to be that insulin pumps were virtually impossible to get covered. Now they usually are not. Continuous blood glucose monitoring devices are the newest tool on the market and there is now resistance to paying for them just as there was to insulin pumps and Chemstrips in the past. That will, of course, change. The way to make it change is to make demands on health care plans along the lines I did to get Chemstrips.

Legal Improvements: Laws Now Provide Explicit Support in Most States

After the DCCT ended and it became indisputable that tight control of diabetes results in fewer long-term complications, many persons assumed that health insurance carriers would promptly pay for the care proven necessary. Not only would such care improve the health of persons under coverage, it would greatly reduce the health care expenses of persons with diabetes as fewer persons with diabetes would suffer from debilitating complications that are expensive to treat. Simply put, years of Chemstrips and quarterly A1C testing cost far, far less than amputating a foot.

Health insurers do not typically rush to meet the proven health care needs of their customers and obtain the obvious savings. What, they ask themselves, would this do for me? It turns out that persons joining a health plan typically remain on that plan for about 5 years. So if Plan A spends an average of $100 each year to improve care for someone with diabetes; and then that plan member switched to another carrier and then another and perhaps another before the plan member is likely to suffer from severe complications, Plan A would not receive the financial benefit of its investment in its member's long-term health because that member would be under the coverage of a different plan before long-term complications were likely to develop. Why, they ask themselves, should we spend more on improving care for our Plan members if they are going to be on a different plan by the time those improvements save us money?

Complicating the health plan cost-benefit analysis further is the fact that many persons with diabetes don't suffer long-term complications until they are retired and on Medicare. Thus the savings from years of paying for better health care would be received by the government rather than the plan providing the coverage along the way. And, the plans asked themselves, "Why should we pay for the government to save money?!"

The American Diabetes Association took the lead in trying to end this short-sighted and convoluted way of thinking by proposing requirements in all states that health plans be obliged to pay for the kind of care proven to be medically necessary. As of 2007, 46 states have passed such requirements. The laws differ from state to state and some are significantly better than others. The ADA should be able to assist you if you want to know what is covered in your state; you can contact them at 1-800-DIABETES. The battle is far from over. The plans will often place only older and less-expensive medications on their formularies and thus try to avoid paying for newer medications or charge a far greater co-pay for plan members to receive them. You can fight these restrictions by appeals to your plan.

Legal Roadblocks: Laws Are Too Often Needed to Help Persons With Diabetes

Some years ago, I was on a plane to Chicago pulling articles out of my backpack and scribbling notes on a legal pad. I was asked by the lady seated next to me what I was working on. I told her I was preparing a talk for a diabetes conference. Are you a doctor, she asked. No, I said, I'm a lawyer. She laughed and asked me why a lawyer was speaking at a medical conference. This chapter attempts to answer her question.

If our health care system were better and more fair, and our society more understanding of the needs of persons with a chronic illness, a lawyer would be about the last person anyone would want or need to see to help handle their medical needs. Unfortunately, an attorney does sometimes play a role on a health care team. I wish I were exaggerating. Sadly, I know I am not. Over the years I have been involved with TCOYD and taken part in advocacy for persons with diabetes, it has become clear that there are a significant number of common legal issues and problems related to diabetes.

When TCOYD began, I mostly spoke on getting health care services and medications, while also training people with diabetes needs based on the results of the DCCT. While some real improvements have come about since TCOYD began, and the work of TCOYD has greatly assisted those efforts, the problem of inadequate care remains overwhelming for millions in this country. Indeed, it has likely grown increasingly obvious and well understood why an attorney may be needed in order to obtain proper health care and fair treatment if you have a chronic illness.

Receiving Better Care From a Health Plan.

While advances in science and technology continue, disputes over acceptance of and payment for them do so as well. When TCOYD began, I often received calls from people concerned about getting payments for Chemstrips, glucose meters, and insulin pumps. In later years, I began to receive a lot of calls about getting a health plan to pay for Viagra. Today, I most often hear from folks trying to get coverage for a continuous glucose monitor or for newer medications such as Byetta and Symlin. Recently, I learned of a new type of insulin pump that provides insulin without use of a tube and I have already received two calls from persons seeking to get one paid for by their insurance carrier. The simple fact is that there is an inevitable delay between the discovery and approval of medical improvements in the treatment of diabetes and the willingness of health insurance carriers to pay for them. As these delays continue, health care improvement is delayed as well. The bottom line appears to be that those of us who recognize that health care improvements can improve our own care need to push to get that care covered. The recommendations we made when TCOYD began remain the same today and are summarized here:

- Learn what new tools and treatments are available
- Ask your health care provider about them
- If the new treatment appears to make sense for you, ask your physician to write a prescription
- Send your health insurer whatever articles or information you can obtain to show why this new treatment is likely to benefit your care
- Ask your physician to support your request with a letter or note of some kind (if possible, try drafting it yourself and asking your physician to improve it as he or she thinks best and then get it signed and send it to your insurer)
- Contact the manufacturer of the tool or medication you want and ask what materials they have to support your request
- Send an explanatory letter to your insurer along with these supporting documents and follow-up with calls to find out what is being done and why; take notes of who is saying what at your plan about your request (Remember: explain why you need this particular tool or medicine or treatment. Answer these questions: What is it about this item that will likely improve my diabetes care? Why can the same improvement not be achieved with some other already approved item? If you can answer these questions, you have the basis for a good claim.)
- Appeal any denial to your health plan
- If the denial is not overturned, make sure you understand why and then, if appropriate, appeal to whatever government agency has oversight over your plan. (This can be a State or Federal agency depending on whether you are on a Medicare plan under Federal authority, or an individual or group plan under State authority.)

These steps more often than not achieve the result requested. Most people give up somewhere along the way and, quite frankly, some insurance carriers know this and count on it to save money. It can take real effort to get new treatments approved, but when you refuse to give up on getting something that you need to improve your health care, you are improving health care both for yourself and for others (**Table 23-2**).

Table 23-2

Staying Insured

When a job or other relationship that provided health insurance ends, there are three ways to stay insured other than getting a new job that provides group health coverage:

1. **COBRA**: This 1986 federal law provides continuing health coverage for employees, their spouses, and dependent children when the employee loses a job either voluntarily or involuntarily for reasons other than gross misconduct.

   "COBRA provides certain former employees, retirees, spouses, former spouses, and dependent children the right to temporary continuation of health coverage at group rates. This coverage, however, is only available when coverage is lost due to certain specific events. Group health coverage for COBRA participants is usually more expensive than health coverage for active employees, since usually the employer pays a part of the premium for active employees while COBRA participants generally pay the entire premium themselves. It is ordinarily less expensive, though, than individual health coverage." [Quoted from the US Department of Labor's website at *http://www. dol.gov/ebsa/faqs/faq_consumer_cobra.html*]

   Group health plans for an employer with 20 or more employees on more than 50% of its typical business days in the previous calendar year are subject to COBRA. COBRA lasts for 18 months after the change in employment and that period can be extended in the case of a disability which began within the first 60 days of COBRA coverage if the Social Security Administration approves the application for COBRA extension and this information is timely provided to the health plan.

2. **HIPAA**: This 1996 federal law guarantees the right to purchase new health insurance after coverage under a group plan, such as COBRA, continuation benefits end.

   "HIPAA amended the Employee Retirement Income Security Act (ERISA), to provide new rights and protections for participants and beneficiaries in group health plans. Understanding this amendment is important to your decisions about future health coverage. HIPAA contains protections both for health coverage offered in connection with employment (group health plans) and for individual insurance policies sold by insurance companies (individual policies)." [Quoted from the US Department of Labor's website at *http://www.dol.gov/ ebsa/faqs/faq_consumer_hipaa.html*]

   If you received health care coverage that ended and you apply for an individual plan within 63 days of the prior coverage ending, you cannot be refused coverage under a new individual plan due to a preexisting condition. If you received health care coverage that ended and you apply to be included in a new group plan within 63 days of the prior coverage ending, you cannot be refused coverage for a preexisting condition unless you received treatment for that condition in the 6 months before the new coverage began and then coverage for that preexisting condition can only be excluded for the first twelve months of new coverage (unless you enrolled after the time you were first allowed to begin coverage, in which case the preexisting condition exclusion may be extended to 18 months).

Problem with both COBRA and HIPAA: Cost. Individuals on COBRA coverage must pay the cost of the insurance themselves; plans selling individuals coverage under HIPAA rules are not limited in how much they can charge for coverage. The cost for COBRA coverage is generally not exorbitant but if you are unemployed and have no savings, that cost can be prohibitive. The cost for HIPPA coverage is often exorbitant and grossly unfair—the law says only that coverage must be offered, it does not prohibit a plan from offering coverage at an unfair and excessive rate.

3. **State Plans**: Most states have some type of plan individuals can join if they are refused coverage elsewhere. You need to contact your state's medical insurance oersight agency for information to find out if your state has such a plan and how to apply to join.

Problem with State Plans: Delays in acceptance, expense, and poor or insufficient coverage. These are common problems but not always true. You need to review your state's specific plan to learn more.

Avoiding the Loss of a Driver's License.

I have represented scores of persons trying to end a driver's license suspension as a result of a diabetes-related issue. The key to ending a suspension is always to make sure the suspended driver truly understands diabetes well enough and handles his or her own diabetes well enough to be able to drive safely. Once I believe my client can do so, it is fairly easy for me to prove to the Department of Motor Vehicles (DMV) why I do. I suspect that many of my clients would tell you they had a harder time convincing me they were safe to drive than they did convincing the DMV. By the time I prepare them for a DMV hearing, it should be fairly easy for them to answer questions honestly and accurately in a way that will prove they can drive safely. I may feel sorry for someone who is not allowed to drive, but that is not enough. I need to know they can drive safely before I help them back on the road.

In my fee agreements, I now require my clients to sign a *Safe Driving Agreement* before I will represent them (**Table 23-3**). This part of my fee agreement is not something I could ever enforce. But legal enforcement of this agreement is not the point. I have never represented any one who did not want to drive safely or who was so irresponsible that they did not care. Usually, it was just a matter of making sure my

Table 23-3

Safe Driving Agreement

You acknowledge your understanding that I am not willing to risk my professional reputation and emotional well-being on behalf of a driver who is not willing to operate a motor vehicle safely to the best of his or her ability. You therefore assure me that you will (*you must initial each numbered statement below or I will not represent you*):

_____ 1) Test your blood glucose immediately prior to driving

_____ 2) Test your blood glucose at least every 2 hours on every occasion in which you drive for more than 2 hours

_____ 3) Keep your blood test meter with you at all times while driving

_____ 4) Keep something with you to treat a low blood glucose reaction in sufficient quantities to raise your blood glucose to a safe level at all times while driving

_____ 5) Never knowingly drive with a low blood glucose level that may impair your ability to drive safely

_____ 6) Work with a licensed health care provider to assist you to recognize or regain the ability to recognize low blood glucose reactions if at any time it becomes apparent that you are unable to recognize a low blood glucose level

client was knowledgeable about diabetes and whatever their own personal needs were. Sometimes, it was a matter of getting improved care for some reason, either because my client was not being treated by a physician with adequate knowledge of the best diabetes care practices or because my client was not adequately trained in knowing how to recognize and avoid hypoglycemia (low blood glucose) incidents. Fortunately, in my experience, DMV officers responsible for suspensions are becoming much more experienced and knowledgeable in understanding and handling diabetes-related suspensions. Regardless of the reason for the suspension or what an attorney needs to be able to do to end one, the truth is that all of us can improve our diabetes care and live more safely by paying more attention day to day. My *Safe Driving Agreement* is really just a way to encourage my clients to think a little more about what they are doing and to make sure they understand some simple ways to avoid problems.

Getting and Keeping a Job

Not only do we need to make sure we understand diabetes and our need for proper care and a safe lifestyle, sometimes we need to make sure others also understand these things. This may often include an employer. As advances in the treatment of diabetes occur that help us to manage diabetes better and more safely, there are fewer and fewer jobs where having diabetes should ever be a serious issue. Most often, when I have been asked to assist clients with job-discrimination concerns, my role has been to help my client write a letter about diabetes and what the employer can do to provide reasonable accommodations that will allow the employee to handle the job without difficulty. Most honest and worthwhile employers receive these letters without recrimination or difficulty. Some welcome them and are pleased to assist their employee to handle their job well and safely. That is not always the case.

Should you tell an employer about your diabetes during a job interview? No! Not only should you not mention it (unless, of course, you are applying to work with a pharmaceutical company selling blood glucose meters or something along those lines. In that case, having diabetes might help you get hired so you may as well brag about it and let them know right off!), it is usually unlawful for them to ask.

When and how can an employer learn about your diabetes? After they make the job offer, but only if all applicants for this position are treated equally and only if there is some legitimate work-based necessity for the medical examination (for example, an applicant to be a police officer may need to demonstrate physical fitness before being hired). Some companies may require that you complete a physical and that they will offer you a job pending satisfactory results. This is lawful if the examination is truly job related. If they then refuse to hire you, there will be clear evidence of why they did so and this can be reviewed to make sure it was lawful and not really an excuse to refuse to hire someone with a chronic illness. Any refusal to hire someone because of diabetes must be based on an actual review of the individual job applicant's health and some legitimate reason why that individual cannot safely and adequately perform the job in question.

Diabetes is sometimes simply misunderstood by a supervisor or employer. Diabetes is sometimes resented out of concern that an employee with a chronic illness may cause an increase in insurance rates for the company or that an employee with diabetes might lead to some unsafe event or a lawsuit of some kind. More often than not, these concerns are completely unjustified and a little effort can explain why.

If explanations and discussions don't help, it may become necessary to file a complaint of disability discrimination with a government agency. The federal agency that enforces workplace discrimination laws is the Equal Employment Opportunity Commission (EEOC). The federal disability law the EEOC enforces is known as the Americans With

Disabilities Act of 1990 (ADA). The ADA outlaws workplace disability discrimination by all private employers with fifteen or more employees.

You can contact the EEOC at 1-800-669-4000 and ask them how and where to file a claim. The EEOC will investigate your claim at no charge to you. Remember, you have 180 days from the date the discrimination occurs to file a claim or you lose your right to file a claim under the ADA. (Some states have laws that extend the deadline to 300 days, but filing within 180 days is always a good idea to avoid risking an unintentional loss of rights.)

If the EEOC chooses not to try and prove or resolve your claim of discrimination, it will issue a "right to sue letter" that allows you to file your claim in court. It is often better to have an attorney assist you as you pursue this kind of claim but it is possible for you to pursue your claim directly with the assistance of the EEOC or a state agency. You can read Titles I and V of the Americans With Disabilities Act on the EEOC website: *http://www.eeoc.gov/facts/qanda.html.*

Some states have laws that go further than federal laws in banning workplace disability discrimination. In California, for example, we have a law that explicitly recognizes diabetes as a disability and bans workplace discrimination against persons with this and many other illnesses. An attorney who practices in the area of disability discrimination can assist you in understanding these laws and, if necessary, making claims of discrimination arising from violations of them. But before you file a lawsuit based on workplace disability discrimination, you will always need to file a disability discrimination claim with a government agency first—either with the EEOC or, if one exists where you live, a state agency that enforces workplace discrimination laws.

One aspect of federal disability law is certain: An individual's specific medical history and needs must be considered in order to determine whether or not that person can be considered disabled under federal law. The fact of having diabetes alone will neither support nor end a claim of workplace disability discrimination. Rather, the medical history of the individual with diabetes must be considered—including, for example, whether that person suffers from impairment of a major life activity resulting from diabetes complications or whether the employer unlawfully treats the individual as if he or she does (**Table 23-4**).

It is not comfortable to consider oneself disabled. Most of us do not want to be looked at or treated differently than anyone else. We just want to be given a fair chance to prove our worth and do our job. Most of us do not think of ourselves as in any way disabled, but I know that when I am sitting at my desk and suddenly am unable to think clearly,

Table 23-4
Can a Person on Insulin Drive a Truck?

Currently, federal law in place since 1970 prevents persons on insulin from driving trucks in interstate commerce. A diabetes waiver program began in 1993 giving persons the opportunity to demonstrate they can drive a truck safely even though on insulin. But a federal court found a similar law improper and the waiver program was ended in 1996. In 1999, the Department of Transportation (DOT) commissioned a new group of experts to study the issue and make recommendations. The study found that it would be feasible and safe to allow persons with insulin-dependent diabetes to drive trucks if they could demonstrate their ability to control and monitor their diabetes. The report can be found on the Internet at *http://www.fmcsa.dot.gov/facts-research/researchtechnology/publications/medreports.htm*

A division of the DOT known as the Federal Motor Carrier Safety Administration (FMCSA) is currently reviewing and preparing to announce new rules and regulations that would allow persons with insulin-dependent diabetes to drive trucks in interstate commerce. The FMCSA can be contacted at 1-800-832-5660. (At the time of publication, the contact on this issue at FMCSA is Sandy Zyworkarte at 1-202-366-2987.) A few states already allow, or are considering rules that will allow, insulin-dependent drivers to work as truck drivers within their state.

read, or speak—when I am nervous and shaky and sweating—there is no doubt that at that moment I am disabled. This kind of temporary disability does not prevent me from performing my work. But it does require that my employer understand my needs and provide me with reasonable accommodations to handle and avoid the problem such as allowing me to test my blood glucose, eat a meal, or even take a break for a while if hypoglycemia actually occurs.

The main issue is not whether or not one is disabled; it is whether or not one is being allowed to overcome it or is being prevented from getting a job and doing one's work despite it. And this is an issue we can and will win.

Obtaining Proper Care for Children in Schools

Another situation in which it may be necessary to make sure others understand the need for proper diabetes care and how to provide it is when a child with diabetes is in school. Any school that receives federal funding (including, of course, all public schools but also many private and parochial schools as well) must comply with Section 504 of the Rehabilitation Act of 1973, which provides individuals with disabilities basic civil rights protection against discrimination. The Education for

All Handicapped Children Act of 1975, amended and renamed in 1991 the Individuals With Disability Education Act (IDEA), guarantees a free, appropriate public education for all children with disabilities. Children with diabetes are specifically protected under this law.

Parents have the right to meet with school officials to develop a Section 504 Plan or an Individualized Education Program (IEP) under the IDEA to address a child's specific needs to manage his or her diabetes. This may include eating as necessary, participating in school activities without discrimination, assistance with blood glucose monitoring and injections, and other issues that the family and the child's physician raise and explain to the school. The 504 Plan and the IEP plan are used to make sure these issues are discussed, understood, and addressed so that safety is maintained for the child and discriminatory treatment is prevented.

Most public schools are able and willing to assist with these plans and have the experience to do so. The main thing a parent can do to make certain the plan is properly devised is to understand the child's daily needs by speaking with the child and the child's health care provider, then communicating those needs to the school and making sure the school is handling those needs properly after the plan is created. An attorney can be used if there are difficulties in achieving these goals and some attorneys specialize in creating plans for disabled children. If a school is resistant to meeting and creating and implementing a plan, an attorney may be needed to obtain compliance with the law. Sometimes, however, government officials or agencies that specialize in providing advice about children with disabilities may work just as well; information about how to obtain those free services is provided in **Table 23-5**.

Table 23-5

Aiding Children With Diabetes

The National Information Center for Children and Youth with Disabilities provides free information on handling school issues for children with diabetes. Their phone is 1-800-695-0285. Their Web site is *www.nichcy.org/* and also includes information on how to contact state agencies that may be able to help: *www.nichcy.org/states.htm*

The US Office for Civil Rights provides free information and assistance on handling school issues for children with diabetes. Their phone is 1-800-421-3481. Their Web site is *www.ed.gov/about/offices/list/ocr/index.html*.

Proper Care for Persons Who Are in Nursing Homes or Suffering From a Critical Illness

Persons in nursing homes and person in hospitals suffering from a critical illness frequently are allowed to let their blood glucose level run high. If the person under care is able to make the determination about their blood glucose level preference and allowed to determine their own level of care, this should not be an issue of great significance. But in many instances, the choice is not made by the person being treated; options and consequences are not explained. Simply put, it is far easier for overworked caregivers to allow blood glucose levels to run high in nursing-care and in critical-care settings. Often it is assumed that as long as the person receiving care does not fall too low and risk serious hypoglycemia, everything should be all right. Unfortunately, hyperglycemia is both unpleasant and deadly. Those of us who have experienced elevated blood glucose levels know all too well the miserable feeling of urgently and incessantly needing to urinate; the unpleasant and awful taste in one's mouth; the discomfort of simply running too high. To be obliged to lie in bed in such a state day after day is a horrifying thought. Yet that is the reality for many persons with diabetes whose blood glucose levels are under the control of others.

Not only is the experience unpleasant, it can also lead to increased morbidity and ongoing critical health problems. A study published by the *New England Journal of Medicine* on November 8, 2001, found that after 12 months, well-managed blood glucose levels in critically ill patients reduced mortality from 8% of 1548 patients to 4.6%. That is a nearly 50% decrease in patients dying in the course of 1 year among the group whose blood glucose levels were well managed. Moreover, the improvement in health care success was similarly high across many different areas of care, reducing the need for red-cell transfusions by 50% among well-managed patients, renal failure by 41%, and bloodstream infections by 46%.

Based on this evidence, it is fair to say that allowing blood glucose levels to escalate too frequently, and without a meaningful evaluation and effort to prevent it, may constitute elder abuse or abuse of patients receiving critical care. Of course, such claims need to be reviewed carefully and the evidence of what would constitute proper care under the circumstances seriously considered based on the facts of each case, but this certainly is an area that all of us should be concerned about as all of us are likely to be in this setting at some point in time.

Discussing treatment options with the health care providers who oversee patients in these circumstances is critical. Reviewing blood glucose test results and taking part in how best to manage care is important as well. Persons should not be left to suffer pain or worsened conditions because of laziness and a haphazard approach to managing blood glucose levels—and this is as true for the elderly and the critically ill as it is for those of us still able to care for ourselves.

Legal Conclusions

There have been many improvements in the legal rights of persons with diabetes since TCOYD began. But discrimination continues to exist for many of us... needed coverage is not always provided and the cost of decent coverage continues to be overwhelming for many of us even when it is available. It seems that by educating ourselves and making proper demands for our own care and treatment, we are likely to benefit others unable to help themselves, as well as our society in general.

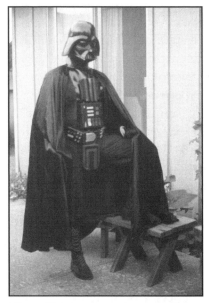

Steve Edelman posing as an
HMO executive on Halloween!

24

Adult Onset Diabetes Becomes a Disease of Our Children and Youth

by Francine R. Kaufman, MD

Excerpts from *Diabesity: The Obesity-Diabetes Epidemic That Threatens America—And What We Must Do to Stop It* by Francine R. Kaufman, MD. Copyright 2005 by Francine Ratner Kaufman. Reprinted by permission of Bantam Books, a division of Random House, Inc.)

My greatest joy as a physician is to be with a patient when they have an "Ah-ha" moment. Watching an epiphany develop and emerge is exciting. I remember a 10-year-old boy with diabetes who decided to do his own experiment about the effect of food on his blood glucose level. He took his shot, ate an egg, and monitored his glucose level hourly over 3 hours. It stayed relatively flat. The next day he ate a hamburger on a bun, and he had a late glucose peak. The third day he ate a candy bar and drank a soda. His glucose level skyrocketed. "Ah-ha," he said, "I get it."

As a physician, I have also had a number of "Ah-ha" moments myself. That moment in time when the right diagnosis flashes into my mind, when I say just the right thing to a family as they watch their child slip away from a devastating illness, and when I realize that there has been a paradigm shift in the world. I witnessed a paradigm shift in diabetes in the mid-1990s. In the middle of a spring day in 1995, I received a call from an emergency department doctor, asking if I could see a 13-year-old patient named Tanesha right away. Tanesha's blood glucose level was 427 mg/dL, at least five times higher than normal for a young teen.

I was already in the diabetes clinic. The waiting room and all of the examining rooms were filled with patients and parents, but that didn't matter. I had to see Tanesha immediately because of her dangerously high blood glucose. Hearing the number, I pictured a typical type 1 patient referred from the emergency department: thin, severely weakened by dehydration, nausea, and fatigue, or even comatose. But I soon learned that Tanesha and her family looked nothing like this picture.

"Tanesha has been hyperglycemic for at least 2 weeks," the ER doctor told me. "I can't figure out why she still looks so good. And you won't believe how big this girl is. She's the largest kid with diabetes I've ever seen." Despite her elevated blood glucose, Tanesha was barely symptomatic. She didn't feel weak or exhausted; she hadn't vomited. Instead, she was hungry. While Tanesha waited in the ER, she had eaten a bag of fries and downed a regular soda. "By the way," the ER doctor added, "Tanesha is African American." This too was puzzling. Type 1 diabetes is rarer in nonwhite children.

Even though I'd been told that Tanesha was overweight, and even though she was not sick after a long bout of hyperglycemia, it didn't dawn on me that she might have type 2 diabetes. Not in 1995. Only when I walked into the examining room did it become apparent that my thinking was all wrong. Tanesha was there with her mother and her grandmother. Each of them weighed at least 250 pounds. I realized that I might be walking into a whole new world.

Tanesha was not merely overweight, she was huge. Her height— 5-foot, 3-inches—was normal for a girl of 13. But she weighed 267 pounds. She had extensive darkening of the skin around her neck. I'd seen this condition, called acanthosis nigricans, in adults with type 2 diabetes. Could this 13-year-old girl have type 2 diabetes? As I questioned Tanesha about her symptoms, her answers confirmed the possibility.

"Are you thirsty?" I asked.

She told me she had been drinking a lot of juice and soda. "My mama told me to stop drinking so much, but I told her I was just thirsty all the time, day and night," she informed me.

"How about urination?" I asked. "Do you have to pee at night?"

"Only 'cause I get up to drink," she explained. "If I didn't need to drink so much, I mightn't need to pee so much."

She actually had it backward. Her body was trying to rid itself of excess sugar by urinating. And because she lost so much water, she was constantly thirsty.

I asked, "How long have you been waking up at night to urinate?" This would tell me how long her blood glucose had been elevated.

She thought and then answered, "At least for this whole year."

Her response crystallized my thinking: Tanesha had type 2 diabetes. How could that be? And then I looked over at her grandmother, and thought: "Just like her grandma."

I didn't need to see blood test results to guess that Tanesha's grandmother, Thelma, had type 2 diabetes. She was obese and sat in a wheelchair. Her face drooped on one side and her left foot turned in, suggesting that she'd had a stroke. People with diabetes have an elevated risk for stroke and heart attack. Her right foot had been amputated, probably a result of the blood circulation and nerve problems that can develop from diabetes.

I asked Thelma about her medical history, half expecting her daughter Joyce, Tanesha's mother, to reply on her behalf. But Thelma's physical problems had not diminished the force of her personality. Joyce stood silently as her mother answered my questions. Tanesha watched and listened.

"They told me I had the sugar in 1966," she said. "They took my foot in 1987. Gangrene." In 1990 she'd had a mild heart attack, followed by a stroke in 1993. The stroke had left her left leg spastic and her left arm paralyzed. "I've been going to therapy for 2 years pretty regular. Still can't open my hand," she said.

"What medications do you take?" I asked.

"Them doctors tried to get me to take insulin. But insulin makes you sick," she said defiantly.

Joyce rolled her eyes at this. She pulled a sheet of paper from her purse and handed it to me. Thelma was supposed to take three medications to control her blood glucose, two more to lower her blood pressure, aspirin to prevent heart attacks and strokes, and a cholesterol-lowering drug. I wondered how many of those pills she actually took.

"Tanesha will be okay, Doc," Thelma continued. "Everybody has a little bit of the sugar in our family, 'cept Joyce. We don't need to pay it no mind. And we don't need to think 'bout putting her on no insulin shots. Don't you worry, Tanish," she said turning to her granddaughter. "You don't need none of those shots, and we don't need to pay the doctor no mind either."

I was shocked. Thelma needed handsful of medicines and had every possible diabetes complication. If that was only a "little bit of the sugar," I thought, what would be a lot? I had not expected her to attempt to thwart me. Tanesha would require insulin injections, at least at the beginning of her treatment.

I turned my attention to Tanesha's mother, Joyce. I needed to inform her and win her over to my side. I also needed to convince Tanesha.

"The blood tests show that Tanesha has diabetes," I explained to Joyce. I quickly turned to Tanesha and added, "Tanesha, there is no doubt about it. A blood glucose level above 400 mg/dL is diabetes. We now must determine what kind of diabetes you have."

"Although almost all children with diabetes have what we call type 1 diabetes, Tanesha may actually have type 2, just like her grandmother," I explained, swinging back to Joyce.

I didn't want to get too technical and lose their attention. "If Tanesha has type 2 diabetes, we may be able to treat her with pills eventually.

But her blood glucose is too high now for the pills to work. The first step is to get her blood glucose level normal, to stop all that drinking and urinating." Then I added, "We must get her well again, so that she doesn't ever have to face what her grandma has faced because of her diabetes."

I looked at Joyce to see if I had made an impression. She remained expressionless for what seemed like a lifetime. Finally, she responded in a quiet but very firm voice: "We will do what you say, Doctor Kaufman. My whole life, I've watched diabetes eat my mother to pieces, because she doesn't take care of herself. No way will I let that happen to Tanesha." Thelma glared at her, but remained silent.

I sighed with relief. The first battle was won; I would be allowed to treat Tanesha with the medications she needed. But that was just one small battle. There was a war yet to win. We would have to get Tanesha to change her eating habits and become more active. She needed to lose weight. I hoped Joyce would do the same for her own sake. It seemed unlikely that Thelma would change, but maybe I could persuade her not to stand in Tanesha's way. Then there would be the constant battle with the rest of the world. Everywhere Tanesha turned, she'd be surrounded by the junk food and soft drinks and candy that threatened her health.

In that clinic room in 1995, I knew that a world of battles would have to be fought for Tanesha. What I didn't know was that this skirmish was the harbinger of a much larger war to come.

The waiting room in my clinic at Children's Hospital is always filled with people—children, parents, nannies, grandparents. When I look at them, I see the changing face of type 2 diabetes. And I see the cause: obesity. Families like Tanesha's are common now: a massively obese child and that youngster's equally heavy relatives, some of whom already show the terrible long-term effects of diabetes. We must do something to try to reverse this trend. But what can we do?

We can all do something—whether we have diabetes or not. Even if we have type 1 diabetes, maintaining a healthy lifestyle and a healthy weight makes a big difference in glucose control and in avoiding diabetes complications; particularly, in avoiding cardiovascular disease.

We can start with our own life and our own home. Commit to a healthy lifestyle. Start to eat healthy portions of healthy foods. Eat fruits and vegetables, whole grains, low-fat, and high-nutrient foods. Stop eating at fast food restaurants and instead eat together as a family. Eating together gives you a chance to touch base and check in with your children and spouse. Eat breakfast, drink water. We weren't meant to drink calories, so get sweetened sodas out of your life. Limit juice; it is nothing but sugar and you are better off eating an orange than drinking a glass of juice. Turn off the TV and the computer games. Get physically active; wear a pedometer and commit to working to get 10,000 steps a day. It might take a long time to get to that many steps, but it is a goal worth achieving. Do this with your whole family. For those with diabetes, those high blood glucose levels may come screaming down. For those without diabetes, but at risk because of family history and other factors, it might be just what is needed since it is the best diabetes preventive.

Make your workplace a healthy environment, too (**Table 24-1**). After all, how much time do you spend there? Each day on your way to work, plan how you can optimize your health. Take a walk at lunch; park far away in the parking lot. Use the stairs; it's a waste of time waiting for the elevator. Be sure water is available, demand healthy food options, stop bringing in junk food and candy, and band together to have a healthy workforce.

We need to be sure our homes, our schools, our communities, and our health care institutions promote health rather than deteriorate it—particularly for people with or at risk for diabetes. To achieve that end, we all have to raise our voice, change our habits, and work toward a healthier future. If not, more and more children like Tanesha will develop diabetes and imperil their life. If we commit now, who knows what the next "Ah-ha" moment might be. If we change our course and opt for health, it might be that we are healthy and vibrant through to old age.

Table 24-1

What to Do at the Workplace

- Wear a pedometer—you need to take 10,000 steps a day and you need to get a lot of them at work
- Park far away—fight for the farthest spot and walk those extra minutes
- Take the stairs—up one and down two
- Take a walk at lunch—you'll have more energy in the afternoon
- Take a walking meeting—your colleagues will be amazed and invigorated
- Don't drink calories—drink only water at work; it will keep you hydrated and alert
- Put resistance bands or 2-lb weights on your wrists and use them when you are on the phone
- Bring your lunch—a salad, healthy leftovers, healthy foods
- Have healthy snacks—don't go to the vending machines
- You need five to nine fruits and veggies a day—get three or more at work
- Make your workplace value health and healthy behaviors

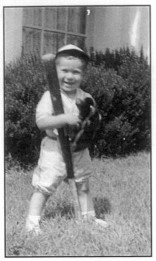

"Play Ball!"… Steve Edelman at 27 months of age.

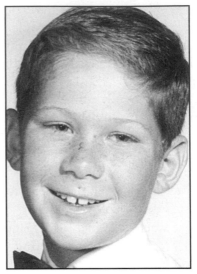

School Days photo of Steve Edelman.

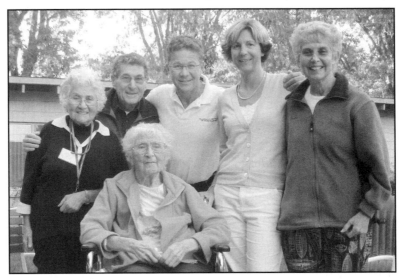

Pictured here *(from left to right)* are Steve Edelman's mother, Joyce, Uncle Allen, Steve, Ingrid, and Aunt Jeanie. Seated in the wheelchair is Steve's 100-year-old grandmother, Lucy.

25

Can Diabetes Be Prevented?

The Answer Is a Resounding, Yes! for Type 2 Diabetes

It dawned on me one day that the best way to prevent the terrible complications of diabetes is to prevent diabetes in the first place. We spend so much of our research efforts and limited health care dollars investigating and treating the eye, kidney, nerve, and heart disease that continue to be so common in our diabetic population. The point is that these complications appear several years after the diagnosis and lead to a tremendous amount of human suffering. Why not put our resources up front and prevent the development of any complications by preventing diabetes altogether? Over the long term, health care costs will be reduced and the quality of many lives will be maintained with this strategy. One of the major obstacles to this strategy is that the people who control the purse strings argue that it will cost more money in the short term. These "bean-counters" commonly say, "Since people change insurance companies every few years on average, why spend money to save the next company from losing money down the road?" This is a strategy for disaster.

One of the more striking facts regarding how we spend our health care dollars these days is that most of the money spent to take care of people with diabetes is for inpatient or hospital charges; namely, heart attacks, strokes, amputations, and dialysis, which are end-stage complications. Only about 13% is spent on drugs and devices such as insulin, pills, glucose meters, continuous glucose monitoring devices, and insulin pumps. I think that all of the health insurance companies should share the costs equally over the long term so they all unite and agree to put money into prevention.

Can We Prevent Type 2 Diabetes? Absolutely, YES!

Prevention strategies are usually based on the etiology or cause of the disease. In the case of type 2 diabetes, prevention strategies have mainly targeted insulin resistance, which is recognized as the main problem. The different types of interventions that have been evaluated or are currently being studied include intensive lifestyle changes (long-term weight-loss and exercise programs) and various medications, such as the "glitazones" (Avandia [rosiglitazone] and Actos [pioglitazone]), carbohydrate absorption inhibitors (Precose [acarbose], and Glyset [miglitol]), insulin secretagogues (Starlix [nateglinide], Glucophage [metformin]), and weight loss agents such as Xenical [orlistat]. **Table 25-1** lists several of the more important type 2 diabetes prevention trials conducted worldwide, which will be discussed more. It is also important to note here that since the causes for type 1 and type 2 diabetes are so very different, the prevention strategies are also completely unrelated.

Definition of Prediabetes

Figure 1-2 shows how we define normal, prediabetes, and diabetes, primarily based on the blood glucose levels at two different times. The fasting blood glucose level, measured first thing in the morning after an overnight fast (nothing to eat for approximately 8 hours), should be less than 100 mg/dL. If the fasting value is 126 mg/dL or greater, that is in the diabetic range. Prediabetes is diagnosed if the value is greater than 100 and less than 126 mg/dL and it basically means that the individual is at high risk for developing diabetes. The medical phrase for prediabetes based on the morning fasting glucose value is called IFG or impaired fasting glucose.

Table 25-1
Primary Prevention Trials of Type 2 Diabetes

Study	Treatment	Relative Risk
FDPS	Intensive diet and exercise vs control	↓ 58%
DPP	Intensive diet and exercise vs placebo	↓ 58%
	Metformin vs placebo	↓ 31%
	Troglitazone vs placebo	↓ 75%*
STOP-NIDDM	Acarbose vs placebo	↓ 25%
XENDOS	Orlistat vs placebo	↓ 37%
DREAM	Rosiglitazone vs placebo	↓ 62%

Abbreviations: DPP, Diabetes Prevention Program; DREAM, Diabetes Reduction Assessment With Ramipril and Rosiglitazone Medication [trial]; FDPS, Finnish Diabetes Prevention Study; STOP-NIDDM, Study to Prevent Non–Insulin-Dependent Diabetes Mellitus; XENDOS, Xenical in the Prevention of Diabetes in Obese Subjects [study].

* Average treatment of 10 months.

The other important time to measure the glucose value in order to diagnose prediabetes is 2 hours after swallowing 75 grams of a very sweet substance. This test is called the 2-hour oral glucose tolerance test or OGTT. This test is primarily used for research purposes; however, because of the rise in type 2 diabetes and the focus on prevention, it is being ordered more frequently by caregivers in the clinic setting. The medical phrase for prediabetes based on the 2-hour value is called IGT or impaired glucose tolerance. These criteria are used to screen potential research volunteers for the prevention trials described below.

Finnish Diabetes Prevention Study

The Finnish Diabetes Prevention Study (FDPS) was one of the first large studies to look at lifestyle modification and how it can prevent someone with prediabetes from converting to full-blown type 2 diabetes. The study was done in Finland (I bet you could have never figured that one out on your own), and after about 3 to 4 years, they demonstrated a significant 58% reduction in the conversion from prediabetes to diabetes compared with the placebo group that did not get lifestyle modification counseling. The active-treatment group was given diet and exercise instructions at baseline and yearly after that and the subjects were given up to seven individual appointments per year. They were asked to exercise 30 minutes a day, cut their total daily fat intake to less than 30%, and eat more fiber in their diet. This study was loosely conducted which really set the stage for one of the more powerful studies called the Diabetes Prevention Program or DPP.

Diabetes Prevention Program

The DPP was a powerful, well-conducted, and highly funded government-initiated (National Institutes of Health) study to prevent the development of type 2 diabetes in people who may be at risk for this condition (prediabetics). The DPP was conducted at 25 major universities around the country. In order to efficiently screen large populations to be potential research volunteers, it is important to identify those individuals who may be at the highest risk. People with diabetes, the lay public, medical students, student doctors (interns and residents), and primary caregivers should be familiar with and knowledgeable about the risk factors for developing type 2 diabetes (**Table 25-2**).

Subjects who were identified with several risk factors for developing type 2 diabetes were brought in for an OGTT. If they had prediabetes, they were asked to volunteer for the DPP. The approximately 4000 subjects who agreed to be in the study were then placed into one of four

Table 25-2

Risk Factors for Developing Type 2 Diabetes

- *Having someone in your family with diabetes, especially a first-degree relative.* Because type 2 diabetes runs so strongly in families, even if a second- or third-degree relative has diabetes, your risk goes up. There is really no such thing as "old-age diabetes," which a lot of people refer to and do not consider a familial risk factor.

- *Being overweight, especially with central obesity, commonly referred to as a "beer belly."* People with insulin resistance develop a certain type of fat in the abdominal area giving the person "the apple shape" or upper-body obesity versus "the pear shape" or lower-body obesity.

- *Having some or all of the other associated conditions commonly seen in type 2 diabetes, such as high blood pressure or high cholesterol levels.* These conditions may appear many years before the diagnosis of diabetes and contribute to the high rate of heart attack and stroke.

- *Being a member of an ethnic group that has a high incidence of diabetes.* These include African Americans, Hispanics, Native Americans, Asian Americans, and Pacific Islanders. We do not know the reason for the high incidence of type 2 diabetes in these ethnic groups, but it is probably related to genetic makeup and our westernized lifestyle.

- *Having had diabetes during pregnancy (gestational diabetes).* It turns out that when a woman develops diabetes during pregnancy, the diabetes goes away shortly after delivery of the baby most of the time. However, the chance of that woman developing diabetes in the next 5 to 10 years is high (25% to 50%), depending on the ethnic group, degree of obesity, and family history.

- *Having had a baby weighing over 9 pounds.* This is because when a woman's blood glucose level is high during pregnancy, the baby becomes large physically, but it is usually developmentally abnormal internally. Not only does having a large baby put the mother at risk for the development of type 2 diabetes, recent research has suggested there may be delayed adverse effects in the offspring.

- *If any caregiver ever told you that you had a "touch of diabetes" or "borderline diabetes."* This is a common scenario. So many caregivers do not take diabetes seriously enough. Most of the time, when a person is told they have a touch of diabetes, his or her diabetes is fairly advanced, and therapy is warranted immediately. Having a touch of diabetes is like having a touch of pregnancy.

groups: intensive lifestyle changes alone, metformin (also called Glucophage) plus minimal lifestyle changes, troglitazone (also called Rezulin) plus minimal lifestyle, or placebo (fake pill) plus minimal lifestyle. The group sent to the intensive-lifestyle-changes group was given lots of attention by nurses, dietitians, exercise trainers, and clinical psychologists in order to help them achieve the goals of losing 7% of their body weight and exercise 30 minutes a day, 5 days a week. The other three groups took their oral medications and were simply given some general recommendations on diet and exercise.

The results were so impressive and convincing that the study was ended early after 2.8 years (originally it was suppose to run for 4 years). The intensive-lifestyle-changes group had a reduced risk of converting from prediabetes to type 2 diabetes by 58% compared with the placebo group. The group that took Glucophage had a 31% risk reduction compared with the placebo group. It is interesting that Glucophage worked primarily in younger (less than 45 years old) and overweight people where intensive-lifestyle-changes group worked to prevent diabetes in all age and weight groups. The other big lesson in this study is that the earlier you can identify people at risk for type 2 diabetes, the better the various interventions work, whether they be lifestyle or oral medications.

DREAM Trial

The DREAM trial is another impressive study that looked at how well a type 2 diabetes drug called Avandia (rosiglitazone) worked to prevent type 2 diabetes in people at risk compared with a fake pill (placebo). Avandia is a drug similar to Rezulin studied in the DPP, but without serious liver toxicity. It is in a class of medications called insulin sensitizers and is currently approved by the FDA as is Actos (also called pioglitizone) for the treatment of type 2 diabetes. Insulin sensitizers reduce insulin resistance. There was not a lifestyle-changes treatment group in this study like there was in the DPP.

The results demonstrated that for those volunteers who took Avandia, there was an impressive risk reduction of converting from prediabetes to type 2 diabetes by 62% when compared with the placebo group. Of the 5269 subjects with prediabetes who entered the study, 658 taking placebo developed diabetes while only 280 taking Avandia developed diabetes. Just think… if they had a group that had intensive lifestyle modification like the DPP plus Avandia.

The Act Now study is an ongoing trial that is similar to the DREAM trial; however, Actos (pioglitizone), a different glitazone, is being given to people with prediabetes versus placebo. I expect the results to be very positive as well.

STOP-NIDDM, XENDOS, and NAVIGATOR Studies

There have been other prevention trials looking at other diabetes and obesity medications. The Study to Prevent Non–Insulin-Dependent

Diabetes Mellitus (STOP-NIDDM) demonstrated that Precose (acarbose), an oral medication that delays the absorption of carbohydrates in the gut and lowers postmeal glucose levels, can reduce the risk of converting to type 2 diabetes by 25% and also reduce the risk factors for heart disease at the same time. In the Xenical in the Prevention of Diabetes in Obese Subjects (XENDOS) study, the obesity drug Xenical (orlistat), which blocks the absorption of fat in the gut, led to an impressive 37% risk reduction as well (**Table 25-1**). There is also the Nateglinide and Valsartan in Impaired Glucose Tolerance Outcomes Research (NAVIGATOR) study, which is looking at how well a blood pressure drug called Diovan (valsartan) and an insulin secretagogue Starlix (nateglinide) can prevent type 2 diabetes.

The number of oral medications currently available that have been proven to prevent people with prediabetes from converting to type 2 diabetes is impressive (Glucophage, Avandia, Precose, and Xenical). There is no question that lifestyle modification with or without one of these safe and well-proven medications can prevent type 2 diabetes. It is important to note that the FDA has not given formal approval to any medication to be used for the prevention of type 2 diabetes. The American Diabetes Association recommends that individuals with a high risk of developing type 2 diabetes consider starting Glucophage if they are below 60 years of age and obese. Please discuss these issues with your caregiver before starting any of these medications. The pros and cons must be explained to you in detail.

What Do You Do if You Are at Risk for Type 2 Diabetes?

First of all, there are no proven medications or other techniques to 100% prevent people from developing type 2 diabetes; however, there are several proven strategies that can help reduce your risk.

1. Improve your eating habits and try to get down to your ideal body weight. There have been two large studies published (the FDPS and the DPP) that have clearly demonstrated that lifestyle intervention (weight loss and exercise) can reduce the incidence of type 2 diabetes in people who are at risk. Although this is easier said than done, making small nondramatic changes in your diet over time is the best strategy. Maybe just cutting out the morning donuts most of the time or switching from regular soda to diet soda. It may not only be your body weight that is important; it could also be the composition of the food you ingest. For example, being overweight and eating a well-balanced diet with limited sugar and fat may also be a preventive measure. The results of the DPP dem-

onstrated a dramatic reduction in the incidence of type 2 diabetes in people at risk just by their participating in mild aerobic exercise 30 minutes a day 5 days a week and losing just a few pounds.

Regular exercise is the key. I recommend doing anything that is enjoyable to you. Don't just join a fancy health club and only go once a year to pay your dues. If you attempt a sport that you must force yourself to do, your chances of following an exercise program over the long term are slim to none. This is why whenever you go to a garage sale, there is always an almost-new, never-used exercise bike, treadmill, set of weights, or golf clubs for sale... cheap.

2. Obtain your own glucose meter. You should get a glucose meter and test yourself occasionally in the morning before breakfast and 2 hours after a heavy meal. Your morning blood glucose should be less than 100 mg/dL and your postmeal value should be less than 140 mg/dL. If your numbers start to approach or go above these values on a regular basis, you should notify your caregiver. Also don't forget that these meters are not always perfectly accurate so don't panic if you get a super high or low value. Just test again.

3. Look for other conditions associated with type 2 diabetes. Make sure you are checked for the other conditions that are commonly associated with type 2 diabetes, such as high blood pressure and high cholesterol levels. As mentioned several times, it is important to control these silent risk factors that lead to heart attack and stroke. It is very common to develop these other conditions before the development of diabetes, so why not treat them aggressively when they appear?

4. Ask your caregiver about taking one aspirin a day. As discussed in the chapter on heart disease, aspirin is a super-effective, cheap, and easy way to prevent heart attack and stroke. Make sure you check with your caregiver first.

5. Consider drug therapy. Consider taking a medication that may help to prevent the initial development of type 2 diabetes. Until recently, there were no proven drugs to prevent diabetes. However, the results of the DPP have demonstrated that Glucophage is effective at preventing type 2 diabetes in people who are at risk and especially those who are 45 years of age or younger and overweight. Every drug has its pros and cons, and a serious discussion with a diabetes expert is definitely a must if one is considering this option. Remember that lifestyle modification is the most powerful tool that we know of to retard or prevent the development of type 2 diabetes. You should never substitute one of these medications

for lifestyle modification but use them in addition to diet and exercise strategies.

6. Consider getting involved in a research program. Consider being a volunteer in a research protocol that is a prevention trial. There may or may not be one going on in your area, but if you live near a university medical center, you can easily find a listing of the various studies being conducted. Also keep your eyes and ears open to the media since many national studies have public-relations firms that work to get the word out. Read the protocols carefully and discuss the details with your caregiver to make sure the study is right for you.

Can We Prevent Type 1 Diabetes? So Far the Answer Is No

You probably cannot find two things more opposite than the causes of type 1 and type 2 diabetes. The cause of type 1 diabetes is not entirely known, but it is believed that for some reason, either genetic, viral, or environmental, antibodies are produced that specifically destroy the insulin-producing beta cells of the pancreas. Antibodies are the cells in the body that normally attack and destroy anything foreign such as bacteria or germs. The strategies to prevent type 1 diabetes are aimed at preventing the immune system from inappropriately destroying the pancreas. It is not within the scope of this book to get into the nitty gritty of type 1 prevention strategies, but unfortunately all of the prevention trials to date have failed to show benefit.

The Diabetes Prevention Trial for Type 1 Diabetes (DPT-1) was a long-term study launched by the National Institutes of Health in early 1994. The goal of the study was to determine whether we can prevent or delay type 1 diabetes in people who have the immune marker (antibodies that attack the pancreas) for the development of type 1 diabetes. Individuals who tested positive for these pancreas-destroying antibodies were eligible to enroll in either of two studies based on their degree of risk for developing type 1 diabetes over the next 5 years listed below (the screening tests can determine who is at a lower or higher risk). The first, Insulin Injection Trial, was found to be not effective at preventing type 1 diabetes. The second oral insulin trial was also unfortunately found to be ineffective.

Despite no proven prevention strategies, we do have excellent screening tests to help identify people who may develop type 1 diabetes. The screening test is a simple blood test that looks for the antibodies (islet cell antibodies) that attack the pancreas. It turns out that if someone has these antibodies in their blood, he or she will have about a 90%

or higher chance of developing type 1 diabetes within the next 5 years. The official recommendations for screening, which should be done every 3 years, are listed in **Table 25-3**. Most diabetes specialists know the locations of the local free-screening centers, or you can call the government-funded DPT-1 (1-800-HALT-DM1).

If you test positive for being at risk for type 1 diabetes, there is no real list of things to do such as there is for people at risk for type 2 diabetes. Lifestyle changes have not been shown to make a difference. Basically, it comes down to being involved in a clinical trial. If you are interested, there is the government program called TrialNet (continuation of the DPT-1), which is continu-

Table 25-3

Who Should Be Screened for Being at Risk for Type 1 Diabetes?

- Age 45 or younger and have a brother or sister, child, or parent with type 1 diabetes
- Age 20 or younger and have a cousin, aunt or uncle, nephew or niece, grandparent, or half-sibling with type 1 diabetes

---

ing to evaluate new prevention strategies for type 1 diabetes. They are on the Internet at *www.diabetestrialnet.org* and can be called using the number given above.

Screening or being involved in a study may not be for you or your child. If your child is at risk for type 1 diabetes, you may or may not want to have your child tested. If you do not want your child to be involved in a clinical trial after carefully reviewing the protocols, then it comes down to personal preference. If you would worry too much if the test is positive, it may not be worth it. If you are the type of person who likes to know and prepare for the eventuality, testing is for you.

Case Presentations

Case #1: Prevention of Type 1 Diabetes

I can tell you my family's story. I have two teenage daughters, Talia and Carina. When Talia was 7 and Carina was 3, my wife and I decided to have them tested for the antibodies that cause type 1 diabetes. We are the type of people who wanted to know if one or both of our children could eventually develop type 1 diabetes. Talia and Carina still both remember getting their arm poked for blood, but I tell my friends that our Christmas present that year (even though we are Jewish) was that they both tested negative. They are suppose to be retested every 3 years but I have not been able to drag them back to the doctor's office.

Even though we did not fully discuss the possibility of enrolling them in the DPT-1 before they were tested, we still wanted to know if they had the antibodies that would lead to type 1 diabetes. There is no charge for the test and in no way does having the test done commit your child to being a study participant.

Case #2: Prevention of Type 2 Diabetes

Peter is a 63-year-old white male who is one of the Regents of the University of California. He came to me many years ago with blood glucose levels in the prediabetic range (morning level in the 110 mg/dL range and the 2-hour postmeal level around 160 to 180 mg/dL). His A1C at that time was in the upper normal range of 5.9%. Type 2 diabetes ran in his family and he also had a weight problem, high blood pressure, and abnormal cholesterol levels.

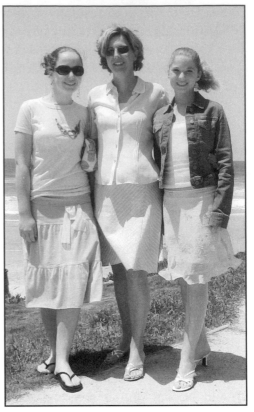

My wife, Ingrid *(center)*, with daughters Talia *(left)* and Carina *(right)*.

Other than that, he was healthy and had an active lifestyle. He came to me because he did not want to get diabetes!

Peter loves to eat and is always fighting to keep his weight from going up. Fortunately he does like to walk. He bought one of those hand held GPS devices and tracked the amount of walking he did meticulously. One clinic visit, he told me he was taking a virtual walk from San Diego to San Francisco and that he was in Pismo Beach near San Luis Obispo right now. In any case, after a long discussion, we decided to start Rezulin (troglitazone) to try and prevent the development of type 2 diabetes. I explained quite clearly to him the pros and cons of taking the drug and that the FDA has not officially approved the use of Rezulin for the prevention of type 2 diabetes. He did well and after a few years, Rezulin was taken off the market and we switched it for Avandia (rosiglitazone), which is a very similar drug that does not cause liver damage. Well, Peter is still on Avandia after many many years with blood glucose levels and A1C values in the upper normal ranges. At least for the past 10 years, we have been able to prevent Peter from developing type 2 diabetes and that is incredible. It was the combination of regular exercise, watching his diet, and medication.

Even if Peter had developed diabetes, he would be on the right track for early treatment and aggressive therapy before any complications became apparent. Remember that the next best thing to preventing diabetes is being the first to know about it.

Summary

The best way to prevent the terrible complications of diabetes is to prevent diabetes in the first place. Diabetes does not have to be a costly and devastating disease. It is not only the health care professionals who must be informed about who is at risk for diabetes; it is also the responsibility of anyone living with diabetes to notify and encourage his or her relatives to be tested for either type 1 or type 2 diabetes. There are no symptoms in the early stages of the development of diabetes, which makes screening programs even more important. We now can say without a shadow of a doubt that type 2 diabetes can be prevented with lifestyle modification and medication. Unfortunately, type 1 diabetes prevention strategies have failed, but more studies are in progress. Even if diabetes is found at the time of screening, or if you develop diabetes while participating in one of the prevention studies, being the first to know you have diabetes is the next best thing to not having it. Early and aggressive treatment of diabetes is the single most important message that I can convey to you.

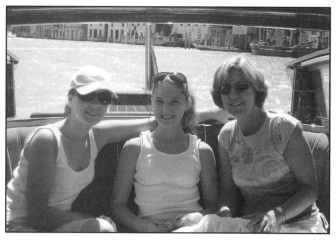

My wife, Ingrid *(right)*, and daughters, Talia *(left)* and Carina *(center)*, in Venice in 2005.

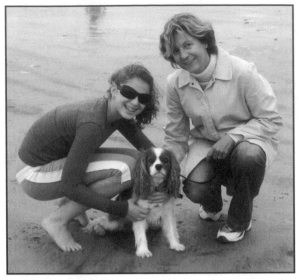

My wife, Ingrid, and youngest daughter, Carina, on the beach in San Diego with my favorite pure bred mutt, Luke.

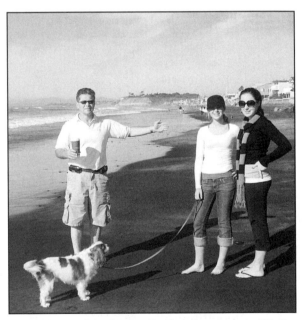

Me with my daughters, Carina *(center)* and Talia *(right)*, and Luke on the beach at Del Mar.

26

Taking Control of Your Diabetes

The Final Word

The Essentials for Taking Control of Your Diabetes

The essentials for taking control of your diabetes can be broken down into these main parts:
1. Blood glucose control
2. Blood pressure control
3. Cholesterol control
4. Following a diabetes warranty program
5. Constantly seeking out new information on how to best control your diabetes.

These basic areas have been covered extensively in this book and should be the backbone of your diabetes care. Controlling your blood glucose level will not only reduce the incidence and severity of the complications of diabetes, but will also allow you to feel better on a day-to-day basis. Since the last edition of this book was published, the goals for glycemic control have been lowered. In fact, all of the major diabetes organizations, such as the American Diabetes Association (ADA), have now said that the ultimate goal is to have the A1C in the normal range (4% to 6%) and not just below 7%, if it can be done safely and without excessive hypoglycemia. We now have so many impressive and effective tools to control our diabetes, including home glucose and continuous glucose monitors, designer insulin analogues, smart insulin pumps, and an even larger variety of new oral and injectable medications that work well alone and in combination with each other and with insulin. I also believe very strongly that continuous glucose monitoring will have a huge impact on the life of people with type 1 and insulin-requiring type 2 diabetes. It truly is the rare individual whose diabetes cannot be controlled with these new medications and devices.

Blood pressure control not only will help reduce the microvascular complications of diabetes (eye and kidney disease), it will also greatly reduce your chance of having a heart attack or stroke. People with diabetes should have a home blood pressure cuff for periodic measurements. High blood pressure is commonly found in people with diabetes and there may be no obvious symptoms. We have many different types of blood pressure medications that work well alone or in combination. The goals for blood pressure control have been lowered (less than 130/80 mm Hg) because of excellent clinical research studies demonstrating major health benefits.

Over the past several years, the bar has also been lowered in terms of acceptable cholesterol levels. Getting a yearly fasting lipid panel or cholesterol screening is of utmost importance. Untreated abnormal cholesterol levels (LDL or bad cholesterol, HDL or good cholesterol, and triglycerides) can lead to heart attack and stroke, which are very common in people with diabetes. Once again, there are no symptoms of abnormal cholesterol levels, which makes screening very important. Experts in the field now advocate aggressive cholesterol control because extensive and well-conducted clinical studies demonstrate that it results in large reductions in the occurrence of these serious life-altering and life-threatening events. One of the more important guideline changes is to get the bad or LDL cholesterol less than 100 mg/dL for all diabetics and less than 70 mg/dL if you already have heart problems. Just as is the case with blood glucose and blood pressure control, there are some fantastic, safe, and powerful drugs to bring the abnormal cholesterol levels into the normal range.

Following a diabetes warranty program helps you stay on top of your health issues in terms of the tests and examinations that you need regularly in order to stay healthy. It follows the same philosophy of the warranty program for your car. If you take your car in for servicing according to the recommended maintenance schedule, your car will most likely run better and last longer. Just replace your body for your car. Make a chart, keep good records, and know what the values mean. The last and most important step is to take action if the values are not in the ideal or near-normal range. In our current era of managed care, you must be super proactive in getting the medications and services you need to stay healthy. This is where education, motivation, and self-advocacy play important roles.

Education, Motivation, and Self-Advocacy

Diabetes control in this country and around the world is still inadequate for the majority of people living with this chronic condition. In addition, there have been numerous advances in the field of diabetes that can potentially wipe out or greatly reduce the amount of human suffering associated with this disease. Why is it that advances in the diabetes medical field have far outpaced care at the community level? I believe one of the greatest missing links is that patient education and motivation have been seriously lacking or nonexistent. We, the people who are living with this condition, need to be the most knowledgeable members of our health care team and take the main responsibility for our health. We are our own best advocates. We need to find out what needs to be done to live a healthy and productive life with diabetes and then go out and do it. Be smart and be persistent.

Spreading the Important Messages of TCOYD

In my many years of experience as a diabetes specialist, I have rarely met a person with diabetes who did not want to live a long and healthy life. I can't tell you how many times I have heard a doctor say, "My diabetic patients are all noncompliant and they just do not care about their own health." I believe these patients have either never been properly educated and motivated to be their own best advocate and to take control of their diabetes or that their caregivers just do not understand the barriers that these patients face. TCOYD is a not-for-profit organization whose mission is to educate and motivate people with diabetes and their loved ones to take a more active role in their condition in order to live a healthier, happier, and more productive life. TCOYD promotes its mission through several information portals. These include a national series of conferences, the new TCOYD television show, an award-winning *MyTCOYD* newsletter, this 3rd edition of the TCOYD book, a membership program, and one-of-a-kind Making the Connection continuing medical education (CME) programs that offer the caregivers of our country cutting-edge advances in diabetes care, as well as providing them with an understanding of what it is like to live with diabetes on a day-to-day basis.

TCOYD Conferences and Health Fairs

TCOYD was founded on the core principle that when it comes to education, motivation, and self-advocacy, nothing replaces face to face interactions. This is why our ongoing national series of conferences remain the foundation of how TCOYD fulfills its mission. The TCOYD conferences and health fairs are held in major convention centers in cities across America and, to date, we have touched the lives of well over 150,000 people. The conferences are normally held on Saturdays from 8 AM to 5 PM and consist of general sessions for all attendees in the morning, a banquet lunch with an inspirational speaker, a variety of afternoon workshops, hands-on sessions offering one-on-one time between experts and patients, exercise programs, an extensive health fair, and a closing general session to end the day on a hopeful and motivating note. These conferences have changed the lives of countless people with diabetes, empowering them to be on the diabetes offensive. You can view an 8-minute documentary on the TCOYD conferences and learn more about them on our Web site *(www.tcoyd.org)*. I would encourage you to try to not only attend a conference, but also to bring your loved ones and other friends and relatives living with diabetes. You can help spread the word as well.

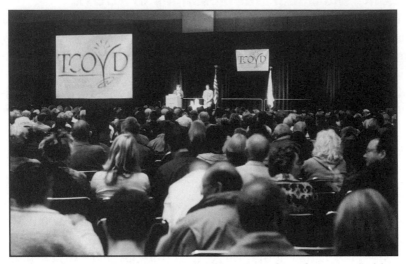

TCOYD crowd at one of our national series of conferences held around the country.

TCOYD Television Show

The first season of the new TCOYD-TV show aired in 2006/2007 and has been the culmination of over 8 years of thinking without having the time to act on those thoughts. The TV show has finally become a reality and it will continue to grow in the future. Although the live conferences are the mainstay of our organization, we are not able to reach the large numbers of people that we can via television. Our current TCOYD-TV show reaches a potential of 11.5 million viewers on the University of California television network that is uploaded to DISH satellite network television. Yours truly is the handsome host. Our topics range from the basics of diabetes care (exercise, diet, medications, insulin therapy, foot care, etc) to more advanced and cutting-edge topics, including con-tinuous glucose monitoring, the always-interesting cooking episodes with Chris Smith (The Diabetic Chef), legal issues, and much more. TCOYD pulls together the top professionals in the field of diabetes as well as real folks who have been successfully living with this condition.

Real, substantive content presented in our taking-control format is the main difference between our show and others that have come and gone. Thinking outside the box is our norm and we have fun shows on the horizon, such as Pimp Your Diabetes; Kids with Diabetes Say the Sweetest Things; Professionals With Diabetes Working in the Field of Diabetes; Intimacy, Sex, and Diabetes, etc. Please visit our Web site (*www.tcoyd.org*) for 24-hour global viewing of all of our previously aired programs and to find out how you can view TCOYD-TV on your television or computer.

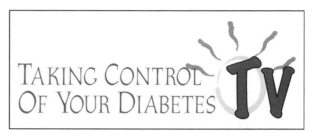

Look for our TCOYD-TV logo on our Web site to get more information on the show and to watch previously aired programs.

The MyTCOYD Newsletter

The *MyTCOYD* newsletter is in its 7th year and continues to fill an important role for our *MyTCOYD* membership. When we visit a city in America to present one of our live conferences, the participants are so motivated at the end of the day that they are happy they have diabetes! We may not return to that city for 1 or 2 years, so the newsletter helps to keep our taking-control messages current throughout the year. *Dr. Edelman's Corner* is a regular newsletter feature. I use this opportunity to say what is pertinent, provocative, controversial, and critical to our members. Some people say I am on some type of hallucinogenic drug when I write *Dr. Edelman's Corner*, but that is not true. I am always a little off the wall, anyway. Look for *Dr. Edelman's Corner* on the Web site *www.tcoyd.org*.

Additional regular features include *From Your Pharmacist, Know Your Numbers, Question of The Month,* and *Product Theater.* From Your Pharmacist reviews the latest medications for people with diabetes that have recently been approved by the FDA. This information is written in sophisticated lay terms by talented doctors of pharmacy such as Candis Morello and Nina Bean of the UCSD School of Pharmacy and Veterans Affairs Medical Center. Know Your Numbers shows a real logbook from an actual patient with a detailed explanation of what kinds of trends and patterns are evident. The purpose of this section is to educate our members on how to interpret their own numbers in order to achieve their glycemic goals. We receive many questions throughout the year from our members, and we try to answer all of them within a very short period of time, usually less than 24 hours. I pick one of the more important questions to print in each issue of our newsletter, along with a detailed answer, so that all of our members can learn together. Product Theater showcases the latest in products and devices; recently we have spotlighted the new tubeless and disposable Omnipod insulin pump and Dexcom's continuous glucose monitor.

In addition to the regularly featured sections, we have other articles written by experts in the field who have been frequent presenters at our conferences that are held around the country. In order to receive the quarterly *MyTCOYD* newsletter, you need to be a member of MyTCOYD.

The Membership Program

The MyTCOYD membership program is a great way to stay connected to TCOYD and all of our programs. Members enjoy many important advantages, such as being able to e-mail me with their questions and concerns at anytime. We call this the Ask The Expert program and if I do not know the answer, I ask one of my smart friends in the field related to the question. This is why I receive over 150 e-mails a day; I very much enjoy hearing from our members. As a member of MyTCOYD, you will receive our quarterly *MyTCOYD* newsletter with the many interesting and informative sections described. Of course, you will receive the 3rd edition of the TCOYD book that you are currently reading and several other items, such as a fast-food guide for those rare times that you are forced to eat junk food, a carb counter, and other cool things. To become a member, please go online to our Web site (*www.tcoyd.org*) or simply call our office (800-998-2693). You can also join when you attend any of our conferences.

"Making the Connection" Professional Education Program: Educating the Caregivers of This Country on the Day-to-Day Struggles of Living With Diabetes

Taking Control Of Your Diabetes (TCOYD) is taking on a challenge that is rarely attempted. Educating physicians about the most up-to-date strategies in diabetes management is a very difficult and slow process. One of the biggest challenges in improving diabetes care in this country is to improve the attitude of caregivers toward their patients struggling with diabetes and to create an empathetic atmosphere with more open two-way communication.

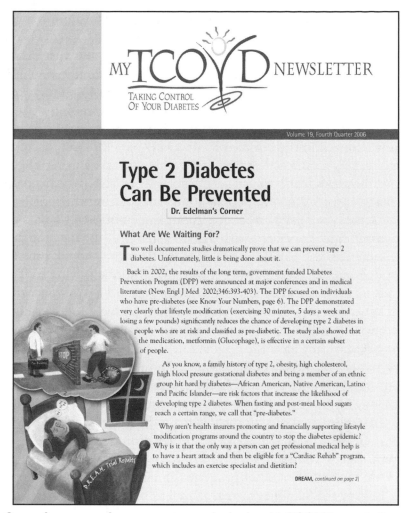

MY TCOYD NEWSLETTER

TAKING CONTROL
OF YOUR DIABETES

Volume 19, Fourth Quarter 2006

Type 2 Diabetes Can Be Prevented

Dr. Edelman's Corner

What Are We Waiting For?

Two well documented studies dramatically prove that we can prevent type 2 diabetes. Unfortunately, little is being done about it.

Back in 2002, the results of the long term, government funded Diabetes Prevention Program (DPP) were announced at major conferences and in medical literature (New Engl J Med 2002;346:393-403). The DPP focused on individuals who have pre-diabetes (see Know Your Numbers, page 6). The DPP demonstrated very clearly that lifestyle modification (exercising 30 minutes, 5 days a week and losing a few pounds) significantly reduces the chance of developing type 2 diabetes in people who are at risk and classified as pre-diabetic. The study also showed that the medication, metformin (Glucophage), is effective in a certain subset of people.

As you know, a family history of type 2, obesity, high cholesterol, high blood pressure gestational diabetes and being a member of an ethnic group hit hard by diabetes—African American, Native American, Latino and Pacific Islander—are risk factors that increase the likelihood of developing type 2 diabetes. When fasting and post-meal blood sugars reach a certain range, we call that "pre-diabetes."

Why aren't health insurers promoting and financially supporting lifestyle modification programs around the country to stop the diabetes epidemic? Why is it that the only way a person can get professional medical help is to have a heart attack and then be eligible for a "Cardiac Rehab" program, which includes an exercise specialist and dietitian?

DREAM, continued on page 2)

Cover from one of our recent award-winning *MyTCOYD* newsletters.

I feel strongly that if the general caregivers in this country really knew what it is like to have diabetes, both emotionally and physically, their level of empathy and genuine understanding would greatly improve. In turn, this would strengthen the communication between the doctor and the patient, and it would diminish the commonly experienced brow-beating and inappropriate labeling of patients as noncompliant.

It is amazing to me that during medical rounds in the hospital, a young resident doctor in training presents a case by starting with something like this: "This patient is a 56-year-old noncompliant male with a 5-year history of type 2 diabetes." After the presentation is completed, I calmly ask the resident, "Why do you say the patient is noncompliant?"

The answer is usually, "The last doctor who saw this patient wrote it in the chart and the blood glucose levels are not under good control." Well, I have never in my life met a person with diabetes who did not want to live a long and healthy life, free of complications like blindness or kidney failure! The residents and interns in the hospital now know very well not to use "that word" when presenting to me... or else!

Our Making the Connection initiative puts the doctors' learning environment smack in the middle of a TCOYD patient conference. Separate from the patient conference, they receive several cutting-edge CME approved lectures from experts in the field. They also join the people with diabetes attending the patient conference during the morning general session to hear a discussion about the emotional barriers that are so commonly associated with diabetes. Later in the day, the doctors have lunch with the patient-conference participants and hear the keynote lunchtime speaker, always a motivational speaker living well with diabetes. During the afternoon, the doctors attend a workshop along with a large group of patients that is led by the psychologist. This is an interactive and enlightening hour for both the patients and the caregivers, because they have the opportunity to express both sides of the doctor-patient relationship and come to an understanding of the frustrations faced by both groups. At the end of the day, the caregivers join together again in their own learning environment to discuss all that they observed and learned during the day from the people who live every day of their life with diabetes. More information on the TCOYD CME programs can be found at *www.tcoydcme.org* or by calling our office.

TCOYD also offers other programs, such as the MiniSeries programs held in the San Diego area, as well as our Latino Initiative led by Dr. Leonel Villa-Caballero.

Please visit our Web site at *www.tcoyd.org* for more information on all of our services or simply call our office. Our target population includes any individual interested in diabetes, including professionals.

Our Continued Challenge

The vision of Taking Control Of Your Diabetes is for all people with diabetes and their loved ones to have full access to proper education and therapy in order to allow for the prevention, early detection, and aggressive management of diabetes and its complications. Our vision statement is our future challenge. TCOYD conferences truly touch the lives of the many people who attend. However, the total number of participants nationwide is only a fraction of the people in this country living with diabetes. Even though we are now reaching more people with our television series and other programs, diabetes education and motivation must be sincerely recognized by our health care industry as an essential part of an effective treatment program. Successful diabetes education programs must be carefully developed and offered to all people with diabetes and their loved ones. Diabetes education must be informative, humorous, practical, adaptable, and compatible with the wide range of ethnic groups and unique individuals that make up our country.

In closing, I want to encourage you to take control of your diabetes. You owe it to yourself and to your loved ones.

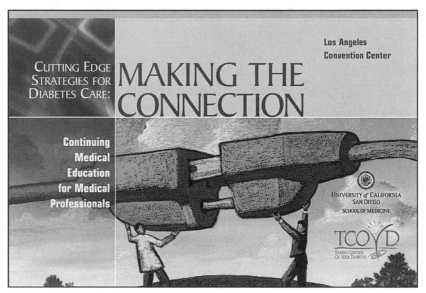

A recent invitation to health care providers to come to one of our Making the Connection programs.

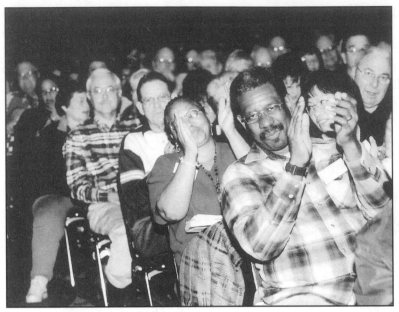

The crowd at a TCOYD conference.

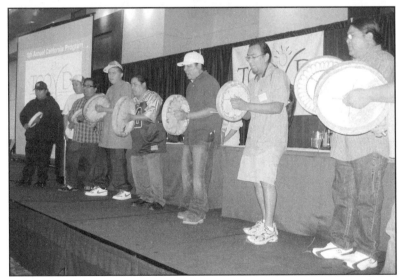

Musicians playing at a TCOYD conference held for Native Americans.

Appendix

Online Medical Resources

These two valuable resources are funded by your tax dollars. They provide a great way to learn about the latest in medical research (Medline Plus) and reliable general information on diabetes (The National Institute of Diabetes and Digestive and Kidney Diseases [NIDDK]):

• Medline Plus: *www.medlineplus.com*
• NIDDK: *www2.niddk.nih.gov*

Diabetes Self-Care on the Internet

New Web sites are going up every day for the necessary and inevitable fact that health care information is going to the Internet. This is especially important in our managed-care environment. Only a few of the excellent sites to list are listed below.

American Diabetes Association (ADA)

(800) DIABETES (342-2383); *www.diabetes.org*
Information in Spanish: *www.portufamilia.org*
The American Diabetes Association is the nation's leading nonprofit health organization providing diabetes research, information, and advocacy. Founded in 1940, the American Diabetes Association conducts programs in all 50 states and the District of Columbia. The mission of the Association is to prevent and cure diabetes and to improve the lives of all people affected by diabetes. To fulfill this mission, the American Diabetes Association funds research, publishes scientific findings, provides information and other services to people with diabetes, their families, health professionals, and the public. The Association is also actively involved in advocating for scientific research and for the rights of people with diabetes.

Rick Mendosa's Diabetes Directory

www.mendosa.com/diabetes.htm; mendosa@mendosa.com
This is a directory of articles, columns, and web pages maintained by Rick Mendosa, a freelance journalist specializing in diabetes. The site includes his annotated directory to more than 800 Web sites about diabetes, which are described and linked in the 15 pages of his online diabetes resources.

Taking Control Of Your Diabetes (TCOYD)

(800) 99-TCOYD (998-2693); *www.tcoyd.org*; *info@tcoyd.org*

The Web site of TCOYD will inform you about the nationwide series of educational and motivational events. TCOYD promotes education, motivation, and self-advocacy by live, one-on-one, and group interactions that are complemented by the Internet information highway. TCOYD also has an informative newsletter, and there is information about upcoming educational programs, publications, and membership. TCOYD offers a Q&A section with Dr. Steve Edelman and other experts in the field.

General Diabetes Resources

Associations

American Association of Diabetes Educators (AADE)
(800) 338-3633; *www.aadenet.org* or *www.diabeteseducator.org*

American Dietetic Association
(800) 877-1600; *www.eatright.org*

Centers for Disease Control (CDC)-Diabetes Home Page
(800) CDC-INFO (232-4636); *www.cdc.gov/diabetes*

Diabetes Exercise and Sports Association (DESA)
(800) 898-4322; *www.diabetes-exercise.org*

International Diabetes Center (IDC)
(888) 637-2675; *www.parknicollet.com/diabetes*

International Diabetes Federation (IDF)
+32-2-538511; *www.idf.org*; *info@idf.org*

Juvenile Diabetes Research Foundation International (JDRF)
(800) 533-CURE (2873); *www.jdrf.org*; *info@jdrf.org*

National Diabetes Education Initiative (NDEI)
(800) 471-7745; *www.ndei.org*; *feedback@ndei.org*

National Diabetes Education Program (NDEP)
(800) 438-5383; *http://ndep.nih.gov*; *ndep@mail.nih.gov*

Diabetes in the Workplace

Job Accommodation Network (JAN)
(800) 526-7234; *www.jan.wvu.edu*

An international toll-free consulting service that provides information about job accommodations and the employability of people with functional limitations. Information concerning the Americans with Disabilities Act can also be found here.

Diet and Nutrition

Calorie King
www.calorieking.com
Setting the food record straight, providing facts that anchor changed thinking about food and result in sustainable behavior improvements and better health.

Nutrition Data
www.nutritiondata.com
Provides complete nutritional information for any food or recipe, and helps you select foods that best match your dietary needs.

Free Diabetes Nutrition Teleconferences
(718) 263-3926; *telediabetes@aol.com*

Information Sources for Diabetes

Behavioral Diabetes Institute
www.behavioraldiabetes.org
An organization dedicated to tackling the unmet psychological needs of people with diabetes.

Children With Diabetes
www.childrenwithdiabetes.com
An online magazine for children, families, and adults living with juvenile diabetes. This is an excellent site for general diabetes information… it is not just for kids!

National Information Center for Children
(800) 695-0285; *www.nichcy.org*
Provides information on handling school issues for children with diabetes.

Prevent Diabetes
www.preventdiabetes.com
An online source of information for diabetes prevention, signs of diabetes, diet, obesity and weight loss, nutritional supplements, foot care, exercise, and treatment. This site also provides links for learning more about blood glucose meters.

Joslin Diabetes Center

(800) JOSLIN-1 (567-5461); *www.joslin.org;*
diabetes@joslin.harvard.edu

Learn about diabetes research and discovery as well as programs for
teens and kids. The Joslin Store offers diabetes management books,
cookbooks, and videos.

MedicineNet

www.medicinenet.com/diabetes/focus.htm

This website states "We bring doctor's knowledge to you," providing
news, signs and symptoms of diabetes, procedures and tests, medications, and information for healthy living. This site also has a medical
terms dictionary.

National Institute of Diabetes and Digestive
and Kidney Diseases (NIDDK)

http://diabetes.niddk.nih.gov

A comprehensive Web site for an introduction to diabetes, complications of the disease, and treatment. Statistics, clinical trials, guidelines,
and research reports are accessible through this site along with additional sources for publications.

The Diabetes Mall

(800) 988-4772; *www.diabetesnet.com*

In addition to information concerning diabetes, this site offers linked
information to technology in diabetes, including insulin pumps and sets,
meters and monitors, and software to be used in controlling diabetes.

TrialNet

www.diabetestrialnet.org

A network of 18 clinical centers working in cooperation with international screening sites and dedicated to the study, prevention, and early
treatment of type 1 diabetes.

US Office for Civil Rights

(800) 421-3481; *www.ed.gov/about/offices/list/ocr/index.html*

Provides information and assistance on handling school issues for children with diabetes.

QuackWatch

www.quackwatch.com

"Your guide to quackery, health fraud, and intelligent decisions."

Pharmaceutical Company Web Sites

Many drug company Web sites have useful information for doctors as well as patients, including complete descriptions of product features and drug prescribing information.

Bristol-Myers Squibb: www.bristolmyers.com
Eli Lilly and Company: www.lilly.com
GlaxoSmithKline: *www.gsk.com*
Merck: *www.merck.com*
Novartis: *www.novartis.com*
Pfizer: *www.pfizer.com*
sanofi-aventis US: *www.sanofi-aventis.us*
Schering-Plough: *www.sphcp.com*

Travel Resources

Center for Disease Control International Traveler Hotline
(877) 394-8747; *www.cdc.gov/travel*
Provides 24-hour-a-day voice and fax information system of international travel recommendations, information on specific diseases, immunizations, and services.

Highway to Health Travel Insurance
(888) 243-2358; *www.highwaytohealth.com*
Provides travelers' assistance, a worldwide physician list, medical evacuation and repatriation, trip planning, and global assistance services.

International Association for Medical Assistance to Travelers (IAMAT)
(716) 754-4883; *www.iamat.org; info@iamat.org*
Provides a list of foreign doctors who speak English in your destination cities and information on food, climate, and sanitary conditions.

Traveler's Emergency Network, Inc.
(800) ASK-4-TEN (275-4836); *www.tenweb.com*

Travelex Insurance Services, Inc.
(800) 228-9792; *www.travelex-insurance.com*
Provides trip cancellation coverage and medical coverage for physicians and hospitalization during a trip.

Universal Travel Protection Insurance
(800) 694-4311; www.utravelpro.com

Worldwide Assistance Services, Inc.
(800) 777-8710; *www.worldwideassistance.com*

Online Stores (e-Commerce)

Diabetes self-care products can be purchased online, including injection kits, meters, pumps, and related accessories and supplies. Just a few online sources are listed here.

Advantage Health Services

(800) 682-8283; *www.advantagerx.com*

CCS Medical

(800) DIABETIC (342-2384); *www.diabetic.com*
A good source for diabetes testing supplies and insulin pumps, specializing in convenient home delivery of health care products.

DrugStore.com

www.drugstore.com
A comprehensive online pharmacy, providing prescriptions, vitamins, and diet and fitness information among many other health-related products and information.

Fifty 50 Pharmacy

(800) 746-7505; *www.fifty50.com*
Donates half of its profits to fund diabetes research.

Publications

Magazines

Diabetes Forecast

www.diabetes.org
Magazine of the American Diabetes Association and comes with a membership. Provides an annual "Resources Guide" of products for use by people with diabetes.

Diabetes Health

www.diabeteshealth.com
Called the information "weapon" against diabetes by the *Wall Street Journal*. Provides cutting-edge, balanced, expert news to the diabetic community.

Diabetes Self-Management

www.diabetesselfmanagement.com
Publishes a bi-monthly magazine, a weekly e-mail newsletter, a number of books, and a blog. Browse magazine archives online.

Books

American Diabetes Association. *Diabetes & Pregnancy: What to Expect.* 4th ed. American Diabetes Association, 2001.

American Diabetes Association. *Gestational Diabetes: What to Expect.* 5th ed. American Diabetes Association, 2005.

American Diabetes Association and Lea Ann Holzmeister. *The Diabetes Carbohydrate & Fat Gram Guide.* 3rd ed. American Diabetes Association, 2006.

Ian Blumer and Heather McDonald-Blumer. *Understanding Prescription Drugs for Canadians for Dummies.* For Dummies, 2007.

Sheri Colberg. *The Diabetic Athlete: Prescriptions for Exercise and Sports.* Human Kinetics Publishers, 2001.

Sheri R. Colberg. *The 7 Step Diabetes Fitness Plan: Living Well and Being Fit with Diabetes, No Matter Your Weight.* Marlow & Company, 2005.

Sheri R. Colberg and Steven V. Edelman. *50 Secrets of the Longest Living People With Diabetes.* Marlowe & Company, 2007.

Lorena Drago. *Beyond Rice and Beans: The Caribbean Latino Guide to Eating Healthy With Diabetes.* American Diabetes Association, 2006.

Francine R. Kaufman. *Diabesity: The Obesity-Diabetes Epidemic That Threatens America—And What We Must Do to Stop It.* Bantam, 2005.

William H. Polonsky. *Diabetes Burnout: What to Do When You Can't Take It Anymore.* American Diabetes Association, 1999.

John Walsh and Ruth Roberts. *Pumping Insulin: Everything You Need for Success on a Smart Insulin Pump.* 4th ed. Torrey Pines Press, 2006.

John Walsh, Ruth Roberts, Timothy Bailey, and Chandra B. Varma. *Using Insulin: Everything You Need for Success With Insulin.* Torrey Pines Press, 2003.

Diabetes Products

Blood Glucose Meters/Data Management Software

There have been several advancements in the development of home glucose meters since the first edition of this book. Many things should be taken into consideration in deciding which blood glucose meter to purchase. These devices come in many sizes and with a varying range of capabilities. Cost of these devices varies as well. Some companies will provide their meter free of charge, since their money is made on the sale of the device's test strips. Sometimes it is more cost-effective to purchase a meter because the strips for it are more economically priced. Test-result returns can come as quickly as 5 seconds or can take as long as 4 minutes. Many meter companies now offer blood letting devices that use the forearm and thus avoid the necessity to prick your sore fingertips. Some meters can store results in memory over a period of time and provide test averages. Others have the ability to download their data to a computer for use with software applications that can further your diabetic control by providing graphs that can help you understand your blood glucose readings and determine patterns in your glucose levels over time. Some applications can even provide help concerning diet and exercise based on your meter's stored results. Research the different meters on the market and ask yourself, "How will I be using this meter?" The best meter is the one that is right for you.

Table A-1 provides a partial list of blood glucose meters currently on the market and their features. A comparison of available blood glucose meters can be found at *www.diabetes.org/diabetes-forecast/resource -guide.jsp*. Contact information for obtaining additional information or making a purchase of these meters can be found in some of the Web sites listed below.

Abbott Diabetes Care, Inc.
(888) 522-5226; *www.abbottdiabetescare.com*

Bayer HealthCare Diabetes Care
(800) 348-8100; *www.bayerdiabetes.com*

Home Diagnostics, Inc.
(888) 777-7357; *www.homediagnosticsinc.com*

LifeScan
(800) 227-8862; *www.lifescan.com*

Metrika, Inc.
(877) 212-4968 x5; *A1cNowMail@Metrika.com; www.metrika.com*

Roche Diagnostics
(800) 858-8072; *www.accu-chek.com*

Continuous Glucose Monitors

Abbott Diabetes Care
www.abbottdiabetescare.com
Maker of the FreeStyle Navigator Continuous Glucose Monitoring System.

Dexcom, Inc.
www.dexcom.com
Maker of the DexCom STS continuous glucose monitoring system.

Medtronic Diabetes
(800) MINIMED (646-4633); *www.minimed.com*
Maker of the MiniMed Guardian continuous glucose monitoring system.

Inhaled Insulin

Pfizer
(800) TRY-FIRST (879-3477); *www.exubera.com*
Maker of Exubera (insulin human [rDNA origin]) Inhalation Powder.

Insulin Pens

Eli Lilly & Company
www.lilly.com
Maker of the Humalog Mix 75/25 Pen and HumaPen Memoir.

Novo Nordisk Inc.
www.novonordisk.com
Maker of the Levemir Flex Pen and NovoPen 3.

sanofi-aventis US
www.sanofi-aventis.us
Maker of the Lantus/Apidra OptiClik and Lantus SoloStar.

Insulin Pumps

Animas Corp.
(877) YES-PUMP (937-7867); *www.animascorp.com*
Maker of the Animas 2020 insulin pump.

Disetronic Medical Systems
(800) 280-7801; *www.disetronic-usa.com*
Maker of the Accu-Chek Spirit insulin pump.

Insulet Corporation
(800) 591-3455; *www.myomnipod.com*
Maker of the OmniPod Insulin Management System.

Medtronic Diabetes
(800) MINIMED (646-4633); *www.minimed.com*
Maker of the MiniMed Paradigm Real-Time insulin pump and continuous glucose monitoring system.

Smiths Medical MD, Inc.
(800) 826-9703; *www.cozmore.com;*
cozcustomerservice@smiths-medical.com
Maker of the CozMore Insulin Technology System, including the Deltec Cozmo insulin pump, CoZmonitor blood glucose module, and CoZmanager PC communications software.

Table A-1

Blood Glucose Monitors: Features

Product (Manufacturer)	Control Solution	Calibration Method	Features
Accu-Chek Active*† (Roche Diagnostics)	Yes	Snap-in code key	Small sample size; two-step procedure; meter turns on automatically when strip is inserted; results are downloadable; alternate site testing; rubber grips; English and Spanish instructions, including a "First Time Guide"; toll-free call center with multilingual reps
Accu-Chek Advantage* (Roche Diagnostics)	Yes	Snap-in code key	Small sample size, capillary action, and large target area for easy dosing; downloadable 100-value memory with time and date; new shape and rubber grips; English/Spanish instructions (see *Accu-Chek Active*)
Accu-Chek Aviva (Roche Diagnostics)	Yes	Code key	Wide-mouth dosing area attracts and holds blood sample allowing patients to fill the strip easily. Large, wide strip and rubber metal grips provide easy handling. Alternate site testing; results are downloadable; 500-value memory; small sample size (0.6 microliter); 7-, 14-, and 30-day averaging
Accu-Chek Compact*† (Roche Diagnostics)	Yes	Automatic	Handle-free test strips; 8-second test time and 1.5-microliter sample size; no manual coding; option to test on six sites, including fingertip, forearm and palm; underdosed strip detection; 100-value memory with time, date, and 7-day averaging; downloads into Accu-Chek Compass software; English/Spanish instructions (see *Accu-Chek Active*)
Accu-Chek Complete* (Roche Diagnostics)	Yes	Snap-in code key	Two-step test procedure; holds up to 1000 values; "ATM-like" push-button selection for information entry; software available for uploading test results; English/Spanish instructions (see *Accu-Chek Active*)
Accu-Chek Voicemate (Roche Diagnostics)	Yes	Snap-in code key	For the blind and visually impaired; step-by-step voice guide; touchable strips; portable; no cleaning required; Lilly brand insulin identification ensures customer of correct insulin formulation; English/Spanish instructions (see *Accu-Chek Active*)

Continued

Product (Manufacturer)	Control Solution	Calibration Method	Features
Advance Intuition (Hypoguard)	Yes	Code chip	Two-step testing; automatic on/off with strip insertion; 3-microliter sample size; 1-button memory recall; stores up to 10 tests; large display screen; Guide-Me-Curve strips guide the finger to application site where blood is wicked onto test strip; 10-second test time
Advance Micro-draw* (Hypoguard)	Yes	Code chip	Test strips wick the blood onto the end of the strip; 1.5-microliter sample size; digital display, 250-test memory with time and date stamp; 14- and 30-day average and downloading capabilities with GlucoBalance Data Management Software
Ascensia Breeze Glucose Monitoring System*† (Bayer HealthCare, LLC)	Yes	Automatic	Disc-based meter requires no coding; underfill detection; each function button does only one thing; eliminates individual strip handling, performing 10 tests without reloading; test strip atuomatically draws amount of blood required; downloadable memory for PC tracking; stores up to 100 results; alternate site testing
Ascensia Contour Blood Glucose Monitoring System† (Bayer HealthCare, LLC)	Yes	Automatic	Automatic accuracy, control marking, and underfill detection; no coding; small sample size (0.6 microliter); 240-test memory with time, date, and 14-day average; easy viewing of sample fill; alternate site testing
Ascensia Dex 2 Diabetes Care System*† (Bayer HealthCare, LLC)	Yes	Automatic	Disc-based meter eliminates individual strip handling; performs 10 tests without reloading; disc automatically calibrates monitor for 10 tests; test strip actively draws amount of blood needed; advanced data managment; downloadable memory for PC tracking; stores up to 100 results with time, date, and averages; alternate site testing
Ascensia Elite Blood Glucose Monistoring System† (Bayer HealthCare, LLC)	Yes	Strip calibration	No buttons; turns on with test strip insertion; blood touched to the tip of test strip is automatically drawn into the test chamber; 20-test memory and 3-minute automatic shutoff; alternate site testing; individual foil-wrapped strips
Ascensia Elite XL Blood Glucose Monitoring System† (Bayer HealthCare, LLC)	Yes	Strip calibration	No operating buttons; turns on with test strip insertion; 120-test memory with date, time, and 14-day average; 3-minute automatic shutoff; alternate site testing; individual foil-wrapped strips

Product			Description
Assure* (Hypoguard)	Yes	Code chip	Two-step testing; large touch screen display; 180-test memory with time and date stamp; download with GlucoBalance Data Management System; Guide-Me-Curve strips guide the finger to application site where blood is wicked onto test strip
Assure II (Hypoguard)	Yes	Code chip	Two-step testing; automatic on/off with strip insertion; 3-microliter sample size; 1-button memory recall; stores up to 10 tests; large display screen; Guide-Me-Curve strips guide the finger to application site where blood is wicked onto test strip; results in 30 seconds
BD Logic Blood Glucose Monitor* (BD)	Yes	Built-in button	Uses Ultra-Fine 33 Lancets; time-specific averaging for adjusting insulin dose based on patterns of blood glucose values; optional memory functions allow for recording insulin type and dose of each insulin delivery; results downloadable to BD Diabetes Software
Focus Blood Glucose Monitoring System* (QuestStar Medical, Inc.)	Yes	Automatic calibration	No-button testing; hands-off automatic calibration; automatic hematocrit and temperature corrections; automatic sample volume check; word prompts for guidance; foil-wrapped test strips with 24-month shelf life; plasma or whole blood referenced; stores up to 165 results with time, date, insulin type, and dosage; averages glucose readings; clock; data port for PC download; prompts in 10 languages
FreeStyle*† (Abbott Diabetes Care)	Yes	Built-in button	Small blood sample (0.3 microliter); various testing sites; large display; strip insertion turns meter on; sample pulled into strip by capillary action; blood can be added, using the same target area on strip, up to 1 minute; 250-test memory with date, time, 14-day average; data downloadable to a PC or managed with FreeStyle Co-Pilot PC data management system
FreeStyle Flash*† (Abbott Diabetes Care)	Yes	Built-in button	Up to four programmable daily alarms; backlight display; test port light; small blood sample (0.3 microliter); offers various testing sites; more blood can be added, using the same target area on the strip, for up to 1 minute; 250-test memory with date, time, 14-day average; data can be downloaded to a PC or managed with FreeStyle Co-Pilot PC data management system

Continued

Product (Manufacturer)	Control Solution	Calibration Method	Features
FreeStyle Tracker*†§ (Abbott Diabetes Care)	Yes	Built-in buttons on PDA	Stores up to 2,500 glucose results in electronic logbook; alternate testing sites; small blood sample (0.3 microliter); 2,500-item food list with carb values per serving size; insulin tables; prescribed regimen table; reminder alarms for checking glucose or keeping appointments; data downloadable to PC or managed with FreeStyle Co-Pilot PC data management system
InDuo*†‖ (LifeScan)	Yes	Built-in single button	Combined blood glucose meter/insulin dosing system; less painful alternate site testing (arm); 5-second test time; tiny blood sample; 150-test memory with date/time; 14- and 30-day test averaging; no cleaning; insulin doser uses 3-mL PenFill insulin cartridges and NovoFine max 8-mm length needles; doses in 1- to 70-unit increments; remembers last dose and elapsed time; data downloading with OneTouch software
OneTouch Basic* (LifeScan)	Yes	Built-in single button	75-test memory with optional display of date and time; simple, 3-step test procedure; large, easy-to-handle test strips; single-button coding; data downloading with OneTouch software
OneTouch SureStep* (LifeScan)	Yes	Built-in single button	Single-button testing; touchable test strip; off-meter dosing; large display; 150-test memory; 14- and 30-day test averaging; data downloading to PC with OneTouch software
OneTouch Ultra*† (LifeScan)	Yes	Built-in single button	Alternate-site testing; small blood sample; easy blood application with Fast-Draw design test strip, including confirmation window; 150-test memory with date and time; 14- and 30-day test averaging; no cleaning necessary; data downloading with OneTouch software
OneTouch UltraSmart*§ (LifeScan)	Yes	Built-in single button	Electronic logbook and blood glucose monitor in one; small blood sample; easy blood application; confirmation window; 3,000+ test and logbook; 7-, 14-, 30-, 60-, and 90-day test averaging; data downloading with OneTouch Software; warning to check ketones at 240 to 600 mg/dL
Prestige IQ* (Home Diagnostics, Inc.)	Yes	Standard strip	Accurate results; data management, including date and time and 14- and 30-day averaging; large digital display; Internet uploading capabilities, allowing patients to track, graph, record, and share test results; test strips are highly absorbent; sample size confirmation on back of test strip

Product (Manufacturer)	Control Solution	Coding/Calibration	Features
Precision Xtra*†‖ (Abbott Laboratories)	Precision high/low and normal	Calibrator in each box of test strips	Measures blood glucose and blood ketone levels; TrueMeasure technology minimizes effects of agents like Tylenol, vitamin C, and uric acid for glucose-specific results; 2-step testing; end-fill/top-fill design; downloadable 450-test memory; luminous case, large backlit display, test port spotlight; Precision Xtra strips use 40% less blood for sample size, 10-second test time; alternate site testing capability
QuickTek* (Hypoguard)	Yes	Built-in button	250-test memory with time and date; data downloading with GlucoBalance Data Management software; large test strip for easy handling; small sample size (3.5 microliter); 2-step testing
ReliOn NewTek (Hypoguard/Wal-Mart Pharmacies)	Yes	Built-in button	Pre-calibrated and pre-loaded with 100 test strips; 1-step test; disposable with no strip handling, calibration, or battery replacement; small sample size; 100-test memory; 10-test averaging and automatic warning system for expired strips or adverse environmental conditions
ReliOn Ultima (Wal-Mart Pharmacies)	No (available toll-free #)	Calibrator on each box of strips	End-fill strips require a 2.5-microliter blood sample size; wallet-sized carrying case contains ReliOn lancing device, 10 lancets, and logbook; stores up to 450 results; individually wrapped test strips
Sidekick Testing System (Home Diagnostic, Inc.)	No	No coding required	Vial of 50 test strips with blood glucose meter built onto top of vial. No coding required. All the basic features of traditional monitor including fingertip or forearm testing, 1-microliter sample size, and test results in <10 seconds. Discard vial when empty (or upon expiration date)
TrueTrack Smart System*†	Yes	Code chip	Biosensor technology; accurate test results in 10 seconds with a 1-microliter blood sample; alternate site testing; Track Ease Smart System also available; for more details go to (Home Diagnostics, Inc.) *www.thesmartchoice.com*

Abbreviations: CLIA, Clinical Laboratory Improvement Amendments; MEMo, Medicines Evaluation and Monitoring Organizations.

Continued

* Downloadable test results.
† Alternate site testing.
‡ Combination blood glucose monitor, lipid, and ketone tests.
§ Electronic logbook.
‖ Combined blood glucose monitor and insulin dosing system.
¶ Combination blood glucose monitor and ketone tests.

Adapted from: *Diabetes Forecast.* 2007;60:RG36-RG51.

Index

Page numbers followed by "f" indicate figures; those followed by "t" indicate tables.

Albumin *(continued)*
 creatinine ratio, to, 240-241
 in diabetic kidney disease, presence of, 239-240
 excretion rates, 240t
 in urine, 240, 242, 244, 274
  life insurance application denied because of, 240
  reducing, 245
  timed collection, tests for, 240
 long-acting basal insulin analogue, bound to, 133
Alcohol, 76-77, 82, 181, 203-204
Aldactazide, 219t
Aldomet (methyldopa), 219t
Aldoril, 219t
Aliskiren (Tekturna). *See* Tekturna (aliskiren)
Alpha
 -blockers, 219t, 220
 cells, 200
 lipoic acid, 233
Altace (ramipril), 219t, 246t, 346t
Altocor (lovastatin), 224t, 248t
Alzheimer's disease, 60f
Amaryl (glimepiride), 94, 105t, 193, 273
American Association of Diabetes Educators (AADE), 368
American Diabetes Association, 25, 98, 216, 243-244, 251, 327, 350, 357, 367
American Dietetic Association, 368
Americans With Disabilities Act, 319, 334, 369
Amitriptyline, 232
Amlactin, 290
Amlodipine/atorvastatin (Caduet). *See* Caduet (amlodipine/atorvastatin)
Amlodipine (Norvasc). *See* Norvasc (amlodipine)
Ammonium lactate, 286
Amputations
 cause of, 27, 229, 340-341
 expenditures on, 345
 fear of, 48, 319
 preventing, 51, 236
 quality of life, impact on, 87
 vascular disease role in, 233
Amylin, 38, 135-136
Anemia, 270
Anger, 46, 46t
Animas
 Corp., 166f, 375
 insulin pump, 166f, 190
Ankle edema, 113, 113t
Antara (fenofibrate), 224t, 225
Antibiotics, 290
Antidepressant medications, 51, 232-233, 269
Antiendomysial antibodies, 270
Antifungal solutions and creams, 284-285
Antigliadin antibodies, 270
Antihistamines, 290
Anti-inflammatory medications, 262, 264
Antioxidants, 222, 226, 233, 243, 244t, 248-250
Antiseizure medications, 232
Antispasmodic medicines, 271
Antitissue transglutaminase antibodies, 270
Antiyeast solutions and creams, 285
Apidra (glulisine), 59f, 64, 100, 131t, 132f, 134, 136, 143t, 144f, 145t, 146-147, 163, 176-178, 180, 182-183, 187, 249
Appetite
 changes in, 48
 loss of, 273, 274
 satiety and, 116f, 117, 136, 138
Aquaphor, 290
ARBs (angiotensin receptor blockers), 218, 219t, 220-221, 239, 244t, 246-247, 247t, 250
 in diuretic combinations, 219t

Arthritis, 96, 261f, 263
Aspart (Novolog). *See* Novolog (aspart)
Aspirin, 59f, 226-228, 287, 351
Atacand (candesartan), 219t, 247t
Atacand HCT, 219t
Atenolol (Tenormin). *See* Tenormin (atenolol)
Atherosclerosis
 family history of, 214
 fatal, 227
 impact of, 213t, 233-234
 overview of, 211
 preventing, 218, 226-228
 risk factors for, 222, 227
Athletes
 case studies of, 190-191
 organizations for, 146, 368
 personal accounts of, 319-320
 publications for, 373
 self-care for, 85, 101, 102
Athlete's foot (tinea pedis), 284f
Atorvastatin (Lipitor). *See* Lipitor (atorvastatin)
Atorvastatin/amlodipine (Caduet). *See* Caduet (amlodipine/atorvastatin)
Atropine/diphenoxylate (Lomotil). *See* Lomotil (diphenoxylate/atropine)
Autoimmune condition, 20, 269
Autoimmune diabetes, 21
Autonomic neuropathy, 97, 99t, 153
Avalide, 219t
Avandamet (rosiglitazone/metformin), 115t
Avandaryl (rosiglitazone/glimepiride), 115t
Avandia (rosiglitazone), 94, 106f, 111-113, 112t, 118, 124-126, 193, 257, 272, 346, 346t, 349-350, 354
Avapro (irbesartan), 219t, 247t
Avastin (bevacizumab), 255, 256f
Axid (nizatidine), 268

Bacterial overgrowth syndrome, 268-269
Bad breath (halitosis), 278, 278t
Basal
 /bolus balance, 164
 /bolus or basal/prandial insulin regimen, 147-148, 150, 151t
 insulin, 131t, 133-135, 146, 148, 151t, 153-154, 154t, 157, 176, 181, 194-195
  doses, 303
  profiles, 164
 rates, 154-155, 157, 160, 166, 184, 186
Bayer Diagnostic Division, 34
Bayer HealthCare, LLC, 378t
Bayer HealthCare Diabetes Care, 374
Behavior, changing, 71, 72-73
Behavioral Diabetes Institute, 369
Belladonna/phenobarbital (Donnatal). *See* Donnatal (belladonna/phenobarbital)
Benazepril (Lotensin). *See* Lotensin (benazepril)
Benicar HCT, 219t
Benicar (olmesartan), 219t, 247t
Bentyl (dicyclomine), 271
Berkson, Richard, 15
Beta
 -adrenergic blocker/diuretic combinations, 219t
 -blockers, 219t, 221
 cells, 21, 38, 157, 199-200, 208
Betaxolol (Kerlone). *See* Kerlone (betaxolol)
Bevacizumab (Avastin). *See* Avastin (bevacizumab)
Biguanides, 104, 107-110, 109t
Bile acid sequestrants, 224t, 225
Bisacodyl (Dulcolax). *See* Dulcolax (bisacodyl)
Bisoprolol (Zebeta). *See* Zebeta (bisoprolol)
Bisphosphonate therapy, 263

Muscle
  cells, glucose taken up by, 87, 93
  diabetic conditions affecting, 263
  infarction, 263
Musculoskeletal system, diabetes impact on, 259-264
MyTCOYD newsletter, 361-362, 363f

Nadolol (Corgard), 219t
Nail, trimming, 235, 236f, 284
Nasal anatomy, 292f
NASH (nonalcoholic steatohepatitis), 272
Nateglinide and Valsartan in Impaired Glucose Tolerance Outcomes Research (NAVIGATOR) study, 350
Nateglinide (Starlix). *See* Starlix (nateglinide)
National Diabetes Education Initiative (NDEI), 368
National Diabetes Education Program (NDEP), 368
National Eye Institute (NEI), 252
National Information Center for Children, 369
National Information Center for Children and Youth with Disabilities, 336t
National Institute of Diabetes and Digestive and Kidney Diseases (NIDDK), 367, 370
National Institutes of Health, 28, 254, 323, 347, 352
Nausea, 118, 137, 139, 265, 267, 273-274, 311-312
NAVIGATOR (Nateglinide and Valsartan in Impaired Glucose Tolerance Outcomes Research) study, 350
NDEI (National Diabetes Education Initiative), 368
NDEP (National Diabetes Education Program), 368
Necrobiosis lipoidica diabeticorum (NLD), 283, 283t, 287-288, 288f, 290
NEI (National Eye Institute), 252
Nephropathy, 28, 90t, 238, 263. *See also* Kidney: disease
Nerve disease (neuropathy). *See also* Peripheral: neuropathy
  causes of, 42
  diagnosing, 231, 232f
  exercise precautions in event of, 90t, 99t
  focus on, 211
  gastrointestinal, 265, 266t, 269-271, 274. *See also* Gastroparesis
  glucose levels, excessive as cause of, 21, 27, 125, 229, 249
  as long-term diabetes complication, 28, 169
  as microvascular diabetes complication, 28, 238
  oral, 278, 278t
  overview of, 229-231, 236
  painful diabetic, 231-233
  preventing, 19, 31, 229, 233
  reducing, 202
  treating, 232-233
  as workplace challenge, 315
Neurontin (gabapentin), 232, 269
Neuropathic
  arthropathy (Charcot's joint), 230-231, 231f, 263
  ulcers, 283t
Neuropathy, peripheral. *See* Peripheral: neuropathy
Neutrogena, 290
Nexium (esomeprazole), 268
Niacin extended-release (Niaspan). *See* Niaspan (niacin extended-release)
Niacin (nicotinic acid), 224t
Niaspan (niacin extended-release), 224t, 225
Nicardipine (Cardene). *See* Cardene (nicardipine)
NIDDK (National Institute of Diabetes and Digestive and Kidney Diseases), 367, 370
NIDDM (non–insulin-dependent diabetes mellitus), 22
Nifedipine
  Adalat. *See* Adalat (nifedipine)
  GITS (Procardia XL). *See* Procardia XL (nifedipine GITS)
Night-time eating, 46, 72
Nimodipine (Nimotop). *See* Nimotop (nimodipine)
Nimotop (nimodipine), 219t
Nisoldipine (Sular). *See* Sular (nisoldipine)
Nizatidine (Axid). *See* Axid (nizatidine)
Nizoral (ketoconazole), 268, 285
NLD (necrobiosis lipoidica diabeticorum), 283, 283t, 287-288, 288f, 290